Volume II

The School Nurse's Source Book of Individualized Healthcare Plans

Issues and Applications
in School Nursing Practice

Editors

Martha J. Arnold   Cynthia K. Silkworth

SUNRISE
River Press

Material from NANDA (North American Nursing Diagnosis Association) used with permission. Copyright © North American Nursing Diagnosis Association. *NANDA Nursing Diagnoses: Definitions and Classification 1999-2000*. Philadelphia, PA: North American Nursing Diagnosis Association, 1999. (Available from: NANDA, 1211 Locust St, Philadelphia, Pa 19107. 800-647-9002; 215-545-1985; fax: 215-545-8107; e-mail NANDA@nursecominc.com).

.

For additional copies of this work, contact:
Sunrise River Press, 11605 Kost Dam Rd.
North Branch, MN 55056, 651-583-3239
                    800-895-4585

Dedication

To Molly Jean, daughter, faithful friend and business partner

MJA

To Duane with thanks for your love, support and encouragement

CKS

Editors

Martha J. Arnold, R.N., B.S.N., P.H.N.

School Nurse, Director of Health Services, Chisago Lakes Area Schools, Lindstrom, Minnesota

Cynthia K. Silkworth, M.P.H., R.N., C.S.N.P., F.N.A.S.N.

School Nurse, Coordinator for School Health Services, White Bear Lake Area Schools, White Bear Lake, Minnesota

Contributors

Sue Boos, M.S., R.N., C.S., A.R.N.P.

Assistant Professor of Nursing, Department of Nursing, School Nurse Advisor, Fort Hays State University, Hays, Kansas

Constance M. Cotter, R.N., B.S.N., M.N.

School Nurse, Nurse Liaison for Specialty Clinics, Wichita Public Schools, Wichita, Kansas

Janice Denehy, R.N., Ph.D.

Associate Professor, University of Iowa College of Nursing, Iowa City, Iowa

Charlotte R. Gorun, R.N., B.S.N.

School Nurse, Phoenix Center, Inc., Little Falls, New Jersey

Margarita Fernan Granthom, R.N.

School Nurse, 504 Coordinator, Sweetwater County School District Number One, Rock Springs, Wyoming

Judith F. Harrigan, R.N., M.S.N., P.N.P., F.N.A.S.N.

School Health Services Coordinator, New York State Education Department, Albany, New York, Adjunct Instructor, School of Nursing, University of Rochester, Rochester, New York

Carolyn F. Holman, R.N., M.S.N., C.S.N., C.R.N.P.

School Nurse, Retired, Mobile County Public Schools, Family Nurse Practitioner, Dept. of Family Practice, College of Medicine, University of South Alabama, Mobile, Alabama

Ann Hoxie, R.N., C.P.N.P., M.S.

School Nurse, St. Paul Public Schools, St. Paul, Minnesota

Patricia S. Latona, R.N., M.S.N.

School Nurse, Alamogordo Public Schools, Alamogordo, New Mexico

Brenda Kay Lenz, R.N., B.S.N, M.S.N.

School Nurse, Secondary, Buffalo School District, Buffalo, Minnesota

Janet Lowe, R.N., M.A., C.P.N.P.

School Nurse, St. Paul Public Schools, St. Paul, Minnesota

Mary Jo Martin, R.N., B.S.N.

School Nurse, Katherine Curren Elementary, Hopkins, Minnesota

Tamara Gonzalez Oberbeck, R.N., B.A., M.S.

School Nurse, Jefferson Junior High School, Columbia, Missouri, Certified Ophthalmic Medical Technologist

Denise Ornelas, R.N., B.S.N., M.S., P.N.P.

School Nurse, St. Paul Public Schools, St. Paul, Minnesota, Former State School Nurse Consultant, Minnesota Department of Health

Susan Poulton, R.N., C.S., M.S.N.

Nurse Consultant, Grant Wood Area Education Agency, Coralville, Iowa

Katherine J. Saffie, R.N.

School Nurse, Lawrence Public Schools, Staff Nurse, Lawrence General Hospital, Lawrence, Massachusetts

Sally Zentner Schoessler, B.S.N., R.N.

School Nurse, Scribner Road School, Penfield, New York

Jeanne M. Sedgwick, R.N., P.H.N., M.S.

School Nurse, St. Paul Public Schools, St. Paul, Minnesota

Mariann Smith, R.N., B.S.N., M.N.

School Nurse, Medical Educational Liaison Nurse, Wichita Public Schools, Wichita, Kansas

Linda L. Solum, R.N., B.S.N.

School Nurse, Heritage Middle School, West St. Paul, Minnesota

MaryAnn Tapper Strawhacker, R.N., B.S.N.

Special Education Nurse Consultant, Heartland Area Education Agency, Johnson, Iowa

Mary A. Swanson, R.N., B.S.N., M.S.

School Nurse, Armstrong High School, Robbinsdale, Minnesota, Adjunct Faculty, School of Nursing, University of Minnesota

Gail Synoground, R.N., A.R.N.P, Ed.D., F.N.A.S.N.

Professor of Nursing, Intercollegiate Center for Nursing Education, Washington State University College of Nursing Spokane, Washington

Jeanette H.Williams, R.N., B.S., M.H.S.

School Nurse, Itinerant Early Childhood Nurse, Special School District of St. Louis County, St. Louis, Missouri

Acknowledgments

First of all we want to thank all our nationally diverse contributors for their expertise, enthusiasm, and prompt attention to details and to time lines.

Second, we want to thank all our school nursing colleagues and users of the award-winning Volume I for their endless encouragement and their requests for Volume II of this book.

Third, we thank publisher Dave Arnold, who always believed Volume II had an important place in the professional world of school nursing. Thanks also to Sylvia Timian, of St. Louis Park, Minnesota, for her patience and copyediting and to the staff at Mori's Studio of Edina, Minnesota, for the book design and typesetting.

Fourth, we want to thank our families for their support and understanding during the endless hours of work on this project.

Finally, and most importantly, we would like to thank the children and adolescents we work with who have taught us very valuable lessons regarding the numerous aspects of their health conditions and the impact each one has on their lives, in and outside of school. We hope the book reflects what they have taught us.

Contents

1 | Individualized Healthcare Plans

Denise Ornelas

INTRODUCTION

School nurses face many challenges as school communities move into the next century. Student achievement, account-ability, and school reform will affect not only teachers but also those professionals that strive to support the educational process. Where will school nursing be? It is time to improve the visibility of school nursing practice to our consumers: students and families, teachers, principals and administrators, community medical providers, and third-party payors. School nurses need to link their services to learning readiness, and ongoing educational achievement and to the broader private and public healthcare delivery systems. An Individualized Healthcare Plan (IHP) is a method to provide such linkages.

The purpose of this book is to help school nurses develop IHPs that help to meet the needs of students and clearly document school nursing practice to our customers. The beginning chapters of this book add to and highlight information from *The School Nurse's Source Book of Individualized Healthcare Plans, Vol. I,* including Using the Nursing Process, Using Nursing Diagnosis, and Individualized Healthcare Plans in the School Setting. The subsequent beginning chapters of this next volume give the reader new and expanded information about nursing lan-

guages, delegation as it relates to IHPs, special education and 504 plans and, for those providing school nursing services to a diverse population of students, pertinent chapters addressing the health needs of homeless children and the health and cultural considerations of immigrant and refugee children. This book also includes chapters on multiple health conditions. Each chapter provides current information on the specific condition and includes a case study and sample IHP that the school nurse can individualize for use with a specific student.

Why Should School Nurses Use Individualized Healthcare Plans

The nursing process has emerged as the scientific approach to the identification and solution of problems in nursing practice. The nursing process consists of a) assessment, b) diagnosis, c) planning, d) implementation, and e) evaluation. These stages are dynamic in nature, changing as more information is received, evaluated, and interpreted.[1] The nursing process is the cornerstone of nursing practice and is applicable to all areas of nursing practice, including school nursing. Readers should refer to *volume 1 of The School Nurse's Source Book of Individualized Healthcare Plans*, chapter 1, "Using the Nursing Process in the School Setting," for detailed information on using the nursing process in the school setting. Utilization of the nursing process in schools results in the development of IHPs for students who have health-related issues.

The IHP provides a format to record each step in the nursing process, where the school nurse summarizes key information from the assessment phase, synthesizes problem statement(s) in the form of a nursing diagnosis, formulates goals, formulates plans of action, and documents interventions and the evaluation of outcomes.[2]

When students at school need ongoing nursing management, it is essential that there be a documented plan of care.[3] Documentation promotes sound planning, coordination, continuity, and evaluation of care.[4] A review of the literature outlines the many purposes of care planning and IHP development for students. Carpenito[5] stated that care plans have two professional purposes, administrative and clinical. These categories can be applied to IHPs.

Administrative purposes of IHPs include:
- defining the focus of nursing, validating the nurse's position in the school
- facilitating the management of health conditions to optimize learning
- differentiating the accountability of the school nurse from others in the school (i.e., paraprofessionals, teachers)
- providing criteria for reviewing and evaluating care-quality assurance
- providing data for statistical reports, research, third-party reimbursement, and legal evidence
- creating a safer process for delegation of nursing care in the school setting

Clinical purposes of IHPs include:
- clarifiing and consolidating health information that is meaningful for students, families, and staff

- establishing the priority set of nursing diagnoses for a student
- providing a method of communication to direct the nursing care needed by a particular student
- building the foundation for documentation
- ensuring consistency and continuity of care as students move within and outside of school districts
- directing specific interventions for the student, family, and other school staff to implement
- providing a means to review and evaluate nursing goals and outcome criteria

Individualized Healthcare Plans—Prioritize your Student Population

Sometimes school nurses are overwhelmed by the pressure (real or perceived) to write an IHP for every student who has a special healthcare need. While nurses in an acute care setting write a care plan for each patient it may not be realistic or an appropriate expectation of school nurses due to the high number of clients in their caseload. Patients are admitted specifically to a hospital for nursing and medical care. Students only receive nursing care that provides the needed and essential support to allow them to participate in their educational pursuits.

School nurses often have high to unreasonable student ratios and in some cases school nurses may only be in a particular school once a week. However, these barriers do not excuse the nurse from her/his responsibility to provide quality nursing services. The nurse working in the school setting may need to set limits as to how much of a student's multiple health issues she/he can manage within the constraints of the assigned student population.[6] School nurses should prioritize students and their needs. Begin by first identifying those students whose health needs affect their daily functioning. Consider the following in setting priorities:

- Students who are medically fragile with multiple health needs
- Students who require extended nursing care or multiple contacts with the nurse/delegatee during the school day
- Students with health needs that are addressed on a daily basis
- Students who must have health needs addressed as part of the IEP or 504 process

School nurses are also encouraged to consult with other school nurses within the school district, community, or state. Remember an IHP does not have to address every health issue of the student. Later in this chapter prioritization of health needs of individual students will be addressed.

Components of the Individualized Healthcare Plan

The IHP provides a format for assessment (summarizing key information), nursing diagnosis (synthesizing a problem statement), development of goals, interventions, and outcomes to meet the health needs of students, and evaluation.

Assessment

Assessment provides the foundation for development of an IHP. An accurate assessment is needed for a meaningful IHP. Include five main areas in your assessment: health history, current health status/management, self-care skills/needs, psychosocial status, and the health issues related to learning.

Most nurses utilize a combination of several methods to complete a comprehensive assessment.

- Interview of student/family
- Review of past medical, nursing, and educational records, such as hospital or outpatient reports, IHP, Emergency Care Plans (ECP), IEP, and 504 plans
- Review of current medical records
- Consultation with other community providers, physician and primary healthcare providers, hospital staff, home care agency, or counseling services
- Physical assessment/measures of pertinent body systems, i.e., sensory functioning, vision and hearing
- Interview of other school staff who interact with student
- Observation of student in classroom

Nursing Diagnosis

Individual pieces of data by themselves have no meaning. It's the method of organizing the data about a particular student and drawing a conclusion that separates professional school nurses from paraprofessionals, teachers, and other school staff. Nursing diagnoses define what school nurses distinctly identify and contribute as autonomous practitioners in the school setting rather than as subordinates to another professional.[3]

A nursing diagnosis summarizes the present status of the student and can include various types of diagnoses, such as actual, high risk, and wellness. The diagnosis should focus on the effects of a health condition as it pertains to the student. A nursing diagnosis usually contains several elements besides the current concern. It also identifies the contributing factors or causes and the student's response to the concern.

The North American Nursing Diagnosis Association (NANDA) developed definitions and a diagnostic classification system to uniformly and precisely identify the health issues for which nurses are accountable. NANDA defines a nursing diagnosis as "a clinical judgment about an individual, family or a community responses to actual and potential health problems or life process. Nursing diagnoses provide the basis for selection of nursing interventions to achieve outcomes for which the nurse is accountable."[7]

In 1994, the National Association of School Nurses (NASN) declared: "It is the position of the NASN to support the use of NANDA diagnosis in the school health setting."[8]   Several resources are available to school nurses to further explain the history, appropriateness, and use of the NANDA Nursing Diagnosis and Classification System.[3,5-13]

Priority Setting of Nursing Diagnosis

The number of nursing diagnoses that may be appropriate for any given student can inundate nurses. Just as school nurses must determine for which students an IHP will be developed, they must determine which health issues can be managed within the limitations of the school environment. When school nurses determine the priority of nursing diagnoses, they can better direct the resources toward goal achievement. Carpenito[5] described priority diagnoses as those nursing diagnoses that, if not managed now, will deter progress to the achievement of outcomes or will negatively affect the client's functional status.

School nurses must be realistic and knowledgeable of resources available when prioritizing nursing diagnoses. Resources, including the time required and skill of the school nurse and any delegates, must be considered. In setting priorities, school nurses should first focus on the health issues that affect safety (physical and environmental needs that are potentially life threatening). Next would be those diagnoses that affect the student's ability to learn and succeed in the educational setting. Finally, overall consideration should be given to those diagnoses that the student, family, and /or teacher perceive as priorities.

Goals

Once the nursing diagnoses have been determined and prioritized, goals are developed. A goal is a hoped-for outcome, a statement of what is desired. It should be realistic in terms of student potential and the nurse's abilities. Goals should be worded in a clear and concise manner that can be understood by all team members. Often it is appropriate for the student and/or family to help in the planning of goals. Goals can be short-term or long-term, but in either case they must be measurable. Student goals should describe a measurable behavior of the student that is evident after nursing interventions have been completed. Measurable behaviors include resolution of a problem or evidence of progress toward an improved health status or continued maintenance of good functioning.

Bulechek and McCloskey[14] define goals as the "guideposts to the selection of nursing interventions and criteria in the evaluation of nursing intervention." Readily identifiable and logical links should exist between the diagnosis and plan of care. The activities prescribed should assist or enable the client to meet the identified expected outcome. During evaluation, student goals are used to determine the success or appropriateness of the IHP. If goals are not achieved or progress is not evident, the school nurse should revise the IHP.

Nursing Interventions

A nursing diagnosis requires that the nurse prescribe the definitive treatment for the situation. A nursing intervention is defined as "any treatment, based upon clinical judgement and knowledge, that a nurse performs to enhance patient / client outcomes."[15] This definition was refined by the Iowa Intervention Project which developed a classification system of interventions (Nursing Intervention Classification /

NIC) performed by nurses in all practice settings. "Nursing interventions include both direct and indirect care; both nurse-initiated, physician-initiated, and other provider-initiated treatment."[15] In the school setting it is important to remember that appropriate interventions may vary across settings and that some interventions may be delegated to other staff. Additionally, some interventions may be shared with other school staff without necessitating delegation. An example of this could be:

Subsequent chapters of this book will describe NIC and the delegation of nursing activities.

Nursing Diagnosis	Goals	Interventions	Outcomes
Alteration in communication due to tracheostomy.	Student has increased independent communication skills.	In-service and encourage staff to utilize methods that promote effective communication. Staff should stand in front of student, use eye contact and good volume.	Student will increase his communication by one verbal or non-verbal cue weekly.

Student Outcomes

An outcome is what the student is expected to do, experience or learn. To be measurable it is paired with a modifier that is the when, where, and how. The essential characteristics of outcome criteria are that they must be:
• long-term or short-term
• in measurable behaviors
• specific in content and time
• realistic and achievable

Measurable verbs are verbs that describe the exact action or behavior of the client that the nurse can validate by seeing or hearing it and, less frequently, touch, taste, and smell. For example: instead of stating "The student will experience less depression," it is better stated "The student will report less depression." School nurses should not choose outcomes that cannot be achieved utilizing the interventions that were selected, in the time frame chosen, or in the context of the school setting.

Increasingly, it will be important to measure student outcomes that can be linked to student achievement, student attendance, student readiness, or student success, all of which can help demonstrate the importance of the role of school nursing.

For the purposes of this book, the chapter authors were directed to use NANDA classification and nursing diagnoses. The Nursing Intervention Classification System (NIC) is a system of standardized language for nursing interventions.[15] The Nursing Outcome Classification (NOC) is a standardized language of nurse-sensitive outcomes.[16] Although the authors were not instructed to specifically use NIC and NOC (due to lack of uniform familiarity) for the IHPs listed, readers are encouraged to move toward use of standardized nursing languages, providing a mechanism for meaningful IHPs.[17]

Figure 1 provides a template for an IHP with abbreviated definitions / explanations.

Figure 1
IHP Components

Assessment Data	Nursing Diagnosis	Goals	Nursing Interventions	Expected Outcomes
Interview of student, family, school staff	NANDA Nursing Diagnoses	Overall desired result	Actions to be taken to achieve the desired outcomes	What the student is expected to do, learn, or experience
Review of pertinent past and current records: nursing, medical educational, IHP, ECP, IEP, 504	Problem statement	Basis for nursing interventions	Goal oriented	Measurable in positive or negative terms
	Summarizes the present status of the student	Basis for student outcomes	May vary across settings	Short-or-long term
Consultation with other providers: MD, hospital, home care, counseling agencies	Types: actual, risk for, wellness	Measurable	Implemented by various school staff	Specific in content and time
	Effects of a given situation on student	Short-or-long term	Direct or indirect	Realistic and achievable
Physical assessment Self-care skills Vision and hearing Psychosocial status	Contains several elements: Current concerns Contributing factors Student response	Clear and concise	Nurse, physician, or other provider initiated	

Evaluation

An IHP is the written plan of care for a student with health needs in the school setting. The IHP is not a one-time event, but is dynamic through the process of evaluation. The evaluation process includes:

a) reviewing the desired student goals and outcomes

b) collecting data to determine the outcomes

c) comparing the actual outcomes to the desired outcomes

d) documenting the outcomes on the IHP

e) relating the appropriateness and effectiveness of the selected interventions to the outcome

f) reviewing and modifying the plan of care as necessary.[13]

Evaluation allows the school nurse to make judgments about the student's progress toward identified goals. Some questions that should be addressed by the school nurse include the following. Is the outcome still appropriate? Does any intervention need to be added or changed to continue progress toward the goal? Is the timeline still appropriate? Can goal achievement be related to the nursing interventions? Are there any barriers to meeting and achieving student outcomes? Were there unexpected beneficial student outcomes? Are the nursing diagnoses still pertinent for the student's health condition?

Usually it is not necessary to rewrite the IHP. Revising the plan, making additions or deletions, as appropriate, and documenting changes by dating and initialing changes to the IHP may be all that is needed. You may need to write an additional progress note to document your assessment, subjective or objective data, which was collected or observed and which prompted the revision.

IHP evaluations should be completed with any significant change in the student's health status or physician-prescribed medication/treatment. If the student has a relatively stable health status, the school nurse may wish to consider establishing a review periodicity so the evaluation is not forgotten till the end of the school year.

Summary

The role of the nurse in the school setting is to assess the health needs of children and to coordinate with staff, families, healthcare providers, and community agencies to provide a comprehensive school health program that facilitates the maximum educational opportunity for students. As school nursing moves into the 21st century, it is increasingly clear that the health needs of students will continue to be complex, that there will be a demand for accountability by school nurses, and that documentation will be a cornerstone of reimbursable nursing services. Individualized Healthcare Plans are and will continue to be essential. In June 1998, NASN developed a position statement on IHPs.[18] The conclusion states, "It is the position of the National Association of School Nurses that each student with a relatively complex health condition or a need for modification of the school environment due to a health condition should have an IHP. It is also the position of NASN that the professional school nurse should be responsible for the writing of the IHP in collaboration with the student, family, and healthcare providers."

REFERENCES

1. Dunn JD. A nursing care plan for the handicapped student. *J School Nurs.* 1984;54(8): 302-335.

2. Luehr RE. Using the nursing process in the school setting. In: Haas MB ed. *The School Nurse's Source Book of Individualized Healthcare Plans Vol I.* North Branch, Minn: Sunrise River Press,

1993:12-13. (Sunrise River Press, 11605 Kost Dam Road. North Branch, MN 55056. 800-895-4585; fax 651-583-2023.)

3. Hootman J. *Nursing Diagnosis: Application in the School Setting.* Scarborough, Me: National Association of School Nurses, 1996:19.

4. Schwab NC, Panettieri MJ, Bergren MD. *Guidelines for School Nursing Documentation: Standards, Issues, and Models.* Scarborough, Me: National Association of School Nurses, 1998:3.

5. Carpenito LJ. *Nursing Diagnosis Application to Clinical Practice* 7th ed. Philadelphia, Pa: JB Lippincott Company, 1997:61.

6. Hootman J. *Quality Nursing Interventions in the School Setting: Procedures, Models and Guidelines.* Scarborough, Me: National Association of School Nurses, 1996:1(3).

7. North American Nursing Diagnosis Association. *NANDA Nursing Diagnoses: Definitions & Classification 1999-2000.* Philadelphia, Pa: North American Nursing Diagnosis Assn, 1999:8. (NANDA, 1211 Locust Street, Philadelphia, PA 19107. 800-647-9002; fax 215-545-8107; e-mail: NANDA@nursecominc.com)

8. National Association of School Nurses. *Nursing Diagnosis Position Statement.* Scarborough, Me: National Association of School Nurses, 1994.

9. Haas MB, ed. *The School Nurse's Source Book of Individualized Healthcare Plans.* North Branch, Minn: Sunrise River Press, 1993. (Sunrise River Press 11605 Kost Dam Road, North Branch, MN 55056. 800-895-4585; fax 651-583-2023.)

10. Lunney M. The significance of nursing classification systems to school nursing. *J School Nurs.* 1996;12(2):35-37.

11. Hootman J. Nursing diagnosis: a language of nursing; a language for powerful communication. *J School Nurs.* 1996;12(4):19-23.

12. Lunney M, Cavendish R, Luise BK, Richardson K. Relevance of NANDA and health promotion diagnoses to school nursing. *J School Nurs.* 1997;13(5):16-22.

13. Denehy J, Poulton S. The use of standardized language in individualized healthcare plans. *J School Nurs.* 1999;15(1):38-45.

14. Bulecheck G, McCloskey J. Nursing interventions: treatments for nursing diagnoses. Philadelphia, Pa: WB Saunders, 1985.

15. Iowa Intervention Project. *Nursing Interventions Classification* (NIC). 2nd ed. St. Louis, Mo: Mosby-Yearbook, 1996:17. (Mosby-Yearbook, 11830 Westline Industrial Drive, PO Box 46908. St. Louis, MO. 63146-9806. 800-426-4545; fax 800-535-9935.)

16. Iowa Outcomes Project. *Nursing Outcomes Classification (NOC).* St. Louis, Mo: Mosby-Yearbook, 1997:22. (Mosby-Yearbook, 11830 Westline Industrial Drive, PO Box 46908. St. Louis, MO. 63146-9806. 800-426-4545; fax 800-535-9935.)

17. Pavelka L, McCarthy AM, Denehy J. Nursing interventions used in school nursing practice. *J School Nurs.* 1999;15(1):29-37.

18. National Association of School Nurses. *Individualized Healthcare Plan Position Statement.* Scarborough, Me: National Association of School Nurses, 1998.

BIBLIOGRAPHY

Bednarz P. The Omaha System: a model for describing school nurse case management. *J School Nurs*, 1998;14(3):24-30.

Bulecheck G, McCloskey J. Nursing interventions: treatments for nursing diagnoses. Philadelphia, Pa: WB Saunders, 1985.

Carpenito LJ. *Nursing Care Plans & Documentation 2nd ed.* Philadelphia, Pa: JB Lippincott Company, 1995.

Carpenito LJ. *Nursing Diagnosis Application to Clinical Practice 7th ed.* Philadelphia, Pa: JB Lippincott Company, 1997.

Denehy J, Poulton S. The use of standardized language in individualized healthcare plans. *J School Nurs.* 1999;15(1):38-45.

Dunn JD. A nursing care plan for the handicapped student. *J School Nurs.* 1984;54(8): 302-335.

Haas MB, ed. *The School Nurse's Source Book of Individualized Healthcare Plans. Vol 1*. North Branch, Minn: Sunrise River Press, 1993. (Sunrise River Press, 11605 Kost Dam Road, North Branch, MN 55056. 800-895-4585; fax 651-583-2023.)

Hootman J. Nursing diagnosis: a language of nursing; a language for powerful communication. *J School Nurs*. 1996;12(4):19-23.

Hootman J. *Nursing Diagnosis: Application in the School Setting*. Scarborough, Me: National Association of School Nurses, 1996.

Hootman J. *Quality Nursing Interventions in the School Setting: Procedures, Models and Guidelines*. Scarborough, Me: National Association of School Nurses, 1996.

Igoe JB. Summary statement on school nurses working with handicapped children. *J School Health* 1980;50(5):287.

Iowa Intervention Project. *Nursing Interventions Classification* (NIC). 2nd ed. St. Louis, Mo: Mosby-Yearbook, 1996. (Mosby-Yearbook, 11830 Westline Industrial Drive, PO Box 46908. St. Louis, MO. 63146-9806. 800-426-4545; fax 800-535-9935.)

Iowa Outcomes Project. *Nursing Outcomes Classification (NOC)*. St. Louis, Mo: Mosby-Yearbook, 1997. (Mosby-Yearbook, 11830 Westline Industrial Drive, PO Box 46908. St. Louis, MO. 63146-9806. 800-426-4545; fax 800-535-9935.)

Luehr RE. Using the nursing process in the school setting. In: Haas MB, ed. *The School Nurse's Source Book of Individualized Healthcare Plans Vol I*. North Branch, Minn: Sunrise River Press, 1993:12-13. (Sunrise River Press, 11605 Kost Dam Road, North Branch, MN 55056. 800-895-4585; fax 651-583-2023.)

Lunney M. The significance of nursing classification systems to school nursing. *J School Nurs*. 1996;12(2):35-37.

Lunney M, Cavendish R, Luise BK, Richardson, K. Relevance of NANDA and health promotion diagnoses to school nursing. *J School Nurs*. 1997;13(5):16-22.

National Association of School Nurses. *Nursing Diagnosis Position Statement*. Scarborough, Me: National Association of School Nurses, 1994.

National Association of School Nurses. *Individualized Healthcare Plan Position Statement*. Scarborough, Me: National Association of School Nurses, 1998.

North American Nursing Diagnosis Assosciation. *NANDA Nursing Diagnoses: Definitions & Classification 1999-2000*. Philadelphia, Pa: North American Nursing Diagnosis Assn, 1999. (NANDA, 1211 Locust Street, Philadelphia, PA 19107. 800-647-9002; fax 215-545-8107; e-mail: NANDA@nursecominc.com)

Pavelka L, McCarthy AM, Denehy J. Nursing interventions used in school nursing practice. *J School Nurs*. 1999;15(1):29-37.

Proctor S, Lordi S, Zaiger D. *School Nursing Practice: Roles and Standards*. Scarborough, Me: National Association of School Nurses, 1993.

Schwab NC, Panettieri MJ, Bergren MD. *Guidelines for School Nursing Documentation: Standards, Issues, and Models*. Scarborough, Me: National Association of School Nurses, 1998.

2

The Unique Qualities and the Similarities of IHPs and Other Educational, Health, and Home Care Agency Plans

Denise Ornelas

An IHP, emergency care plan (ECP), individual educational program (IEP), and Section 504 plan are all used within an educational setting as a process to document preparation and planning for student success. Often the student may require a combination of two or more of these plans. Distinct differences exist between the plans, yet some of the components, assessment, goals, or student outcomes may overlap. It is important for the nurse to understand these similarities and differences.

Both the IHP and ECP are specifically developed to manage health issues and are part of the nursing process, whereas the IEP and 504 plan are developed to deal with learning / educational issues of which there may or may not be a related health issue.

The IHP and ECP are nurse-initiated planning processes, while teachers, parents, and/or administrators initiate IEP and 504 plans.

Although students and families can, and are encouraged to, be involved in the development of an IHP or ECP, the IEP and 504 plan require parent participation. In fact, each has a "due process" component to ensure that the rights of students/parents are not violated.

Professional nursing standards set the expectation of developing IHPs and/or ECPs in order to deliver quality nursing care. Rarely does a state statute require

these plans. In contrast, federal legislation, Individuals with Disabilities Education Act (IDEA) and 504 plans, and subsequent state laws and rules mandate the use of IEP and 504 plans with qualifying students.

Finally, the components of an IHP and ECP have been developed through professional guidelines and nursing research. In order to produce an effective IHP and ECP, all components should be included but are not necessarily required by a state or federal statute. There is some flexibility for professional judgment. However, the IEP and, to a lesser extent, the 504 plan have specific components that must be addressed in entirety with only exceptions authorized by statute or rule.

The IHP and ECP also have specific differences.

Remember the IHP is developed out of the nursing process to address the actual or potential responses of a student to a health condition/s. The ECP also comes out of the nursing process but is developed to deal with a specific potential medical emergency such as hypoglycemia, anaphylaxis, or status epilepticus.

An IHP is an ongoing process in response to a current health need. The IHP may require delegation by the nurse of certain nursing intervention activities in order to achieve the student outcome. However, the ECP is developed for a health need that can only be anticipated.

Also, the entire ECP could be initiated and carried out exclusively by other school staff who respond to the emergency through training and delegation by the school nurse. Because of the difference, it is only logical that the IHP is developed first and the ECP is a specific product of the IHP. An ECP fits as an activity that is completed as one of several possible activities within a nursing intervention. An ECP should never be considered as a substitute for an IHP.[1]

The ECP is a well-defined step-by-step process that proceeds in logical order and provides specific directions about what to do in a particular emergency situation. It is usually written in language that can be understood by persons with limited nursing / medical knowledge. The plan includes specific information about the child's medical condition, current and emergency medications, and appropriate emergency intervention. Not having an ECP could potentially jeopardize the safety of a student in the school setting if a medical emergency occurred due to a known health condition. The ECP must be shared / given to all appropriate building staff and usually involves specific training to ensure a prepared response by staff. Practice or rehearsal may also be needed. The goal is to ensure maintenance of the student's health and safety in any anticipated life-threatening emergency.

An IHP may or may not be shared with building staff, depending upon the student's condition and his or her involvement in the plan. Overall, an IHP does not have the same sense of urgency as an ECP.

Individual Education Program/ 504 Plans

The IEP is written as part of the special education process after it has been determined that the student is eligible and will need special academic or related services to attain academic goals. A 504 plan is written when a student requires accommodations in instruction or environment to attain academic goals, but does not meet eligibility criteria for special education.

When it has been determined that the student has specific health issues, the IHP can often be incorporated or added to the IEP or 504 plan. In some circumstances goals and student outcomes from IHP may be attached to a specific IEP academic goal. In other cases it is simply adopted as an addendum to the IEP. In the case of a 504 plan, the IHP may be the foundation upon which the plan is built. In many situations the development of an IHP may eliminate the need for a 504 plan. Because the implementation of the 504 process varies by state, the school nurse must know the specifics of the district and state where she/he works. Chapters Five and Six deals more specifically with the special education process and 504 mandate.

Emergency Evacuation Plan

An emergency evacuation plan (EEP) is written for a student who has a health condition that requires special considerations for environmental emergencies such as fire, tornado, earthquake, hurricane, or bomb scare. It is similar to an ECP in that it is a well-defined, step-by-step process that proceeds in a logical order dependent upon the previous action in response to an event that can only be anticipated.

School nurses and educational staff develop an EEP with knowledge about the student, physical layout of the school building, school district policies and procedures, and the community's emergency response system. Often this plan is developed in consultation with community agencies such as fire or police departments. An intervention activity in an IHP may be the development of an EEP. However, an IHP or ECP is not a prerequisite, for an EEP, and an EEP cannot substitute for an IHP or ECP.

An IHP for students who are accompanied to school by a nurse from a home care agency

As students with increasingly complex health needs enter schools, they often are accompanied by a nurse from an outside agency, such as a home care agency. This situation raises many issues and questions. How are nursing roles differentiated? What type of healthcare plan is needed and who is responsible? There are also many legal and potential ethical questions that are beyond the scope of this book. For the purposes of this book we will examine roles, and responsibilities as they pertain to healthcare planning in the school setting.

School Nurse Role

The school nurse is responsible for health services to all students enrolled in the school. Because the school nurse will not be providing direct care to the student, the IHP will reflect case management or care coordination activities. The following are some general guidelines:

1. The school nurse meets with home care case manager and staff who will accompany student to school prior to starting school.
2. School nurse helps to determine where and when student's medical needs will be met in the school setting.
3. School nurse orients agency staff to health office, use of phone, OSHA guidelines for schools, and emergency supplies or procedures.
4. School nurse obtains nursing care plan from home care agency initially and periodically when renewals / reviews are completed. This care plan is part of the pupil health record and may be part of the IHP.

5. School nurse obtains necessary release of information needed between home care agency and school, assuring student confidentiality.
6. The school nurse is not usually responsible for primary / direct nursing care to the student, but in the event of an emergency may provide nursing support.
7. The school nurse should develop an ECP and / or EEP if appropriate.
8. The school nurse facilitates storage of needed equipment such as oxygen, suctioning machine, humidity, or IV pole.
9. The school nurse is a member of the IEP team and provides health information needed for special education planning.
10. School nurse Fosters communication between primary care provider, home care agency, school staff, and parents.
11. School nurse instructs agency staff to keep any incidental information on other students confidential.
12. School nurse collaborates with classroom staff and home care agency to provide information to classmates / parents, if appropriate.

Home Care Agency Role

The role of the agency staff is to attend to the medical needs of the individual student, provide direct nursing care, and work cooperatively with school staff for the benefit of the student. Some general guidelines for home care agency staff include:

1. Provide name, address, and telephone number of agency and case manager. Also provide name / title of those attending school with the student.
2. Have case manager meet initially with school nurse to provide care plan, and each review thereafter. Keep school nurse informed of any changes in health status or procedures performed during the school day.

3. Work with school nurse and classroom staff to decide when and where nursing procedures will be performed to avoid classroom disruption.

4. Indicate the distance the home care staff should be from the student, such as on call outside the classroom or within the classroom.

5. Clearly describe behaviors / conditions which require medical attention.

6. Responsible to assist only the students assigned by the home care agency. School insurance does not cover agency involvement with other students or staff.

7. Maintain confidential any information derived from parent or home situation. In those cases where it is the judgment of the agency staff that it is in the interest of the child for information to be shared, parental written permission will be obtained.

8. Collaborate with school nurse and classroom staff to provide information or in-service to classmates / parents, if appropriate.

9. May attend IEP meetings or educational conferences by invitation of parent, following due process procedures.

10. Does not act as conduit of communication between parent and school about educational concerns, but instead encourages the parent to communicate directly with school staff, so as to avoid misunderstandings.

11. Provide orientation to school nurse and staff regarding agency structure, and roles and responsibility of agency staff.

The components in the IHP for the student who comes to school with home care nursing stay the same: Nursing Diagnosis, Goal, Interventions, and Outcomes. The following is a small example of such an IHP.

Nursing Diagnosis	Goals	Interventions	Outcomes
Disuse syndrome related to congenital myophathy/ immobility	Student will maintain health status while achieving educational goals	Direct care provided by home care nurse (see attached home care plan) Multidisciplinary conference. To identify health needs, roles and responsibilities of school staff and home care nurse. Develop emergency evacuation plan Develop emergency care plan in collaboration with home care nurse/ parent Provide orientation to home care nurse re: school space for care & privacy, phone, equipment storage	Student will maintain present level of physical functioning Student will experience continuity of care to meet needs Student will experience safety (physical & environmental) in the school

The Nursing Intervention Classification (NIC) system has identified several interventions that would be appropriate to use in the IHP of a student who is accompanied to school by a home care nurse. These include Environmental Management for Safety, Delegation, Family Involvement, Emergency Care, Multidisciplinary Care Conference, Referral, and Documentation.[2]

REFERENCE

1. National Association of School Nurses. *Emergency Care Plans for Students with Special Health Care Needs Position Statement.* Scarborough, Me: National Association of School Nurses, 1998.
2. Iowa Intervention Project. *Nursing* Interventions Classification (NIC). 2nd ed. St. Louis, Mo: Mosby-Yearbook, 1996. (Mosby-Yearbook, 11830 Westline Industrial Drive, PO Box 46908, St. Louis, MO 63146-9806. 800-426-4545; fax 800-535-9935.)

BIBLIOGRAPHY

Allen BS, Ball J, Helfer B. (1998). Preventing and managing childhood emergencies in school. *J School Nurs.* 1998;14(1):20-24.

American Academy of Pediatrics Committee on School Health. (1990). Guidelines for urgent care in schools. *Pediatrics.* 1990;86:999-1000.

EMSC Task Force on CSHCN. (1997). Coordinating care for children with special health care needs. *Ann Emerg Med.* 1997;30(3):274-280.

Haas MB. Individualized healthcare plans. In: Haas MB. ed. *The School Nurse's Source Book of Individualized Healthcare Plans.* North Branch, Minn: Sunrise River Press, 1993:41-44. (Sunrise River Press, 11605 Kost Dam Road, North Branch, MN 55056. 800-895-4585; fax 651-583-2023.)

Haas MB. Constructing an Individualized healthcare plan. In: Haas MB, ed. *The School Nurse's Source Book of Individualized Healthcare Plans.* North Branch, Minn: Sunrise River Press, 1993:45-54 (Sunrise River Press, 11605 Kost Dam Road, North Branch, MN 55056. 800-895-4585; fax 651-583-2023.)

National Association of School Nurses. *Emergency Care Plans for Students with Special Health Care Needs Position Statement.* Scarborough, Me: National Association of School Nurses, 1998.

Parette HP, Bartlett CR, Holder-Brown L. The nurse's role in planning for the inclusion of medically fragile and technology dependent children in public school settings. *Issues Comp Pediatric Nurs.* 1994;17:61-72.

University of Colorado Health Sciences Center, School of Nursing. *Safe at School: Planning for Children with Special Health Care Needs.* Lawrence, Kan: Learner Managed Designs, 1996.

Valluzzi JL, Brown SE, Dailey BD. Protecting the rights of children with special health care needs through the development of individualized emergency response plans. *Infant Young Children.* 1997;10(2):66-80.

3 Delegation of School Nursing Activities

Denise Ornelas

Overview

School nursing is a specialty branch of nursing that seeks to prevent or identify client health or health-related problems (primary and secondary prevention) and intervenes to modify or remediate these problems (secondary and tertiary prevention).[1] These purposes are accomplished through the provision or facilitation of health services and health education in, or as part of, the school. In so doing, school nursing contributes directly to the student's education, as well as to the health of the family and the community.[2]

Today, school nurses are often faced with decisions as to how to provide the needed healthcare services within the constraints of the school system. Financial and human resources are limited, while student needs are increasing. Therefore, many school nurses need to delegate some of the intervention activities to unlicensed assistive personnel. This chapter discusses the standards, concepts, and guidelines to delegation decision making and the application to IHP development.

Standards and Regulations

School nursing, like all nursing practice, is governed by professional and regulatory agencies. Professional agencies set the standards of practice and determine the scope of practice for nurses. According to the American Nurses Association,[3] standards are authoritative statements by which the nursing profession:

- describes the responsibilities for which its practitioners are accountable
- provides direction for professional nursing practice
- defines the nursing profession's accountability to the public
- defines the client outcome for which nurses are responsible

Regulatory agencies determine the minimum level of preparation for licensure, enforce the agreed upon scope of practice language of the state Nurse Practice Act, and enforce the laws in order to protect the public. In fact, the state Nurse Practice Act is one of the most crucial elements that the school nurse must understand when delegating intervention activities. The Nurse Practice Act, regulations, and declaratory statements of the state of practice usually take precedence over all other professional guidelines.

Definition and Concepts

Delegation is the transfer of responsibility for the performance of a task from one person to another, with the former retaining accountability for the outcome.[4] Delegation presumes that the delegator has greater knowledge, experience, and judgment and that the delegated task is only a subcomponent of the total student care process. In delegating, the school nurse uses professional judgment to decide what nursing care may be delegated and to whom.

The National Council of State Boards of Nursing[5] established the premises that constitute the basis for the delegation decision-making process. Included are:

- A licensed nurse must have ultimate responsibility and accountability for the management and provision of nursing care.
- A licensed nurse must be actively involved in and be accountable for all managerial decisions, policymaking, and practices related to the delegation of nursing care.
- Unlicensed assistive personnel (UAP) are equipped to assist, not replace, the nurse.
- The practice-pervasive nursing functions of assessment, evaluation, and nursing judgment must not be delegated.
- The UAP cannot redelegate a task delegated to an unlicensed person.

When the school nurse is deciding to delegate an intervention activity, she/he must remember that the school nurse retains the accountability for the student outcome. Many administrators and parents want to decide which nursing tasks school nurses can and cannot delegate and even to whom to delegate. While non-nurses may suggest which nursing acts may be delegated, it is the school nurse who ultimately decides the appropriateness of the delegation. This delegation is to a selected person for a specific task to a specific child in a specific situation. Once the task has been delegated, the unlicensed person cannot redelegate that task.

Deciding to Delegate

The American Nurses Association Code of Ethics[6] states, "The nurse exercises informed judgment and uses individual competency and qualifications as criteria in seeking consultation, accepting responsibilities, and delegating nursing activities." It continues with " Inasmuch as the nurse is accountable for the quality of nursing care rendered to clients, nurses are accountable for the delegation of nursing care activities to other health workers. Therefore, the nurse must assess individual competency in assigning selected components of nursing care to other nursing service personnel. The nurse should not delegate to any member of the nursing team a function for which that person is not prepared or qualified. Employer policies or directives do not relieve the nurse of accountability for making judgment about the delegation of nursing care activities."

When deciding to delegate, school nurses must consider professional standards and meet the obligations of the state Nurse Practice Act. To help nurses make appropriate delegation decisions, the Five Rights of Delegation[5] can be utilized.

The Right Task

Determination of the task, procedure, or function that is to be delegated. Is the procedure reasonably routine with a reasonably predictable outcome?

The Right Person

Staff availability. Who is available to do the nursing task, at the required time? Are enough trained staff available?

The Right Direction

Assessment of the potential delegate's competency. What kind of training has this UAP had? Is the UAP able to understand the limitations of this delegation? Is this a reliable person? Will they seek appropriate help? Will they complete the appropriate documentation?

The Right Supervision

Consideration of the level of supervision available and a determination of the level and method of supervision required assuring safe performance. How much initial and ongoing supervision does this procedure for this specific student require? How will the school nurse document and assure that adequate training and supervision have occurred? By what method and how frequently does the school nurse need to assess for the student's safety and appropriate outcome?

The Right Circumstances

Assessment of the client needs including age and vulnerability. Is this child particularly vulnerable due to age, developmental level, cognitive abilities, gender, or special health need?

Steps to Safe Delegation

In 1995, the National Association of State School Nurse Consultants[7] identified nine steps to safe delegation of nursing care. They are as follows.

1. The RN validates the necessary physician orders, parent/guardian authorization, and any other legal documentation necessary for implementing the nursing care.
2. The RN conducts an initial nursing assessment of the student's healthcare needs.
3. Consistent with the state's nurse practice act and the school nurse's assessment, the nurse determines what level of care is required.
4. Consistent with the state board of nursing regulations, the RN determines the amount of training required for the UAP. If the individual has not completed standardized training, the RN must ensure that the UAP obtains such training in addition to receiving child-specific training.

5. Prior to delegation, the nurse must have evaluated the competence of the individual to safely perform the task.
6. The RN provides a written plan of care to be followed by the unlicensed staff member.
7. The RN indicates, within the written care plan, when RN notification, reassessment, and intervention are warranted, due to a change in the student's condition, the performance of the procedure, or other circumstances.
8. The RN determines the amount and type of RN supervision necessary.
9. The RN determines the frequency and type of student health reassessment necessary for ongoing safety and efficacy.
10. The RN trains the UAP to document the delegated care according to the standards and requirements of the state's board of nursing and agency procedures.
11. The RN documents activities appropriate to each of the nursing actions listed above.

Supervision

Inherent in the decision to delegate is the obligation to provide supervision to the UAP. The American Nurses Association, which sets the standards of professional nursing, defines supervision as "The active process of directing, guiding and influencing the outcome of an individual performance of an activity."[4] Supervision is generally categorized as on-site (the nurse physically present or immediately available while the activity is being performed), or off-site (the nurse has the ability to provide direction through various means of written and verbal communications).

What is a reasonable level of supervision of a UAP in the school setting? Little has been written or researched about this component of nursing delegation. In 1990, Haas[8] stated that "a specific amount of time will depend upon the abilities, training and type and number of delegated nursing care tasks. However, a best practice would be to have on-site direct supervision of health aides by professional nurses for 50% or better of the health aide's work time. This means that the nurse is observing the care given by the health aide and training the health aide. Some time will be spent carrying out other professional activities with students and staff as well.

A minimum level of supervision would be an overlap of 20% of the health aide and professional work time at each school site. Of course, paraprofessionals should have access to professional nurses 100% of the time by phone should problems develop with particular students. If the nurse is present on-site for less than 20% of the health aide work hours, it is not likely that the nurse can adequately monitor the performance of the health aide, delegate, and train for additional tasks, or monitor students' responses to treatment.

Rights and Responsibilities

The school nurse delegator has the responsibility to make a proper act of delegation by giving clear specific directions to a person who can perform safely and competently. The burden of determining the competency of the person who will perform the tasks and ongoing evaluation rests with the nurse. The delegator is accountable for the act delegated and may incur liability if found to be negligent in the process of delegating and supervising.

The delegate has the responsibility of carrying out the delegated act or function correctly and is accountable for accepting the delegation and for his/her own actions in carrying out the act.

Based on a review of the literature, the following is a list of rights and responsibilities that could be used with UAPs as a guideline that would assure quality and safety while meeting the needs of children with special healthcare needs.

The UAP has:

- The right not to assume responsibility for a nursing task or acknowledge delegation from anyone other than an RN. Depending upon the state, this may constitute practicing nursing without a license.
- The right to training education, support, supervision, and monitoring on a regular basis for any delegated task.
- The right to ask for support, counseling, and teaching from the school nurse.
- The right to refuse delegation if you cannot competently perform task.
- The right to expect a written plan of care including emergency information.
- The right to expect a health delegation policy at your district level.
- The responsibility to maintain health data as confidential.
- The responsibility to support student's healthcare plan as developed by the licensed school nurse.
- The responsibility when performing task to make sure it is done correctly, at the right time and to report any concerns to the professional nurse.
- The responsibility not to transfer the performance of a nursing task from one student to other students without specific delegation for each student.
- The responsibility not to redelegate any task to another UAP.

IHP and Delegation Documentation

The IHP provides an effective vehicle for the documentation of nursing delegation. When describing the interventions needed to meet the student's goals and objectives, the school nurse can identify those activities that will be delegated on the IHP. The following is an excellent example by Denehy and Poulton.[9]

Figure 1. A sample IHP for a child with spina bifida.

Delegation (NIC 7650)

- Teach associate to do catherization procedure at the beginning of the school year.
- Review procedure with associate every two months.
- Teach associate the signs and symptoms of urinary tract infections.

This documentation should not be confused with the documentation of the training and supervision of the UAP. Documentation of training should include dates and times of training, a summary of training techniques employed, evaluation of the UAP's readiness, and appropriate signatures.[10] Documentation of supervision must be completed each time it is performed, as well as methods of supervision, a statement about UAP performance, and any necessary remedial measures.[10] In many situations, the use of a checklist or flow sheet is appropriate.

Summary

It is the role and responsibility of the school nurse to develop Individual Healthcare Plans to meet the health needs of students. School nurses often must rely on the help and cooperation of others in the school setting to help meet those needs. Appropriately, the nurse can choose to delegate intervention activities. The documentation of these delegated activities can easily be incorporated into the IHP. When delegation is documented, the quality of nursing care and the safety of the student are assured.

REFERENCES

1. National Association of School Nurses. *Philosophy of School Health Services and School Nursing.* Scarborough, Me: National Association of School Nurses, 1988.
2. Proctor S, Lordi S, Zaiger D. *School nursing practice: Roles and Standards.* Scarborough, Me: National Association of School Nurses, 1993:11.
3. American Nurses Association. *Standards of Clinical Nursing Practice.* Washington, DC: American Nurses Publishing, 1991:1.
4. American Nurses Association. *Registered Professional Nurses & Unlicensed Assistive Personnel.* Washington, DC: American Nurses Publishing, 1994:11.
5. National Council of State Boards of Nursing. *Delegation: Concepts and the Decision Making Process.* Chicago Ill: Natl Council of State Boards of Nursing, 1995:1, 2, 4.
6. American Nurses Association. *Code for Nurses with Interpretive Statements.* Washington, DC: American Nurses Association, 1985:1.
7. National Association of School Nurse Consultants. *Position Paper: Delegation of school health services to unlicensed assistive personnel. Am J School Nurs.* 1995;11(2):17-19.
8. Haas M. (1990). Standards of Practice: Delegation of Care and Supervision of Health Aides. In: *Healthy Children Healthy Schools.* Minneapolis, Minn: Minnesota Dept of Health, 1990:18.
9. Denehy J, Poulton S. The use of standardized language in individualized healthcare plans. *J School Nurs.* 1999;15(1):38-45.
10. Panettieri MJ, Schwab N. Delegation and supervision in school settings. *J School Nurs.* 1996;12(2):11-18.

BIBLIOGRAPHY

American Federation of Teachers. *The Medically Fragile Child in the School Setting: A Resource Guide for the Educational Team* 2nd ed. Washington, DC: American Federation of Teachers, 1998.

National Association of School Nurses. *Philosophy of School Health Services and School Nursing.* Scarborough, Me: National Association of School Nurses, 1988.

American Nurses Association. *Standards of Clinical Nursing Practice* Washington, DC: American Nurses Publishing, 1991.

American Nurses Association. *Registered Professional Nurses & Unlicensed Assistive Personnel.* Washington, DC: American Nurses Publishing, 1994.

American Nurses Association. *Code for Nurses with Interpretive Statements.* Washington, DC: American Nurses Association, 1985.

Cohn SD. Legal issues in school nursing practice. *School Nurse* 1988;4(1):9-12.

Cronenwett LR. The use of unlicensed assistive personnel: when to support, oppose or be neutral. *Journal of Nursing Administration,* 1995;25(6):11-12.

Denehy J, Poulton S. The use of standardized language in individualized healthcare plans. *J School Nurs.* 1999;15(1):38-45.

Essex N, Schifani J, Bowman S. Handle with care your school's tough new challenge: educating medically fragile children. *Am School Board J,* 1994;181:50-53.

Guidelines and Procedures for Meeting the Specialized Physical Health Needs of Pupils. Sacramento, Calif: California State Dept of Education, 1990. (Available from 1-800-346-2742.)

Haas M. Standards of Practice: Delegation of Care and Supervision of Health Aides. In: *Healthy Children Healthy Schools.* Minneapolis, Minn: Minnesota Dept of Health, 1990:18.

Heater B, Becker A, Olson R. Nursing interventions and patient outcomes: a meta-analysis of studies. *Nurs Res,* 1988;37(5): 303-307.

Holvoet JF, Helmstetter E. *Medical Problems of Students with Special Needs: A Guide for Educators.* Boston, Mass, College-Hill Press, 1989:110-114, 311-312.

Irvine D, Sidani S, Hall L. Linking outcomes to nurses' roles in health care. *Nurs Economics,* 1998;16(2):58-64.

Johns G. *Organizational Behavior: Understanding Life at Work.* New York, NY: Harper Collins, 1992.

Jones EH. PL 94-142 and the role of school nurses in caring for handicapped children. *J School Health,* 1979;49(3):147-156.

Josten L, Smoot C, Beckley S. Delegation to assistive personnel by school nurses. *Am J School Nurs.* 1995;11(2):8-16.

Luckenbill D. *The School Nurse's Role in Delegation of Care: Guidelines and Compendium.* Scarborough, Me. National Association of School Nurses, 1996.

Lynch EW, Lewis RB, Murphy DS. Educational services for children with chronic illnesses: perspectives of educators and families. *Exceptional Children,* 1992;59(3):210-220.

McGrew K, Algozzine B, Spiegel A, Thurlow M, Ysseldyke J. *The Identification of People with Disabilities in National Databases: A Failure to Communicate.* Minneapolis, Minn: University of Minnesota, College of Education, National Center on Educational Outcomes, 1993. (Technical Report no.6)

Minnesota Nurses Association. (1997). *Position Paper: Delegation and Supervision of Nursing Activities.* St. Paul, Minn: Minnesota Nurses Association, 1997. (Available from 1-800-536-4662.)

National Association of School Nurse Consultants. *Position Paper: Delegation of school health services to unlicensed assistive personnel.* Am J School Nurs. 1995;11(2):17-19

National Council of State Boards of Nursing. *Delegation: Concepts and the Decision Making Process.* Chicago, Ill: Natl Council of State Boards of Nursing, 1995.

National Education Association. *Providing Safe Health Care: The Role of Educational Support Personnel.* Washington, DC: National Education Association, 1998. (Available from 202-822-7131.)

National Standards of Nursing Practice for Early Intervention Services. Supported in part by project MCJ-215052 from the Maternal and Child Health Bureau (Title V, Social Security Act), Health Resources and

Services Administration. 1994 (This award was administered through the University of Kentucky College of Nursing Grant Leadership Development for Nurses in Early Intervention, University of Kentucky Chandler Medical Center, Lexington, Kentucky, 40536-0232.) (Available from 606-323-6687.)

Nursing Standards for Children with Special Health Care Needs: Guidelines for Practice. Screening and Assessment Manual, Newborn-Six Years and their Families. Seattle, Wash: Family Centered Nursing Graduate Specialty, Dept of Parent-Child Nursing, U of Washington, 1990. (Available from 206-685-1288.)

Palfry JS, Haynie M, Porter S, Bierle T, Cooperman P, Lowcock J. Project School Care: integrating children assisted by medical technology into educational settings. *J School Health*, 1992;62(2):50-54.

Panettieri MJ, Schwab N. Delegation and supervision in school settings: standards, issues, and guidelines for practice (part 2). *J School Nurs*. 1996;12(2):19-27.

Petr CG , Barney DD. Reasonable efforts for children with disabilities: the parents' perspective. *Social Work*, 1993;38(3):247-254.

Proctor S, Lordi S, Zaiger D. *School Nursing Practice: Roles and Standards.* Scarborough, Me: National Association of School Nurses, 1993.

Schwab N. Liability issues in school nursing. *School Nurse*, 1988;4(1):13-21.

Schwab N, Haas M. Delegation and supervision in school settings. *J School Nurs.* 1995;11(1):26-34.

Standards of Nursing Practice for the Care of Children and Adolescents with Special Health and Developmental Needs. Supported in part by project MCJ-215052 from the Maternal and Child Health Bureau (Title V, Social Security Act), Health Resources and Services Administration. 1994 (This award was administered through the University of Kentucky College of Nursing Grant Leadership Development for Nurses in Early Intervention, University of Kentucky Chandler Medical Center, Lexington, Kentucky, 40536-0232.) (Available from 606-323-6687.)

Todaro AW, Failla S, Caldwell TH. A model for training community-based providers for children with special health care needs. J School Health, 1993;63(6):262-265.

Standardized Languages in Nursing: Integrating NANDA, NIC, and NOC into IHPs

Susan Poulton and Janice Denehy

INTRODUCTION

In the last decade, nursing has come to realize the importance of standardized languages to advance the profession of nursing. This awareness has developed for a number of reasons. First, nurses realized that even though their practices were the same or similar in many situations, the words they used to describe their activities differed considerably from nurse to nurse, from region to region, and from one specialty to another. This lack of consistency hindered communication among nurses in their attempts to share information about nursing practice and caused confusion when communicating with other health professionals.

Second, as nursing entered the information age where healthcare records are computerized, it was essential that a standardized system be used to meet the requirements of the computerized patient record. It is important for common terminology to be used to enter information into a computer and to develop databases used to aggregate data. Such standardized information is also essential for reimbursement of services that nurses perform.

Another advantage of standardized languages is that even though nursing care is a major component of healthcare, there has been little documentation of what nurses do, the nursing actions or interventions they implement on behalf of school-age children and their families. In fact, nursing's contribution to healthcare and school health has been largely invisible. Standardized languages give nurses a tool to clearly describe their role in promoting health in a common language to school administrators, other health providers, and the public.

Finally, developing a knowledge base for nursing practice is critical to the profession. In order to do research on nursing practice, there needs to be some consensus on how nurses describe their practice. The development of standardized languages in nursing is an important step toward meeting these challenges faced by the profession.

So, what are standardized languages, and why are they important to school nurses? Standardized languages encompass a group of carefully developed classifications that describe the phenomena that comprise nursing practice – nursing diagnoses, nursing interventions, and nursing outcomes. A number of standardized languages have developed in nursing over the last 25 years. The North American Nursing Diagnosis Association (NANDA) developed a classification of nursing diagnoses that is widely used and accepted in the nursing profession.[1] Karen Martin developed the Omaha System of diagnoses and interventions used by nurses in community and home care settings.[2] More recently, the Iowa Intervention Project created the Nursing Interventions Classification (NIC) in response to the need for a common nomenclature to describe what it is that nurses do on behalf of clients.[3] The Iowa Outcomes Project constructed the Nursing Outcomes Classification (NOC) to assist nurses in measuring the outcomes of the care they deliver.[4]

These well-coordinated classifications not only developed standardized terminology to describe the diagnoses, interventions, and outcomes included in their classifications, but also defined these phenomena and operationalized each diagnosis, intervention, and outcome. For example, the new NANDA nursing diagnosis *Risk for Altered Development* includes four clusters of Risk Factors—Prenatal, Individual, Environmental, and Caregiver—each of these includes specific risk factors related to the diagnosis.[1] The NIC intervention *Developmental Enhancement* lists 47 activities the nurse might carry out to implement the intervention.[3] This provides information to the nurse about what this intervention entails and provides a certain amount of standardization of care. However, because the nurse may use only a few of these activities or can add other activities as appropriate, it allows for individualized care. The NOC outcome *Child Development: 3 Years* includes 16 indicators to evaluate in determining the developmental status of a 3 year-old child.[4] From these examples, it is evident that these classifications not only promote the use of standardized language, but also provide valuable information about what these diagnoses, interventions, and outcomes are to include. Such information will not only serve to improve nursing practice, but has the potential to enhance communication among nurses and to promote research on nursing practice.

Standardized language has the power to assist school nurses to clearly communicate what they do and to articulate their value to the health of children. The use of a standardized language in Individualized Healthcare Plans (IHPs) is helpful in communicating with other health professionals and the education team. IHPs usually include a nursing diagnosis, a goal, and interventions designed to reach the identified goal. The use of NANDA diagnoses, NIC interventions, and NOC outcomes assists school nurses in using a common language to describe what they do to meet student goals as outlined in the IHP. Linkages among NANDA, NIC, and NOC are included in the appendices of the NIC and NOC books.[3,4] These linkages facilitate the selection of interventions and outcomes appropriate for the nursing diagnosis made for the child. In addition, the NIC interventions and NOC outcomes are coded and can be written in a manner that can be entered into computerized information systems, information needed for potential reimbursement for services delivered to children with special healthcare needs in school settings.

We live in an era in which healthcare costs are a major concern, and cutting these costs by cutting personnel or services is common. This makes it imperative that school nurses have a language to articulate clearly what they do daily so their activities will be visible. This is particularly important as schools attempt to do more with fewer resources and difficult decisions about prioritizing limited educational funding often mean trimming or cutting existing programs. Particularly challenging to school nurses is articulating their contribution to the educational mission of the schools in terms educators can understand and appreciate. Using standardized language that clearly and succinctly identifies and defines components of care, as well as simply listing how these components are operationalized, will assist in this process.

A number of authors have written about standardized languages and their importance for school nurses.[5-9] This chapter gives an overview of standardized languages and shows how they can be integrated into IHPs.

Individualized Healthcare Plans

As school nurses know, well-written IHPs provide documentation of students' health needs, actual nursing care to be provided to meet these needs, and a plan to evaluate the outcomes of this care. IHPs also provide information for delegation and determining staffing needs in each school. The use of IHPs helps all school staff better understand the health condition of a student and improves communication among the people working with the student by clearly articulating each component of care. In addition, the documentation of nursing services provided to students is information needed for determining staffing. The use of standardized language in IHPs is useful in communicating with other health professionals and the education team about the special healthcare requirements of students. The use of NANDA nursing diagnoses, NIC interventions, and NOC outcomes assists school nurses to clearly articulate in a common language what they do to meet the student health goals.[8] In addition, the diagnosis, intervention, and outcome labels are coded and written in a manner that can be entered into computerized information systems and used for reimbursement. Linkages among NANDA diagnoses, NIC interventions, and NOC outcomes assist the school nurse to choose appropriate interventions for the diagnoses identified, and NOC outcomes measure the effectiveness of those interventions.

NANDA Nursing Diagnoses

The North American Nursing Diagnosis Association (NANDA) began its pioneering work in 1973. The work of this association has set the stage for the use of standardized language for the profession. The NANDA nursing diagnoses have gained widespread acceptance and use in nursing. The 1999-2000 NANDA classification has 158 nursing diagnoses.[1] A nursing diagnosis is defined as "A clinical judgment about individual, family, or community responses to actual and potential health problems/life processes. A nursing diagnoseis provides the basis for selection of nursing interventions to achieve outcomes for which the nurse is accountable."[1 (p. 49)] Nursing diagnoses have a label or name, a definition, related factors which describe conditions antecedent to or associated with the diagnosis, and defining characteristics which are observable signs and symptoms that are manifestations of the diagnosis.

There are three types of nursing diagnoses. The first type is an *actual* diagnosis which describes existing health conditions in a client, family, or population (e.g., *Ineffective Individual Coping*). The second type is a *risk* diagnosis that describes a health condition that may develop in a vulnerable person (e.g., *Risk for Injury*). The third type of nursing diagnosis is a *wellness* diagnosis that describes levels of wellness and the potential for enhancement to a higher level of functioning (e.g., *Potential for Enhanced Spiritual Wellbeing*). The classification has developed over the years as nurses have suggested and created new diagnoses related to their practice area and submitted them for review by the NANDA Diagnosis Review Committee for consideration into the classification. The latest edition of the NANDA classification added 31 new diagnoses.[1] An additional 37 diagnoses were revised on the basis of feedback by nurses interested in updating existing diagnoses to reflect current practice. School nurses have an opportunity to add to the nursing diagnoses in the NANDA classification by creating new diagnoses that reflect the needs identified in the school population. An example identified by the author (JD) is *Risk for Unintended Pregnancy*, which would be an appropriate diagnosis for sexually active adolescents.

The nursing diagnoses in the NANDA classification have been organized into a taxonomy according to nine patterns. This taxonomic structure, based on Martha Roger's patterns of unitary persons, provides structure to retrieve diagnoses. Diagnoses are numbered in a basic outline format. Since this numbering system was developed, computerization has changed the parameters of numbering systems. NANDA's Taxonomy Committee has tentatively approved a new taxonomic structure adapted from Marjorie Gordon's Functional Health Patterns.[10] Work continues on this new structure and codes for computerization of nursing diagnoses.

NANDA Nursing Diagnoses in IHPs

In the IHP, the nursing diagnosis describes the identified problem area that will be addressed in the school setting. The nursing diagnoses are developed by the school nurse using clinical judgment and are based on the assessment data gathered about the student. The nurse may come up with one or more nursing diagnoses for a particular student. Each diagnosis will lead to specific student goals and expected outcomes and appropriate interventions to reach those goals and outcomes. The use of NANDA provides a common language to define the student's problem areas. The written nursing diagnosis includes the diagnostic label, etiology, related or risk factors, and defining characteristics. A fourth

component, secondary to, may be used if needed to clarify the diagnosis to users of the IHP. Sometimes this component may help explain to teachers and parents why the identified problem is a concern for this student. For example, the diagnosis *Constipation related to immobility, characterized by hard, infrequent stools, secondary to cerebral palsy*, includes all four components.

The Nursing Interventions Classification

The Nursing Interventions Classification (NIC) is a comprehensive, standardized language describing treatments that nurses perform in all settings and in all specialties.[3] It was developed by a research team formed in 1987 at The University of Iowa College of Nursing, including nurses representing a wide range of clinical specialties and practice settings. NIC was created on the basis of existing research and clinical practice. The structure of NIC is easy to use with language that is familiar and clinically useful. "It has been implemented in numerous clinical and educational settings and is currently being field tested in a variety of clinical agencies from tertiary care and long-term care settings to ambulatory settings and schools. NIC is included in the Methathesaurus for a Unified Medical Language by the National Library of Medicine, has been added to the index of the Cumulative Index to Nursing & Allied Health Literature (CINAHL), and listed by the Joint Commission on Accreditation of Healthcare Organizations (JCAHO) as one classification that can be used to meet the standard on uniform data."[8 (p. 40)]

The NIC includes 433 interventions which are grouped into a taxonomy to facilitate access by the practicing nurse. A nursing intervention is defined as "Any treatment, based upon clinical judgment and knowledge, that a nurse performs to enhance patient/client outcomes."[3] [(p. xvii)] Each nursing intervention has a name or label, a definition, a set of activities that a nurse does to carry out the intervention, and a short list of background readings. NIC contains interventions that reflect the wide scope of school nursing practice.[7] It includes interventions for illness management (e.g., *Seizure Management*), disease prevention (e.g., *Immunization/Vaccination Administration*), and health promotion (e.g., *Health Education*). There are also interventions for individuals (e.g., *Tube Care: Gastrointestinal*), for families (e.g., *Family Integrity Promotion*), as well as aggregates and communities (e.g., *Health Education and Environmental Management: Safety*). In addition to direct care interventions, those interventions "performed through interaction with the patient(s)" (e.g., *Medication Administration and Oxygen Therapy*), there are indirect care interventions that are "performed away from the patient but in behalf of the patient" (e.g., *Delegation, Documentation and Referral*).[3] [(p. xvii)] The given NIC label and definition are to be used as stated in NIC, but the activities listed under each NIC label are only suggestions. Any of these suggested activities can be selected if needed for the individual student, or other additional activities may be created as appropriate.

The structure of NIC has been designed for easy accessibility, going from an abstract level to a more concrete level. The highest and most abstract level of the taxonomy is the domains. The six domains of NIC are: "Physiological: Basic, Care that supports physical functioning; Physiological: Complex, Care that supports homeostatic regulation; Behavioral, Care that supports psychosocial functioning and facilitates life-style changes; Safety, Care that supports protection against harm; Family, Care that supports the family unit; and Health System, Care that supports ef-

fective use of the healthcare delivery system."[3] [(pp. 56-57)] The six domains are organized into 27 classes which further group related interventions. For example, the Safety domain includes two classes, "Crisis Management, Interventions to promote immediate short-term helping both psychological and physiological crises" and "Risk Management, Interventions to initiate risk-reduction activities and continue monitoring risks over time."[3] [(p. 66)] The Crisis Management class lists 10 interventions, and Risk Management includes 36 related interventions. A coding system is used to identify each intervention, based on the domain, class, and the specific intervention. This coding system will facilitate the use of NIC interventions in a computer information system. This classification has been enthusiastically accepted by the profession. It is currently being used in practice, education, and computer information systems. In addition, clinical validation has begun in numerous settings, ranging from large hospitals and long-term care settings to ambulatory settings and schools.

NIC Nursing Interventions in IHPs

In the IHP, the NIC intervention label describes and categorizes the care delivered. After the label, specific activities to implement the intervention are listed. These activities are to be individualized to the student and carried out by the school nurse or other designated person. Interventions implemented in the school setting and listed in the IHP include both direct and indirect care. The interventions may be specific prescribed orders (e.g., *Medication Administration* and *Urinary Catherization: Intermittent*), nursing care and ongoing monitoring of health status, delegating and teaching of nonlicensed personnel, supervision of these staff members, and follow-up and ongoing communication with parents, the education team, and healthcare providers. It is important to include both direct care (e.g., *Tube Care: Gastrointestinal*) and indirect care (e.g., *Delegation* and *Multidisciplinary Care Conference*) interventions in the IHP. Also included with the intervention activities is the title or name of the person delegated to carry out the activity in the school setting. Remember that delegation includes consideration of the person's willingness to complete the task, the competency level and scope of practice, training and supervision of that person, and safety of the student/potential for harm.

The listed activities in NIC are suggestions that fit with the particular intervention. If appropriate, these activities may be chosen and individualized to meet student needs. Of course, additional activities should be included, if necessary, to meet the needs of the student. The authors of NIC recommend six factors to consider when choosing a nursing intervention.[3] These same factors can be applied to the process of choosing interventions to include in the IHP. First, consider what is the desired student outcome already identified and which interventions can be undertaken to help the student reach the stated goals. Second, consider the nursing diagnoses and what interventions will change the related factors or treat the signs and symptoms. Third, think about the research base of the interventions and choose those that have proven to be effective. Fourth, consider the feasibility of actually completing the intervention and what is pertinent to the student's health status. Fifth, choose interventions that will be acceptable to the student and parents, and perhaps to the staff involved in the care of the child. Sixth, consider the capability and competence of the staff carrying out the intervention. After consideration of each of the above factors, the nurse can determine what interventions are needed

to meet the student goals and outcomes and optimize the student's health.

School nurses bring a vast knowledge and experience base to their practice. They often know what interventions need to be initiated for students with special healthcare needs. It is just a matter of using a classification system to put the interventions on paper, using the standardized language provided by the classification. With repeated usage, patterns will develop and many of the same intervention labels will be used for groups of students with similar health concerns, as with the linkages among diagnoses, interventions, and outcomes.

NOC Nursing Outcomes

Like NIC, the Nursing Outcomes Classification (NOC) was developed by a research team at The University of Iowa College of Nursing. This classification consists of 190 nurse-sensitive outcomes which "define the general patient state or perception resulting from nursing interventions."[4 (p. 22)] The procedures used by the Iowa Outcomes Project to develop NOC were similar to NIC. In NOC, each outcome has a neutral label or name and a definition, followed by a list of indicators which describe the client behavior or the patient status. NOC outcomes are stated in *neutral terms*. The reason for this is that client status may move in the desired direction, however, it may remain unchanged or deteriorate. Therefore, a neutral outcome label is able to accurately characterize the actual behavior, whatever the direction. It is important to note that NOC outcomes differ from desired patient outcomes or goals in that goals are stated as the *desired* end results or behavior and are not neutral in nature.

Each NOC outcome also includes a five-point scale to rate indicators. For example, the outcome *Risk Control: Sexually*

Transmitted Diseases (STD) uses the 5-point scale, never, rarely, sometimes, often, and consistently demonstrated, to measure the related indicators; the outcome *Parenting* uses the 5-point scale, not, slightly, moderately, substantially, and totally adequate, to measure the indicators related to parenting.[4] The scales can be used to determine baseline status prior to intervention, and to compare with client status at different points after interventions have been implemented. By making this comparison, the nurse can determine the effectiveness of the intervention and modify it accordingly.

NOC has developed 16 different scales to measure outcomes. The outcomes in the first edition of NOC were designed for individuals and their caregivers; the second edition, to be published in 2000, will add outcomes for groups, families, and communities. When using NOC outcomes, one must use the NOC label and definition as written. Outcomes can be customized, however, by choosing indicators that are relevant to the specific child's goals or by developing additional indicators.

The NOC outcomes have been organized into a taxonomy. The taxonomy consists of six domains: "Functional Health, Outcomes that describe capacity for and performance of basic tasks of life; Physiological Health, Outcomes that describe organic functioning; Psychosocial Health, Outcomes that describe psychological and social functioning; Health Knowledge & Behavior, Outcomes that describe attitudes, comprehension, and actions with respect to health and illness; Perceived Health, Outcomes that describe impressions of an individual's health; and Family Health, Outcomes that describe health status, behavior, or functioning of the family as a whole or of an individual as a family member."[4 (p. 1)] The six domains contain 24 classes: for instance, the Functional Health domain contains the following classes: Energy Maintenance, Growth and Development, Mobility, Self-Care, and Sensory Function. At the next level, each class groups related outcomes (e.g., Growth and Development contains 17 outcomes related to an individual's physical, emotional, and social maturation). NOC is currently beginning the process of validating the outcomes as well as field testing the outcomes in clinical practice. The NOC outcomes have been coded with a unique six-digit number reflecting the domain, class, and outcome. In addition, each indicator, scale, and scale value can be added to the code to facilitate the computerization and analysis of outcome data.

NOC Outcomes in IHPs

The use of NOC in the IHP assists the nurse to identify and evaluate the student outcomes. The IHP is reviewed at least yearly and when there is any change in the student's health status. Basically, when evaluating the IHP, the nurse must decide if the stated goal was achieved. "The evaluation process includes: a) reviewing the desired student outcome, b) collecting data to determine the outcome, c) comparing the actual outcome to the desired student outcome, d) documenting the outcome on the IHP, e) relating the appropriateness and effectiveness of the selected interventions to the outcome, and f) reviewing and modifying the plan of care as necessary. The use of NOC outcomes provides a quantitative measure of student progress that is easy for all healthcare providers to use and understand."[8 (p. 44)] The language used in NOC outcomes is easily understood by other members of the healthcare and the education team.

To review, when writing the actual IHP, the school nurse determines the nursing diagnosis based on assessment data; from this diagnosis the nurse writes goals for the student; the interventions are then designed to meet the goals articulated; and finally, the outcomes are measured to determine the effectiveness of the interventions and progress toward meeting student goals. The NOC outcome label indicates the area of concern to be monitored. The outcome is directly related to the nursing diagnosis; the nurse may identify one or more outcome statements per nursing diagnosis. Each NOC outcome has a scale and a list of indicators. These indicators can be tailored to the individual student needs. The outcome statement is neutral, written at a more abstract level using the NOC terminology. The individual student goal in the IHP may be written using the NOC terminology by determining the desired condition on the measurement scale of the outcome. When it is time to complete the evaluation of the IHP, the actual outcomes can be evaluated using the NOC outcome scale. The NOC scales can be included right in the written IHP (see Sample IHP) and used before or after the intervention. By including the NOC scales in the IHP, members of the team can see how student outcomes will be measured and can observe student progress toward reaching the goals established in the IHP.

Summary

School nurses know that it is important to document their delivery of special healthcare services to students in IHPs. To make the IHP a useful document, it is best to write the IHP in a consistent way that can be easily communicated to other members of the healthcare team and members of the education team. By using standardized language in IHPs, school nurses will be doing just that—documenting the provision of special health services to individual students consistently in a form that is easily communicated to others involved in the care of the student. The use of a standardized language also provides data on the care provided and the outcomes of that care. This information can then be entered into computerized information systems for data collection and research. A survey of computer technology utilization in school nursing in 1992 found that only 4% of the 188 school nurses sampled used computers to develop IHPs; by 1996 the number had increased to 24%.[11] By computerizing the data included in IHPs, school nurses have the potential to develop large databases. This information can be used to show school nurses' contribution to the health of children with special needs.

This data also will provide the impetus for research on interventions that school nurses use and how they use their time. It can also be used to examine the linkages between interventions and outcomes — which interventions are most effective in reaching the desired outcome. When coupled with student demographic and educational data, school nurses will be able to track the academic progress of children with special healthcare needs. This data has the potential to show the value of school nurses in promoting optimal health and maximizing learning in children with special healthcare needs. Such data may help make the case for additional nurses or personnel to assist nurses in their work with students. In this age of budget cuts and the replacement of nurses with nonlicensed personnel, it is even more important for school nurses to document what nursing interventions, both direct and indirect, are necessary to meet the special healthcare needs of children. This process is assisted through the use of standardized languages. Finally, it is essential for this information to be entered into databases that show in a tangible way what school nurses do to contribute to the health of the children they serve.

Individualized Healthcare Plan*
Asthma

Assessment Data	Nursing Diagnosis	Student Goals	Interventions	Outcomes
12-year-old diagnosed asthma at age 9	**Risk for Ineffective Breathing (NANDA 1.5.1.3)** Characterized by shortness of breath, coughing, and/or wheezing related to asthma	ˉ. Student will demonstrate appropriate use of inhaler at the beginning of school year.	**Airway Management (NIC 2K-3140)** **Activities:** • Review use of inhaler with student at the beginning of the school year. (Nurse)	**Symptom Control Behavior (NOC 4Q-1608)** **Indicators:** Recognizes symptom onset Never 1 Rarely 2 Sometimes 3 Often 4 Consistently 5
Carries Proventil inhaler at all times		2. Student will initiate treatment when symptoms appear throughout the school year.	• At the beginning of the school year, review with teacher, and other appropriate staff, the signs and symptoms of asthma exacerbation and when student should use his inhaler.	Uses preventive measures Never 1 Rarely 2 Sometimes 3 Often 4 Consistently 5
Independent in identifying symptoms and need for treatment		3. Student will keep record of peak flow meter readings if required throughout the school year.	• Every two months, obtain student's record of inhaler use for documentation in health file. Report increased use of inhaler to parents/physician. (Nurse)	Uses relief measures Never 1 Rarely 2 Sometimes 3 Often 4 Consistently 5

M.D. order normal P.E. program	4. Student will keep record of use of inhaler for health office throughout the school year. 5. Student will avoid having an emergency asthma attack during this school year.	**Emergency plan:** See STUDENT ASTHMA ACTION CARD[12] located in classroom, locker room, and health office.	Reports controlling symptoms Never 1 Rarely 2 Sometimes 3 Often 4 Consistently 5

I have read and approve of the above plan for school healthcare:

Parent signature_____   Date reviewed by the educational team_____

Nurse signature_____   Physician signature (optional)_____

*See Appendix for student profile information to include on an IHP form.

Individualized Healthcare Plan*
Diabetes

Assessment Data	Nursing Diagnosis	Student Goals	Interventions	Outcomes
	Altered Health Maintenance (NANDA 6.4.2)		**Hyperglycemia Management (NIC 2G-2120)** **Activities:**	**Treatment Behavior: Illness or Injury (NOC 4Q-1609).** **Indicators:**
12-year-old with diabetes diagnosed 3 years ago, history of poor control	Related to lack of independence in diabetes management and poor control of diabetes	1. Student will administer insulin injections independently 50% of the time during this school year.	• Assist student to check blood sugar 30 minutes before lunch per protocol. (Nurse/trained staff)	Complies with recommended treatment Never 1 Rarely 2 Sometimes 3 Often 4 Consistently 5
On Insulin three times per day (one time at school)		2. Student will use glucometer independently 50% of the time during this school year.	• Review use of glucometer with student at the beginning of the school year and as needed. (Nurse)	Complies with medication regimen Never 1 Rarely 2 Sometimes 3 Often 4 Consistently 5
Needs assistance with diabetes management			• Monitor urine for ketones if blood sugar >250. (Nurse/student)	Performs self-care consistent with ability Never 1 Rarely 2 Sometimes 3 Often 4 Consistently 5

Missed 20 days of school last year because of illness related to diabetes		• Assist student to draw up and administer insulin before lunch per protocol.(Nurse)
		• Review insulin administration with student at the beginning of the school year and as needed. (Nurse)
		• Instruct dietary staff on appropriate food choices for student at the beginning of the school year and review every semester. (Nurse)
Regular P.E. with some restrictions if blood sugar is > 250 and urine with ketones present. (See management protocol in classroom and health office)	3. Student will select appropriate foods and comply with diet 50% of the time during this school year.	• Instruct student on appropriate diet at the beginning of the school year and review as needed after review of blood sugars (see food list). (Nurse)
	4. Student will record blood sugars and insulin on log during this school year.	• Instruct teachers on appropriate food choices for student, signs of hypo/ hyperglycemia and appropriate response at the beginning of the school year and review every two months (see food list and emergency plan). (Nurse)

Individualized Healthcare Plan*
Diabetes (continued)

Assessment Data	Nursing Diagnosis	Goals	Interventions	Outcomes
		5. Student will recognize signs and symptoms of early insulin shock and report to staff immediately during this school year.	• Instruct student on signs of hypo/hyperglycemia and appropriate response at the beginning of the school year and review as needed depending on level of control. (Nurse)	Monitors changes in disease status Never 1 Rarely 2 Sometimes 3 Often 4 Consistently 5
		6. Student will be absent from school fewer than 2 days per month during this school year.	• Review with student her available sources of sugar. (Nurse) • Instruct student on urine ketone testing per attached protocol and review as needed. (Nurse) • Assist student in adjusting insulin dose, carbohydrate/fluid intake, and exercise program as indicated per protocol. (Nurse) • Report adjustments in management plan, blood sugars, and signs/ symptoms of hypo/ hyperglycemia to parent/ physician. (Nurse)	Balances treatment, exercise, work, leisure, rest and nutrition Never 1 Rarely 2 Sometimes 3 Often 4 Consistently 5

Self-Responsibility Facilitation (NIC 3O-4480)

Activities:
- Set up contract with student at the beginning of the school year to promote independence with diabetic management, review with student monthly. (Nurse)
- Encourage independence and provide positive feedback to student at each interaction as appropriate. (Nurse)
- Report student's progress to parents at least monthly and encourage their support. (Nurse)

Self-Esteem Enhancement (NIC 3R-5400)

Activities:
- Reinforce student's positive aspects at each interaction as appropriate. (Nurse/staff)

7. Student will participate in two extracurricular activities this school year

Self Esteem (NOC 3M-1205)

Indicators:
Description of success in work or school

Never	1
Rarely	2
Sometimes	3
Often	4
Consistently	5

Individualized Healthcare Plan*
Diabetes

Assessment Data	Nursing Diagnosis	Student Goals	Interventions	Outcomes
			• Provide student access to private place (health office) for checking blood sugars and administering insulin. (Nurse/staff)	Description of success in social groups Never 1 Rarely 2 Sometimes 3 Often 4 Consistently 5
			• Encourage participation in school activities as appropriate. (Nurse/staff)	Description of pride in self Never 1 Rarely 2 Sometimes 3 Often 4 Consistently 5
			• Monitor self esteem regularly, i.e. negative comments about self, interactions with peers, involvement in activities, etc., and refer to school counselor as indicated. (Nurse/staff)	Expresses positive feelings about self-worth Never 1 Rarely 2 Sometimes 3 Often 4 Consistently 5

I have read and approve of the above plan for school healthcare:

Parent signature_____   Date reviewed by the educational team_____

Nurse signature_____   Physician signature (optional)_____

*See Appendix for student profile information to include on an IHP form.

REFERENCES

1. North American Nursing Diagnosis Association. *NANDA Nursing Diagnoses: Definitions & Classification 1999-2000*. Philadelphia, Pa: North American Nursing Diagnosis Assn, 1999. (NANDA, 1211 Locust Street, Philadelphia, PA 19107. 800-647-9002; fax 215-545-8107; e-mail: NANDA@nursecominc.com)

2. Martin KS, Scheet NJ. *The Omaha System: Applications for Community Health Nursing*. Philadelphia, Pa: WB Saunders Company, 1992.

3. Iowa Intervention Project. *Nursing Interventions Classification (NIC)*. 2nd ed. St. Louis, Mo: Mosby-Year Book, 1996. (Available from Mosby-Year Book, 11830 Westline Industrial Drive, PO Box 46908, St. Louis, Mo 63146-9806. 800-426-4545; fax 800-535-9935.)

4. Iowa Outcomes Project. *Taxonomy of Nursing Outcomes Classification (NOC)*. Iowa City, Iowa: Iowa Outcomes Project, 1997. (Available from Mosby-Year Book, 11830 Westline Industrial Drive, PO Box 46908, St. Louis, Mo 63146-9806. 800-426-4545; fax 800-535-9935.)

5. Hootman J, Nursing diagnosis — a language of nursing; a language for powerful communication. *J School Nurs.* 1996; 12(4):19-23.

6. Lunney M. The significance of nursing classification systems to school nursing. *J School Nurs.* 1996;12(2):35-37.

7. Pavelka L, McCarthy AM, Denehy J. Nursing interventions used by school nurses. *J School Nurs* 1999;15(1): 27-31.

8. Denehy J, Poulton S. The use of standardized language in individualized healthcare plans. *J School Nurs.* 1999;15(1):38-45.

9. Cavendish R, Lunney M, Luise BK, Richardson K. National survey to identify the nursing interventions used in school settings. *J School Nurs.* 1999;15(2):12-19.

10. Gordon M. *Nursing Diagnosis Process and Application*. 3rd ed. St. Louis, Mo: Mosby-Year Book, 1994.

11. Smith CE, Young-Cureton V, Hooper C, Deamer P. A survey of computer technology utilization in school nursing. *J School Nurs.* 1998; 14(2): 27-34.

12. Asthma and Allergy Foundation of America. 1123 15th Street NW, Suite 502. Washington, DC 20005.

Using Individualized Healthcare Plans with 504 Plans and Accommodations

Jeanne M. Sedgwick

INTRODUCTION

What Is Section 504?

Historically the main interpretation and enforcement of Section 504 of the Rehabilitation Act of 1973 has centered around employment issues for individuals with disabilities. In recent years more emphasis has been given to the enforcement of Section 504 in the area of education of individuals with disabilities. This statute prohibits discrimination against individuals with disabilities, including students, by public school districts receiving federal financial assistance. Unlike Individuals with Disabilities Education Act (IDEA), Section 504 does not have state or federal funding provided to assist districts in complying with its implementation . All costs are the obligation of the local school district. [1,2]

Section 504 protects the rights of persons with disabilities. It prohibits agencies or organizations which receive federal funds from discrimination against otherwise qualified individuals solely on the basis of disability. Under Section 504, individuals are determined to have a disability if they:

1) have a physical or mental impairment which substantially limits one or more major life activities (walking, seeing, hearing, speaking, breathing, *learning,* working, caring for oneself, performing manual tasks).

2) have a record of such impairment, or;

3) are regarded as having such an impairment.

For example, this can mean that a school-age child who has attention deficit disorder (ADD) or some other disability and does not qualify for special education services may still be entitled to accommodations or other services in regular education under Section 504 (see Chapter Appendix I). The learner is regarded as having a disability by a medical doctor. The disability limits the major life activity of learning. The learner must have an accommodation plan under Section 504 if he or she is substantially limited by the disability within the educational setting.

School districts are required annually to take appropriate steps to identify and locate every qualified individual who has a disability, even if that individual does not qualify for special education services. If determined eligible for consideration of a 504 Plan, the team must outline current levels of performance and what services and/or accommodations are necessary for the student to benefit from his/her educational program. These steps must be taken even though the student is not covered by the IDEA special education provisions and procedures. The evaluation and accommodation plan must be developed by the building review team, not the special education team [1,2] (see Chapter Appendix II).

The rational for the school nurse to be involved in this process lies within the very definition of eligibility for consideration for 504: the student must have a physical or mental impairment which substantially limits a major life activity. The school nurse's assessment skills are an essential part of that evaluation to determine the student's physical or mental impairment. In some cases, the school nurse's services may involve direct nursing care, interventions in specific types of primary prevention, and case management, as well as assessment.

How to Develop a 504 Plan

1) Referrals are received from parents, individual teachers, learners, and/or community agencies.

2) Presenting problem(s) and previous interventions are considered and reviewed. The summary includes all current information and recommendations for additional evaluation.

3) The school notifies the parent(s) of the school's reason and intent to conduct an evaluation. This notice includes due process rights and a description of the evaluation. (At this point, some districts require the individual school team to notify the district coordinator of intent to evaluate under 504.)

4) Section 504 requires that a school district evaluate each identified learner with a disability before making an initial placement or any subsequent, significant change in her/his placement.

5) Parental consent is not required by Section 504, but is best practice.

6) In cases where services and/or accommodations are necessary, the school plans a 504 team meeting and identifies all staff and parent(s) who should be included in the meeting. (Some school districts require that the district's Section 504 coordinator be invited to this meeting.)

7) The following factors are considered:
   a) Results of assessment/evaluation
   b) The learner's unmet needs
   c) Needed services and/or accommodation(s)
   d) Possible staff in-service

8) Necessary accommodations and/or services are planned and implemented. Best practice dictates a written accommodation plan. The plan is developed by a multidisciplinary team knowledgeable about the learner and it is reviewed periodically. [3] An annual review is strongly recommended but not required. The frequency of reevaluation and the designation of a case manager (not required, but recommended) can also be stated in the 504 Plan. This helps to ensure compliance and accountability.

First priority must be given to providing this program in the regular education classroom, with a written plan for related aids, services, and accommodations. [4] In 1992, the Department of Education issued a clarification paper that stated that special education and related services as defined under IDEA are required by Section 504 if the child's education cannot be achieved satisfactorily in the regular education classroom with modifications.

Section 504 requires that districts designate an employee to be responsible for assuring district compliance with Section 504 and provide a grievance procedure for parents, learners, and employees. It also requires that the parent have an opportunity to participate and be represented by counsel. Section 504 requires periodic review. The details of due process are left to the discretion of the school district. The Office of Civil Rights investigates Section 504 complaints.[3]

What to Include in 504 Plans

The chapter Appendix III includes samples of 504 plans. Although there are many variations of 504 plans, each 504 plan should address these basic elements:

1) Description of the nature of the concern

2) Description of the basis for the determination of disability

3) Description of how the disability affects a major life activity

4) Description of supplementary aids, services, and accommodations that are necessary

5) Review/Reassessment date

6) Participants' names and titles

7) Case manager

The IHPs that are used by school nurses across the country can become variations of 504 plans. An IHP should include information about the student that would easily fit into a 504 format (see Chapter Appendix IV for example). Both 504 plans and IHPs can help to insure that modifications and accommodations are made in the regular education program.[5]

Individualized Healthcare Plan*
504 Accommodation Plan

Assessment Data	Nursing Diagnosis	Goals	Nursing Interventions	Expected Outcomes
Description of the nature of the concern. Description of the basis of the determination of the disability.	Description of how the disability affects a major life activity.		Description of instructional and supplemental aids, services and accommodations.	

*See Appendix for student profile information to include on an IHP form.

Appendix I. Special Services for Students

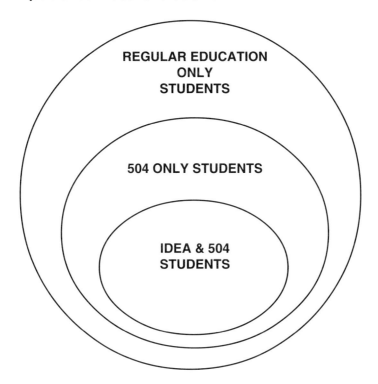

IDEA/504 STUDENTS
Are qualified under one or more of thirteen (13) IDEA disabling conditions. Specially designed individual education programs are planned for each student by IEP teams.

SECTION 504 STUDENTS ONLY
substantial mental or physical impairments that limit one or more of the student's major life activities, special accommodations to the student's program are required. A 504 accommodation plan is designed for each student according to individual need. Examples of potential 504 handicapping conditions not typically covered under IDEA are:
- communicable diseases – HIV, tuberculosis
- medical conditions - asthma, allergies, diabetes, heart disease
- temporary medical conditions due to illness or accident
- Attention Deficit Disorder (ADD, ADHD)
- behavior difficulties
- drug/alcohol addiction
- other conditions

NOTE: IDEA refers to students in special education.

Appendix II. IDEA/504 Flow Chart

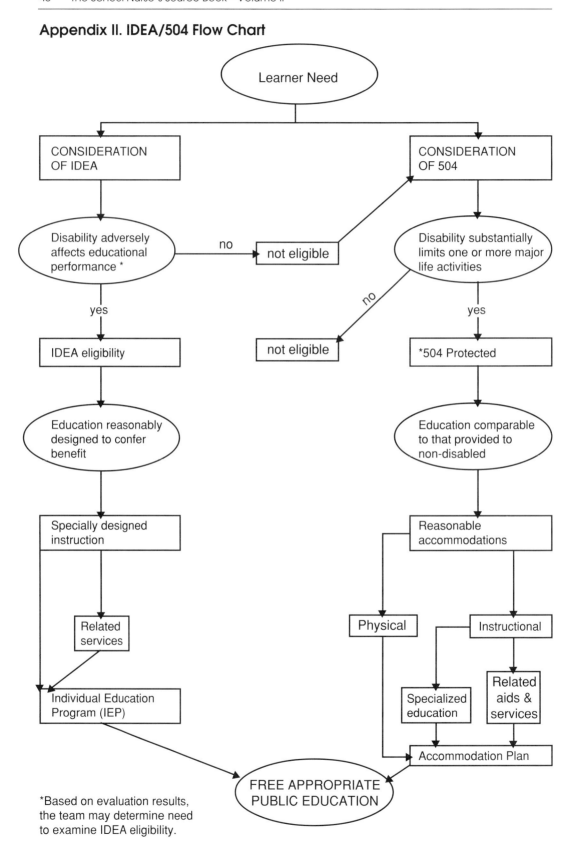

*Based on evaluation results,
the team may determine need
to examine IDEA eligibility.

Appendix III. Sample Section 504 Plans

**REGULAR EDUCATION PLAN
SECTION 504**

Student_____   School_____
Date of Birth_____   Grade_____

1. Describe the nature of the concern: _____
    _____
    _____

2. Describe the basis for the determination of disability:_____
    _____
    _____

3. Describe how the disability affects a major life activity:_____
    _____
    _____

4. Describe the services and/or accommodations that are necessary:_____
    _____
    _____
    _____
    _____

Review/Reassessment date:_____

Signatures

_____   _____
                                        Title

_____   _____
                                        Title

_____   _____
                                        Title

_____   _____
                                        Title

Cc   Cumulative File

STUDENT ACCOMMODATION PLAN
SECTION 504

Student _____   School _____
Date of Birth_____   Grade _____

PART I: JUSTIFICATION FOR SERVICES

1.   Is the student disabled under Section 504?

    ( ) Yes   ( ) No

  ( ) The student has a physical or mental impairment which substantially limits
     one or more of his/hers major life activities.

( )	caring for one's self	( )	hearing
( )	performing manual tasks	( )	speaking
( )	walking	( )	working
( )	seeing	( )	learning
( )	breathing	( )	other

     How does the disability affect a major life activity? _____
     _____
     _____

OR

  ( ) Has a record of such a disability?_____
     _____
     _____

OR

  ( ) Is regarded (perceived) as having such a disability?_____
     _____
     _____

2.   Briefly document the basis for determining the disability?

     _____
     _____
     _____
     _____

PART II: STUDENT ACCOMMODATIONS

Accommodation 1:   _____
                    _____
        Objective   _____
                    _____
        Objective   _____
                    _____
Accommodation 2:   _____
                    _____
        Objective   _____
                    _____
        Objective   _____
                    _____
Accommodation 3   _____
                    _____
        Objective   _____
                    _____
        Objective   _____
                    _____
                    _____

DURATION OF ACCOMMODATION(s) From_____   To_____

Review/Reassessment date: _____

Participants

Name   Title   Date

_____   _____   _____

_____   _____   _____

_____   _____   _____

cc: Student's cumulative file

**504 ACCOMMODATION PLAN
SAMPLE FORM**

NAME _____ DATE _____

STUDENT ID# _____ DATE OF BIRTH _____ CA _____

SCHOOL_____ TEACHER_____ GRADE _____

1. Describe the manner of the concern_____
    _____

2. Describe the basis of the determination of handicap (if any)_____
    _____

3. Describe how the handicap affects a major life activity_____
    _____
    _____

4. The Child Study Team/Intervention Assistance Team has reviewed the files of the above named student and concludes that he/she meets the classification as a qualified handicapped individual under Section 504 of the Rehabilitation Act of 1973. In accordance with the Section 504 guidelines, the school has agreed to make reasonable accommodations and address the student's individual needs by:

PHYSICAL ARRANGEMENT OF ROOM:
_____ seating student near the teacher
_____ seating student near a positive role model
_____ standing near the student when giving directions or presenting lessons
_____ avoiding distracting stimuli (air conditioner, high traffic areas, etc.)
_____ increasing the distance between the desks
_____ additional accommodations_____

LESSON PRESENTATION:
_____ pairing students to check work   _____providing written outline
_____ writing key points on the board   _____allowing student to tape record lessons
_____ providing peer tutoring   _____having student review key points
_____ visual aides   _____orally teaching through multi-sensory modes
_____ providing peer note taker   _____modes using computer assisted instruction
_____ making sure directions are
_____ including a variety of activities during each lesson
_____ breaking longer presentations into shorter segments
_____ additional accommodations_____

ASSIGNMENTS/WORKSHEETS:
_____ giving extra time to complete tasks   _____using self monitoring devices
_____ simplifying complex directions   _____reducing homework assignments
_____ handing worksheets out one at a time   _____not grading handwriting
_____ reducing the reading level of the assignments
_____ requiring fewer correct responses to achieve grade

_____allowing student to tape record assignments/homework
_____providing a structured routine in written form
_____providing study skills training/learning strategies
_____giving frequent short quizzes and avoiding long tests
_____shortening assignments; breaking work into smaller segments
_____allowing typewritten or computer printed assignments
_____additional accommodations_____

TEST TAKING:
_____allowing open book exams   _____allowing extra time for exams
_____giving exam orally   _____reading test item to student
_____giving take-home tests
_____using more objective items (fewer essay responses)
_____allowing student to give test answers on tape recorder
_____giving frequent short quizzes, not long exams
_____additional accommodations_____

ORGANIZATION:
_____providing peer assistance with organizational skills
_____assigning volunteer homework buddy
_____allowing student to have an extra set of books at home
_____sending daily/weekly progress reports home
_____developing a reward system for in-school work and homework completion
_____providing student with a homework assignment notebook
_____additional accommodations_____

BEHAVIORS:
_____praising specific behaviors   _____allowing legitimate movement
_____using self-monitoring strategies   _____contracting with the student
_____giving extra privileges and rewards _____increasing the immediacy of rewards
_____implementing time-out procedures   _____keeping classroom rules simple and clear
_____making "prudent use" of negative consequences
_____allowing for short breaks between assignments
_____cueing student to stay on task (nonverbal signal)
_____marking student's correct answers, not his or her mistakes
_____implementing a classroom behavior management system
_____allowing student time out of seat to run errands, etc.
_____ignoring inappropriate behaviors not drastically outside classroom limits
_____additional accommodations_____

SPECIAL CONSIDERATIONS:
_____suggesting parenting program(s)   _____alerting bus driver
_____monitoring student closely on field trip _____suggesting agency involvement
_____providing group/individual counseling _____in-servicing teacher(s) on student's
_____providing social skills group experiences   handicap
_____developing intervention strategies for transitional periods (e.g., cafeteria, physical
       education, etc.)

MEDICATION:
Physician_____Phone_____
Medication(s)_____Schedule_____
_____Schedule_____
Monitoring of medication(s)_____daily_____weekly_____as needed basis
Administered by_____Title_____

COMMENTS:_____

_____

_____

Participants

Name	Title	Date
_____	_____	_____
_____	_____	_____
_____	_____	_____
_____	_____	_____

Case Manager's Name _____

REFERENCES

1. Department of Education. A clarification of state and local responsibility under Federal law to address the needs of children with attention deficit disorder. *Ofc Special Educ Rehab Services News.* 1992; Winter:7-29.

2. Maroldo RA. Educating students with ADD/ADHD: what are your responsibilities? *Special Educator.* 1992;7: 225-228.

3. Minnesota Department of Education. *Section 504: Educational Modifications and Accommodations.* Minneapolis, Minn: Minnesota Dept of Education, 1994.

4. Horowitz IW, King TB, Meyer WC. Legally mandated options available to children with ADHD within public education. *Clinical Pediatrics.* 1993; 32: 702-70.

5. Sedgwick JM. *Implementation of Section 504 Guidelines in the School Setting for Children Diagnosed with Attentional Disorders.* Mankato, Minn: Mankato State University, 1995.

Using Individualized Healthcare Plans in Special Education—IEPs and In Reimbursement Processes

Janet Lowe

INTRODUCTION

There has been a continual increase in recent years in the number of students with chronic health conditions who are also eligible for and receiving special education services. For some school nurses, working with special education students is a full-time practice. For others, it may be a portion of the myriad of responsibilities they have as part of their school nursing practice.

The range of health conditions among special education students has also increased. Some special education students do not have health-related conditions that impact their ability to learn. Other students have conditions that vary widely from mild health conditions to severe, multiple health conditions that have a profound and direct impact on their ability to learn. The school nurse plays a critical role in the special education process, especially when the health and /or physical needs of the student, if left unattended, would prevent or restrict the student from full participation in his or her educational program.

An Individualized Healthcare Plan (IHP) is a valuable tool that can assist school nurses to accomplish their role in the special education process. IHPs can be integrated into the Individual Education Program (IEP), ensuring that the health needs of the student are addressed and saving the school nurse time.

This chapter gives school nurses guidelines for their role in the special education process. It also provides a description of how the IHP can be used and integrated into the process.

Special Education Procedure

By federal law every school district shall have some type of procedure, or process, for determining if a student is eligible for special education.[1] The exact process and procedure is individualized by each school district. Committees that manage the special education referrals may be called multidisciplinary teams, special education teams, child study committees, or school support teams. These committees are comprised of a multidisciplinary team consisting of regular education teachers, special education teachers, the principal, a psychologist, and related service providers, such as a school nurse, occupational therapist, physical therapist, and speech therapist.

This interdisciplinary team has a responsibility to follow federal and state laws and determine if a student who is having difficulty learning is eligible for special education and, if eligible, to outline the current level of performance, special education needs, goals and objectives, and any services and related services that are necessary for the student to benefit from his/her educational program.

The school nurse's role on this committee is critical. The school nurse brings a unique and valuable perspective on how each child's health may, or does, impact his or her ability to learn. The school nurse may be involved as a related service provider for nursing services on the IEP.

Referral Process and Initial Screening

Learners who are having difficulty in school are referred to the committee that determines special education eligibility. Parents, teachers, or others who are concerned and involved with the student can make referrals. This initial evaluation must include the consent of the parent.[2] or guardian, and some states require listing at least two prereferral interventions. (Prereferral interventions are planned, systematic efforts by regular education staff to resolve apparent learning or behavioral problems.[3])

After a referral is submitted and before conducting an assessment, the team conducts a review of the student's performance in the following areas: intellectual functioning, academic performance, communicative status, motor ability, vocational potential, sensory status, physical status, emotional and social development, and behavioral and functional skills.

The school nurse's role is to review information in the categories of physical and sensory status:

- Chronic health concerns, or problems, that are educationally significant
- Medical diagnosis
- Health conditions affecting strength, endurance, alertness, attendance, organization in the classroom, and activity intolerance

- Medications, or treatments
- Current vision and hearing screenings
- Attendance problems related to health

If the school nurse has already completed an IHP on a student, this information should be readily available.

Notice of an Educational Assessment/Reassessment Plan

The child is assessed in all areas of suspected disability.[4] for an initial assessment and a three year reassessment. According to law, a student who is receiving special education must be reassessed every three years. The special education committee makes a decision, based on concerns related to education needs, about whether an assessment is needed in any of the following areas: intellectual functioning, academic performance, communicative status, motor ability, vocational potential, sensory status, physical status, emotional and social development, and behavior and functional skills.[5]

Federal law[6] requires that a notice be sent to the parent that describing any evaluation procedures the agency proposes to conduct. This notice must include information about the area(s) to be assessed, personnel who will assess the student, including name and title, and the plan for the assessment. The areas to be assessed must be completed by qualified, trained, and knowledgeable personnel. Qualified means that a person has recognized certification, licensing, registration, or other requirements that apply to the area in which he or she is providing special education, or related services.[7] The school nurse is the most qualified person available to complete the health/physical and sensory status areas. Listed below is an example that the school nurse may use when completing this notice.

> *The school nurse will complete a health assessment to determine the learner's health needs that are relative to academic performance and will include: a review of health history, a review and interpretation of medical records, hearing and vision assessment, a review of school health records, parent or guardian interview, classroom observation, and attendance patterns.*

Once the parent or guardian has signed this notice, there are strict regulations, according to law, regarding timelines for when the reports, or assessments, need to be completed. To be compliant with the law, all team members must adhere to these guidelines.

Health Assessment

The purpose of the health assessment is to identify how health problems, or conditions, impact the student's ability to learn and participate in his or her educational program.

If the student has an IHP, the school nurse may already have much of the information accessible for a special education health assessment.

The health assessment may include the following:
- Family health history
- Pregnancy/labor/delivery/neonatal histories
- Developmental history
- Childhood illness/injury/lead poisoning
- Hospitalizations/surgeries
- Review of systems (eyes, ears, nose, throat, respiratory, cardiac, endocrine, neurologic, gastrointestinal, genitourinary, skin)
- Social/emotional history
- Culture issues
- Family issues
- Chemical use issues
- Self-care skills
- Mobility
- Nutrition
- Sleep patterns
- Activity tolerance
- Transition issues/school and work/level of independence
- School attendance patterns
- Allergies
- Current medications and treatments (home and school)
- Current medical diagnosis/healthcare provider(s)
- Nursing diagnosis
- Current IHP/emergency care plan (ECP)
- Vision and hearing
- Insurance access to care

The school nurse should summarize these results in a concise summary for the Assessment Team Summary Report (ATSR).

Assessment Team Summary Report

The ATSR is a summary of all the assessments and a determination is made by the special education committee[8] makes a determination:

1) Whether the student is *eligible for a particular category of special education*

2) Regarding the child's *present levels of performance and educational needs*

3) Whether the child needs special education and *related services*

4) Whether any *additions, or modifications,* to the special education and related services are needed to enable the child to meet the measurable annual goals set out in the child's individualized education program (IEP)

The essential components for the school nurse to include in the ATSR are:
- **Interpretation of Results and Present Level of Performance**

Describe the student's general health status, vision and hearing status, and current health conditions, and their implications on the student's ability to learn and participate in his or her educational program and the impact they have in the student's academic environment (e.g. classroom, field trips, job site).

- **Special Education Needs**

"Special educational needs" means the necessary nursing services required by the student to benefit from special education to attain IEP goals and objectives.

Nursing services is considered a related service. It is the school nurse's responsibility to determine if nursing services as a related service are necessary for the student to benefit from his or her special education program.

The special education needs should be described as the nursing interventions needed during the school day to maintain the current health status and will allow the student to benefit, or be able to participate, in the special education program. Any special adaptations, or supports, that eliminate health-related barriers to learning, such as preferential seating, use of elevator, and self-help skills, also need to be listed and described.

The school nurse may refer to the student's IHP when describing nursing interventions and adaptations. However, summarize briefly, avoiding medical/nursing jargon, when writing your report for the ATSR.

Examples of information to include on the ATSR are listed below. Consult with the case manager as to how she or her would like this information submitted to the ATSR.

Student with Asthma

John was diagnosed with asthma when he was 2 years old. Other than his asthma, he has been in good general health. His vision and hearing status is within normal limits. Currently, his asthma has been stable. Coughing and tightness in his chest are John's main symptoms when he is having problems with his asthma. He is aware of these symptoms and his triggers. The main triggers of his asthma are strenuous exercise, and colds, and he is allergic to cats and dogs. John uses an inhaler daily 15 minutes before physical education, and every 4 to 6 hours as needed. John will need nursing service as a related service for medication administration, assessment for signs and symptoms of exacerbation of asthma, and an emergency plan. The teacher should notify the school nurse of any field trips planned as he will need to bring his inhaler. John may need some adaptations in physical education for certain skills, such as the mile run. The teacher should avoid having John exposed to any animals in the classroom and on field trips.

Student with Attention Deficit Hyperactivity Disorder (ADHD)

Sally has a history of being in good general health. Her vision and hearing status is within normal limits. She was diagnosed two years ago as having ADHD. When she is not on medication, she exhibits symptoms of distractibility and impulsivity. She is currently on Ritalin, 15mg, at 8am and 12 noon daily. With this medication regime, the teachers have noted increased attending to task and less impulsive behaviors; however, she continues to have problems with work completion. Sally will need adaptations in her classroom that include a reduced workload in her assignments, and well-defined coping skills to continue dealing with the impulsive behaviors. Sally will need nursing services as a related service for daily administration of medication and for assessment of medication effectiveness and side effects. She will also need her medication on field trips.

Special Education Categories of Eligibility

The special education committee makes a determination about whether a student is eligible for special education and documents this information on the ATSR.

Listed below are categories of eligibility for special education. Each category has specific criteria that the student must meet to be eligible to receive special education services[9]

A child with a disability means a child with:

1. Mental impairments
2. Hearing and vision impairments
3. Speech or language impairments
4. Deaf-Blindness
5. Emotional disturbances
6. Autism
7. Traumatic brain injury
8. Physically impairments
9. Other health impairments
10. Learning disability
11. Developmental delays (ages 3 to 9)

Physical development, cognitive development communicative development, social and emotional development, adaptive development)

It is the school nurse's responsibility to *become familiar with the criteria* for those areas of eligibility that may involve health-related issues that pertain to nursing, in particular, numbers 2, 4, 5, 7, 8, 9, and 11. Each school nurse needs to check state statutes and rules regarding these categories. The nurse's assessment is crucial in assisting the child study team to determine if a student is eligible for special education services for certain categories.

Many categories of eligibility, such as emotional disturbances, other health impairments, physical impairments, and traumatic brain injury, will need documentation of a medical diagnosis. The school nurse can assume this responsibility to *assist the team in obtaining the medical diagnosis and other medical documentation and to interpret the information received.*

Related Services

"Related services" means transportation and such developmental, corrective, and other supportive services as are required to *assist a student with a disability to benefit from special education.*

A student must be eligible for special education before they can be eligible for nursing as a related service on the IEP[10] *School health services* are considered a related service. Other examples of supportive related services include speech pathology and audiology services, early identification and assessment of disabilities in children, medical services for diagnostic or evaluation purposes, occupational and physical therapy, parent counseling, recreation, counseling, psychological services, rehabilitation counseling services, and social work.[11]

School health services are defined as services provided by a qualified school nurse, or other qualified person.[12] Qualified means that a person has the approved certification, licensing, registration, or other comparable requirement that applies to the area in which he or she is providing special education, or related services.[13]

It is the school nurse's responsibility to determine if nursing services as a related service is a *necessary* service for the student to benefit from his or her special education program. It is considered *necessary* if the student cannot attain his or her IEP goals or participate in the educational program without the supportive service. Related services must be documented on the IEP.

Individual Education Program (IEP)/ Individual Family Service Plan (IFSP)

An IEP is a written statement for each child with a disability that is developed, reviewed, and revised at least annually for a student in accordance with federal and state laws. An IFSP is a written statement for providing services for toddlers and infants with disabilities, and their families through interagency agreements.[14] Procedural and program requirements for the IEP also apply to the educational components of the IFSP.

The IEP must include[15]:
• A statement of the child's present levels of educational performance
• A statement of annual goals, including short-term instructional objectives
• A statement of specific special education and related services provided
• Projected dates for initiation of services and the anticipated duration of the services
• Evaluation procedures
• Transition services

Components of the IEP/IFSP Documentation for School Nursing

Statement of Related Service Needed—The IEP/IFSP should include a general statement regarding the supportive and related services needed. Listed below are some examples of general statements describing why nursing as a related service is necessary for the student.
• Student with ADHD
  Nursing service is a necessary related service for medication administration and management to control neurobehavioral status to allow the student to benefit from his or her special education program.

• Student with learning disability and asthma
  Nursing service is a necessary related service for nebulization treatments to maintain respiratory status and attendance patterns to allow the student to benefit from his or her special education program.
• Student with a gastrostomy tube feeding
  Nursing service is a necessary related service for gastrostomy tube feeding to maintain nutritional status and attendance patterns to allow the student to benefit from his or her special education program.
• Student with seizures
  Nursing service is a necessary related service for medication administration and management to maintain neurologic status and attendance patterns to allow the student to benefit from his or her special education program.

Goals and Objectives— IEP goals and objectives are educationally based. School nurses are usually not required to write educational goals and objectives on the IEP unless a student is learning a behavior, or task, related to his or her health condition (e.g., glucometer testing, self-catheterization, nebulization procedure). For students requiring extensive nursing services, your school district may want you to attach an IHP to the IEP.

Listed below is an example of what the school nurse may use if he or she is required to write educational goals and objectives. Using the Expected Student Outcomes in the IHP examples will assist the school nurse with writing student-based objectives.

Present Level of Performance Area: John has severe persistent asthma and requires daily nebulization treatments at school to maintain respiratory status. With consistent daily treatments his attendance patterns have been good. He has missed only 2 days of school in 3 months due to illness. He is interested in learning more about his asthma and is ready to learn the tasks of the procedure to do the nebulization treatments.

Pupil-Based Special Education Need:
John needs to learn a healthcare procedure that assists him in staying healthy to maintain optimal attendance patterns. John also needs to learn more about managing his asthma.

Annual Goal:
Increase from being dependent on someone else for the nebulization treatment and management of his asthma to being independent in self-care of the nebulization treatment and more knowledgeable regarding management of his asthma.

Objectives:
1. Demonstrate proper administration techniques of the nebulization procedure during 90% of the attempts by the end of the school year as charted by the school nurse.
2. John will be able to describe his triggers and symptoms in 3 out of 4 tries by the end of the school year as charted by the school nurse.
3. John will be able to initiate and follow his prescribed asthma action plan in 3 out of 4 attempts by the end of the school year as charted by the school nurse.
4. John will be able to list motivators and barriers to compliance with the asthma action plan in 3 out of 4 attempts by the end of the school year as charted by the school nurse.
5. John will have minimal disruptions in his education program due to asthma and have a good school attendance pattern (absent fewer than 10 days per school year) as documented by the teacher on the attendance card.

Document Direct and Indirect Nursing Service Time—The IEP must list the special education services and related services provided. The school nurse's name, title, and nursing time must be documented on the IEP. For reimbursement purposes, documentation of nursing service time on the IEP is required.

- Direct Nursing Service – examples include:
  - Administration of medications
  - Administration of nebulization treatments
  - Administration of a gastrostomy feeding
  - Teaching a student a health-related procedure

- Indirect Nursing Service – examples include:
  - Nursing management activities, such as communication with teachers, parents, other disciplines (occupational or physical therapy)
  - Writing of IHPs and emergency plans
  - Teaching educational staff

Periodic/Annual Reviews—There must be procedures for evaluation of the IEP annually. The school nurse's responsibility is to provide an update of the student's health status and health needs. If there are changes in the IEP regarding services needed, services provided, direct or indirect health services time, they need to be documented in the periodic/annual review.[16]

Transition Services

The IEP for each student, beginning no later than age 16 (and at a younger age, if determined appropriate by the state mandate), must include a statement of the needed transition services.[17]

Transition services are a coordinated set of activities that promote movement from school to postschool activities, including postsecondary education, vocational training, integrated employment, continuing and adult education, adult services, independent living, or community participation.

The coordinated set of activities must be based on the individual student needs and include instruction, community experiences, development of employment and postschool objectives and, if appropriate, the acquisition of daily living skills and functional vocational evaluation. Transition services may be specially designed instruction, or related services, if they are required to assist a student with a disability to benefit from special education.

Health Assessment—When

completing the health assessment for a student who is in need of transition services, the school nurse must consider that the student is transitioning from school into postsecondary activities that may include job sites, independent living, and community involvement. The school nurse must assess the related health needs and the student's level of independence in these new environments. In addition to the health assessment, the school nurse should assess the student's independence and level of healthcare skills. Listed below are examples of healthcare skills.[18] Can the student:

- Describe his or her chronic illness or disability
- Understand the implication of chronic illness/disability on daily life
- Describe the needs and accommodations for work or for school
- Identify the healthcare provider and insurance coverage
- State the health need at school, or to teacher

- Know what medication he or she is taking and for what, or carry information in wallet
- Be responsible for taking own medication
- Be responsible for doing own treatments
- Call for medical appointments and keep a calendar of medical/dental appointments
- Access transportation for medical/dental appointments
- Obtain sex education materials/birth control/family planning information as needed
- Fill a prescription, if needed

Assessment Team Summary Report—The school nurse

must summarize the results of the health assessment and assessment of the healthcare skills in the ATSR. The summary should include the interpretation of results, the current level of performance, and the special education needs, including any health-related services, or teaching, needed for transitioning.

IEP Documentation for Transition Services— The IEP must

include a statement of the needed transition services, including any special education or related services needed. If the IEP team determines that transition services are not needed in any of the areas, the IEP must include a statement and rationale to that effect.[19]

Summary of School Nurse's Role in the Special Education Process

1. Being involved on special education committee
2. Initial screening
3. Conducting initial health assessment

and three-year health assessments, and determining whether health problems are significant in the academic environment, including transition planning

4. Conducting annual/periodic reviews
5. Being knowledgeable about the criteria for eligibility for categories of special education that may be health-related
6. Determining if "school health services" are needed for the student to benefit from his or her special education program
7. Documenting school health/nursing services on the IEP/IFSP

Conclusion

The number of children and adolescents with chronic health conditions continues to increase. Newacheck and Taylor [20] found that 31% of 17,110 children under 18 years of age were affected by chronic health conditions and over two-thirds of these children required medications. Many of these students will be eligible for special education.

Students who are in special education have an even higher incidence of chronic health conditions. Palfrey and associates [21] found that 47.8% of special education students are reported to have at least one health condition and 17.8% were reported to have more than one. All students who are in special education are required to have an Individualized Education Program (IEP) and a large number of these students will require healthcare services that are outlined in Individualized Healthcare Plans (IHPs) and Emergency Plans.

Individual Healthcare Plans must be integrated into the IEP process.[22] This integration, and documentation of services provided, will be beneficial to school nurses, school districts, and students for several reasons:

First, school districts are being financially strained to provide healthcare services to students. To receive reimbursement for these services, the services must be documented and outlined on the IEP and the IHP. Third party payers, upon parental consent, may request documentation of these services.

Second, school districts may use the amount of time and service documented on IHPs and IEPs as indicators for the numbers of nursing personnel needed and the distribution of nursing services in a school district. By having this documentation, school nurses may be able to increase the numbers of nurses in a school district and the amount of time assigned to a school.

Third, knowledge of how to integrate IHPs into the IEP process will update school nursing practice to meet mandated state and federal laws and standards of practice.[23] With ensuing litigation in the United States, school nurses are prudent to be knowledgeable of the special education mandates and their role in this process.

Finally, and most important, the integration of the IHP into the IEP process will ensure that children and adolescents receive the necessary healthcare services that will contribute to their educational success.

REFERENCES

1. Individuals with Disability Education Act, 20 USC §1414 (1998).
2. 20 USC §1414 (a.1.C) (1998).
3. Minnesota State Board of Education. Children with a disability. Minn.R. 3525.2550 (1.B) (1998).
4. 20 USC §1414 (a.3.C) (1998).
5. Minn.R. 3525.2750 (1.A) (1998).
6. 20 USC §1414 (b.1) (1998).
7. Individuals with Disability Education Act. 34 CFR 300.115 (1998).
8. 20 USC §1414 (c.1.B.i-iv) (1998).
9. 20 USC §1401 (3.A.B) (1998).
10. 34 CFR 300.17 (note 1) (1998).
11. 34 CFR 300.16 (1998).
12. 34 CFR 300.17 (b.11) (1998).
13. 34 CFR 300.15 (1998).
14. 20 USC §1401 (11,12) (1998).
15. 34 CFR 300.346 (a,b) (1998).
16. 34 CFR 300.146 (1998).
17. 34 CFR 300.46, 300.18 (1998).
18. West MA, ed. *Assessment with Special Needs: A Guide for Transition Planning*. Seattle: University of Washington Press, 1988.
19. 34 CFR 300.346 (1998).
20. Newacheck PG, Taylor WR. Childhood chronic illness: prevalence, severity, and impact. *Am J Public Health*. 1992;82:364-371.
21. Palfrey JS, Singer JD, Walker, DK, Butler JA. Health and special education: a study of new developments for handicapped children in five metropolitan communities. *Public Health Reports*. 1986;101:379-388.
22. Denehy J, Poulton S. The use of standardized language in individualized healthcare plans. *J School Nurse*. 1999;15(1):38-45.
23. Proctor ST. *School Nursing Practice: Roles and Standards*. Scarborough, Me: National Association of School Nurses, 1993.

BIBLIOGRAPHY

The Bluebook: A Uniform System of Citation Cambridge, Mass: Harvard Law Review Association, 1996.

Denehy J, Poulton S. The use of standardized language in individualized healthcare plans. *J School Nurs*. 1999; 15(1): 38-45.

Haas MB, ed. *The School Nurse's Source Book of Individualized Healthcare Plans. Vol 1*. North Branch, Minn: Sunrise River Press, 1993.(Sunrise River Press, 11605 Kost Dam Road, North Branch, MN 55056. 800-895-4585; 651-583-3239; fax 651-583-2023).

Individuals with Disability Education Act, 34 CFR §300 (1998).

Minnesota State Board of Education. Children with a disability. Minn. R. 3525 (1998).

Individuals with Disability Education Act, 20 USC §1400 (1998).

Lowe J, Miller W. Health services provided by school nurses for students with chronic health problems. *J School Nurs*. 1998;14(5):4-16.

Newacheck PG, Taylor WR. Childhood chronic illness: prevalence, severity, and impact. *Am J Public Health*. 1992; 82:364-371.

Palfrey JS, Singer JD, Walker DK, Butler JA. Health and special education: a study of new developments for handicapped children in five metropolitan communities. *Public Health Reports*. 1986; 101:379-388.

Proctor ST. *School Nursing Practice: Roles and Standards*. Scarborough, Me: National Association of School Nurses, 1993.

West M A, ed. *Assessment with Special Needs: A Guide for Transition Planning*. Seattle, Wash: University of Washington Press, 1988.

RESOURCES

Internet access:

Code of Federal Regulations.—Available at: http://www4.law.cornell.edu/cfr 34p300.htm#start

Minnesota Rules.—Available at: http://www.revisor.leg.state.mn.us/arule/3525/

United States Code.—Available at: http://www4.law.cornell.edu/uscode/

Medically Fragile Children in the School Setting

Brenda Kay Lenz

INTRODUCTION

Who are the medically fragile children?

The concept "medically fragile" is frequently heard in educational circles, especially among school nurses. This concept, without a definition, can be very abstract. An initial step, before planning educational programming, is to define the concept and understand who are the medically fragile children.

In reviewing the literature, two terms can be found to define the same group of children. The educational literature most often uses the term *medically fragile*. In May of 1997 the American Federation of Teachers published a manual entitled, *The Medically Fragile Child in the School Setting*. The manual defines medically fragile children as students with specialized healthcare needs that require specialized technological healthcare procedures for life support and/or health support during the school day. These students may not require special education. Medically fragile children have also been described as persons with complex medical care needs who require technology, specific services, or some form of ongoing medical or nursing support for survival. [1]

The healthcare community frequently uses the term technology-dependent child. There now exists a population of technol-ogy-dependent children who, from infancy to adolescence, require specialized medical care and equipment to support them while they grow. These same children were previously cared for in hospitals, oftentimes in the intensive care unit, because they required special equipment and nursing care. [2, 3]

In 1988 the Task Force on Technology-Dependent Children reported to Congress that a technology-dependent child is a child between the ages of birth to 21 years with a chronic disability that requires the routine use of a medical device to compensate for the loss of a life-sustaining body function; daily ongoing care and/or monitoring is required by trained personnel. [4] The technological equipment required to care for these children may include tracheostomy tubes, ventilators, nebulizers, monitors, gastrostomy or other specialized enteral feeding tubes, and hyperalimentation. [5]

Prevalence

Few studies of prevalence have been done. In 1994, Palfrey and associates[5] released data from surveys conducted in 1987 and 1990 in Massachusetts. The surveys were conducted to determine the size, pattern of distribution, and trends in the population of children assisted by medical technology. The authors obtained an unduplicated count of all Massachusetts children from 3 months to 18 years of age who used one or more of the following: tracheostomy, respirator, oxygen, suctioning, gastrostomy, jejunal or nasogastric feedings, ostomies, urethral catheterization, ureteral diversion, intravenous access, or dialysis. They found an overall prevalence estimate of 0.16 percent and applied this rate to the United States child population, which yielded an estimate of 101,800 children assisted by medical technology nationwide.

The number of children that are technologically-dependent continues to grow. New medical techniques and technology have resulted in more children surviving illnesses, including increased survival rates of very low-birth-weight babies and children experiencing major trauma. [3] Also, equipment is now suitable for out-of-hospital care for these children. This has allowed children to be discharged to a home environment. [2]

Pathophysiology

There are a number of etiologies assigned to the disabilities associated with technology-dependent or medically fragile children. Included are congenital anomalies, chronic conditions, perinatal factors, hereditary-genetic conditions, and injuries and infections. [5, 6]

Congenital anomalies

Congenital anomalies, or birth defects, can arise at any stage of prenatal development and show wide variability in etiologic factors as well as in type, extent, and frequency of defects. About 2% to 3% of all births are associated with a major anomaly, mental retardation, or genetic disease. These disorders are associated with chromosomal abnormalities, and others are produced by intrauterine environ-

ment factors. Some disorders are associated with a multifactorial inheritance. A recognized pattern of malformations due to a single specific cause is called a syndrome, such as Down syndrome or fetal alcohol syndrome. [6]

Chronic conditions

A chronic illness is a condition that interferes with daily functioning for more than three months in a year, causes hospitalization of more than one month in a year, or is likely to do either of these. Some of these conditions include malignancies, cerebral palsy and other neuromuscular disorders, seizure disorders, immunodeficiency syndrome, asthma, chronic respiratory disorders (excluding bronchopulmonary dysplasia), congestive heart failure and other noncongenital heart conditions, renal disorders (for example, chronic renal failure, glomerulonephritis), malabsorption, chronic malnutrition, hydrocephalus, and gastroesophageal reflux. [6]

Perinatal factors

Perinatal factors can be associated with prematurity, bronchopulmonary dysplasia, meconium aspiration, perinatal asphyxia, and necrotizing enterocolitis. [6]

Hereditary-genetic conditions

Hereditary-genetic conditions include the following examples: cri du chat syndrome; trisomy 18, trisomy 21, or Down syndrome; cystic fibrosis; Duchenne type muscular dystrophy; mucopolysaccharidoses; other inborn errors of metabolism; Werdnig-Hoffmann disease; Tay-Sachs disease; sickle cell anemia; thalassemia; hemophilia; and inherited immunodeficiencies. [6]

Injuries and Infections

Injuries can include unintentional injuries such as motor vehicle crashes, near-drowning, head trauma, spinal cord injuries, cardiopulmonary arrest, and burns. Infections include congenital viral infections, osteomyelitis, meningitis, viral encephalitis, and acquired immunodeficiency syndrome (AIDS). [6]

Management

Medically fragile children receive treatment intervention based on their particular condition. Interventions may include:

- respiratory management—oxygen, aerosol therapy including bronchodilators, steroids, decongestants, chest percussion, tracheostomy care, suctioning, respiratory and cardiac monitors
- dietary management—feedings, tube feedings, nutritional supplements
- physical activity management—range of motion, frequent repositioning
- elimination management—diapering, maintaining intake and output records, catheterization, ostomy and colostomy care
- neurological management—seizure monitoring, seizure medications
- psychosocial management—family support and coping, education, staff needs

INDIVIDUALIZED HEALTHCARE PLAN

Assessment

History

- What are the diagnoses (may be multiple) and when were they made?
- What is the history related to the diagnoses? Or etiology?
- Prognosis?
- Bodily systems involved in diagnoses? What is the degree and pattern of physical disabilities related to diagnosis? Has there been any change in the disabilities? What was the amount of change and why was there a change?
- Recent hospitalizations and/or surgery? When? What? How does it affect current care?
- Are there existing growth and developmental delays? What are they?
- What healthcare providers are involved in management, including home care and nursing?
- What technologies, equipment, and medication have been needed to manage needed healthcare in the past?

Current Status and Management

- Current medical management plan: technologies, equipment, response in an emergency
- Current medications and side effects
- Assessment of bodily systems including:
  1) Gross and fine motor development, muscle tone, reflexes, mobility needs
  2) Self-care and abilities
  3) Nutrition including feeding method
  4) Respiratory/Cardiac
  5) Elimination
  6) Neurologic/Seizures

7) Activity tolerance
8) Communication
9) Sensory—vision, hearing, taste, touch
10) Mental functioning

- How is care provided in the home—family, nurse, personal care attendant, or other? Is a home care agency involved?
- How does the family pay for this care? Will the school be able to bill the insurance carrier for services rendered while at school?
- What equipment is necessary to care for the student? Who will provide the equipment at school? How will the equipment get to school?
- Transportation needs of the student to/from school?
- Lifting needs? Weight of student, does student participate in transfers, number of adults needed to transfer student?

Self-care

- Student's understanding of medical/health management
- Student's ability to participate in medical/health management and what, if any, can be managed on student's own
- Family or healthcare provider's understanding of needs
- Activities tolerated (dependent on treatments and condition)
- Mobility needs (independent and dependent functioning)

Psychosocial

- Age and developmental level
- Student's perception and feelings of condition(s) and technologies
- Student's perception of what friends, students, and family members think and feel about him/her and his/her condition
- Student's support systems: family, friends, home care, respite care, other
- Outside activities—school-related, sports, church, community
- Mental health concerns

Academic Issues

- Academic or cumulative school records, patterns of academic performance
- Teacher's perception of student's performance and classroom needs
- Comparison of student's performance to peer norms
- School attendance pattern
- Transportation needs: to and from school, field trips
- Need for special education, transportation, classroom adaptations, occupational or physical therapy, vocational guidance
- Amount and type of school health services needed to support the student during school day
- Amount and type of any additional educational support needed during day
- Equipment necessary to care for the child in the school setting. Who will provide the equipment, how will it get to school?
- School environment: privacy and space for needed healthcare activities, storage area for supplies

Nursing Considerations

During the process of developing an IHP, the school nurse and administration will need to make some decisions based on careful consideration of the student's needs.

Staffing Needs

- Based upon the student's needs a determination will be made as to the level of nursing care the student will need. Can the school nurse, in addition to her or his other obligations, provide the nursing care at the frequency and amount that the student needs? Will the school nurse decide to delegate those cares? To whom can she/he delegate? A paraprofessional? Do the cares require skilled nursing services such as an LPN or an RN?
- If hiring additional nursing staff to support the student, consider your options: 1) The school could hire and employ the nurse, 2) The school could contract with a home care agency to provide all services, including direct nursing care and case management, 3) The school could contract with the home care agency to provide the nurse while the school nurse provides case management of the student and supervision of the home care nurse.
- Points to consider when making this decision:
  1) If the student is frequently absent, what will the school-employed nurse do? Will you continue to pay her or him or assign other work?
  2) Schools usually have two pay scales—teacher and paraprofessional contracts. On what pay scale will you hire the licensed nurse? Will you be able to find a nurse to work at that pay level?
  3) If you hire a school-employed nurse and he/she is sick, who will cover the care during the absence?
  4) If you cannot find a school-employed nurse for an extended period, who will cover the cares during this period? Or if your school-employed nurse resigns her or his position, what will you do until you can hire another nurse?
  5) Will this nurse provide educational services in addition to the nursing care as   directed by the Individual Educational Program (IEP) and the licensed teacher? The nurse's contract and job description will need to reflect this issue.
- The school nurse will need to train and supervise staff and substitutes working with the student. Training and supervision need to be documented. Make arrangements for when staff are absent and the student comes to school.
- The school nurse is responsible for any delegated nursing care and staff need to have access to his or her decision-making abilities in a timely fashion, at all times. The school nurse may need to carry a pager or cell phone.

Working with the physician

- Physician orders for any medications, medical treatments, and healthcare procedures to be done at school need to be obtained. This may include physical or occupational therapy, chest percussion, oxygen levels, amount and timing of feedings, medications, when and what type of suctioning, and others.
- If the school bills the insurance carrier or Medical Assistance, the physician will need to sign a Report of Professional Worker (RPW) every two months to continue care. The school nurse is usually the case manager and writes the RPW. See below.

Payment of nursing services

* Arrange for payment of the nursing care. Frequently, skilled nursing services can be billed to Medical Assistance or another insurance carrier. See individual state regulations, supreme court rulings, and healthcare policy about billing options and requirements.
* Insurance providers require detailed records of care completed and periodic reports (usually bimonthly) to the physician for his/her signature. These reports are sometimes referred to as the RPW. Care delegated to a paraprofessional cannot be billed but the licensed nurse's time to train and supervise the paraprofessional can be.

Preparing the school site

* Arrange for a secure place to store any needed equipment and medication. This will need to be close enough to allow for easy access, but out of the reach of other students.
* Make arrangements to get needed equipment to school. This may include: oxygen, humidifiers, nebulizers, and others. Options: parents provide equipment, school bills provider for additional equipment and orders through a durable service goods company, school provides extra equipment.
* Plan on the unexpected. The student's condition may deteriorate and he or she may need more nursing care. What if the oxygen doesn't get delivered or the humidifier quits working?
* Develop an emergency plan and train those involved in working with the student.
* Provide a place for healthcare procedures to be performed which is private and away from the rest of the students—especially if the medically fragile student receives rectal medications, diapering, catheterizations, or experiences periods of dyspnea, etc.

DNR/DNI orders, a special concern

* Do not resuscitate (DNR) or do not intubate (DNI) are orders a physician makes after a serious and lengthy discussion with the family. This can be quite a traumatic decision for families and always indicates the seriousness of the child's condition and the child's prognosis and his/her future quality of life.
* When a child with a DNR/DNI order enrolls at the school, the nurse will want to review the district's DNR/DNI policy. Districts vary on their policy. Some districts do not honor DNR/DNI orders while other honor them, and other districts haven't considered a policy. The school nurse plays a key role in the district's policy as well as in working with the family and meeting the family's needs and the needs of the student. See options concerning DNR/DNI on the next page.

Individualized Healthcare Plan

The medically fragile child brings a complex set of nursing needs to the school and the care plan for the child can be lengthy and detailed. The IHP should include any emergency care plans (ECP) and emergency evacuation plans (EEP) that are needed. Nurses writing an IHP should consult other chapters in Volume I and II, such as spinal cord injury, asthma, seizure disorders, respiratory dysfunction, cardiovascular disease, gastrostomy, ventriculoperitoneal shunts, and cerebral palsy.

OPTIONS CONCERNING DNR/DNI INCLUDE:

Option 1: The district does not honor DNR/DNI orders. If a life-threatening emergency happens, school staff, including the school nurse, will provide CPR until the paramedics arrive. The paramedics may honor the DNR/DNI order if the family has made these arrangements beforehand.

Districts usually have this policy for two reasons. First, staff and the school board are concerned about the trauma associated with allowing a student to die during a school day. They worry about the other children who observe this happening as well as teachers. Second, only the school nurse has a medical background and can assess the student's health status and make a determination to not intervene as ordered by the physician. When the nurse is out of the building, this will fall to the educational staff who are not able to access and provide medical treatment as ordered by a physician. They can, however, administer CPR.

Points to think about -

The school nurse may be vulnerable to legal action in this situation because she has not followed a direct physician order, especially if the child is rescued and his/her condition has deteriorated severely. The school nurse should consult legal counsel.

The school nurse may want to encourage the family to file a copy of the DNR/DNI order with the paramedics prior to an emergency. The school nurse might also want to provide a copy of the order to the paramedics when they arrive.

Option 2: The district honors DNR/DNI orders. If a life-threatening emergency happens, school staff would not provide CPR. Paramedics would be called to transport the child to emergency services. Staff would make the student comfortable until paramedics arrive but would not administer CPR.

Points to think about -

How will the school nurse delegate care in this situation? Only a registered nurse can make assessments followed by a decision about medical treatment or nontreatment. If the school nurse is unavailable, who will assess the health status of the child and make the decision not to provide CPR? If the school nurse is already delegating care for the child to a registered nurse, this point is mute. How will the school nurse delegate this if the nurse is an LPN? Or a paraprofessional?

Option 3: The district doesn't honor CPR but has made an exception in the case of this child. The district, after hearing from the physician and family, decides that providing CPR to this child would severely injure the child and so have allowed an IHP to include no CPR or rescue breathing.

Points to think about -

These would be the same as noted in number two above.

REFERENCES

1. American Federation of Teachers. *The Medically Fragile Child in the School Setting.* 2nd ed. Washington, DC: American Federation of Teachers, 1997.
2. Storgion S. Care of the technology-dependent child. *Pediatr Ann.* 1996;25(12):677-684.
3. Kirk S. Families' experiences of caring at home for a technology-dependent child: a review of the literature. *Child Care, Health Dev.* 1998; 24(2): 101-114.
4. US Department of Health and Human Services. *Fostering Home and Community-Based Care for Technology Dependent Children.* Washington, DC: US Government Printing Office, 1988.
5. Palfrey JS, Haynie M, Porter S, et al. Prevalence of medical technology assistance among children in Massachusetts in 1987 and 1990. *Pub Health Rep.* 1994; 109(2): 226 - 233.
6. Wong D, Whaley L. *Essentials of Pediatric Nursing.* 5th ed. St. Louis, Mo: Mosby, 1997.

Homeless Students with Special Health Needs

Gail Synoground

INTRODUCTION

Homelessness among children is an increasing problem. Its manifestations include children in poor physical and psychosocial health, lack of academic success, and many other health-related issues. The following three cases illustrate some of the problems this population faces.

Recently, a family of three children and their mother was brought to the attention of the local school officials. The children had not been attending school for the past three months. The father of the children had been in and out of jail for domestic violence; however, the mother returns to him after each release. Eight-year-old Johnny, who is the youngest of the three children, is being registered at the school today. He is a pale, frail-looking child whose eyes focus on the floor, making very little eye contact. His hair had been crudely cut with very short hairs in places and other areas where the scalp appeared shaved. Live lice were noted along with several scabbed over and bleeding lesions covering the entire scalp. Occipital lymph nodes were swollen. In observing the rest of the child it was noted that he had a rash over most of his body. He complained of intense itching, especially at night.

Linear threadlike lesions were noted between his fingers. The child had not been seen by a medical professional since he was 3.

Ten-year-old Darlene presents continually to the school nurse complaining of stomach pain. Her father has been jailed for domestic violence and the mother, who appears very depressed, is not able to provide basic, emotional, or medical care for her child. Darlene is having difficulty focusing on her schoolwork and is about one grade behind for her age.

Six-year-old Mark is the son of a 52-year-old single father. The father was previously married and has two children in their 30s. His first wife passed away. Mark is the product of a brief affair between the father and a woman he met in a bar. Although she delivered the child she did not wish to keep Mark and left him with the father. Mark was diagnosed with fetal alcohol syndrome and was labeled a "crack baby" as well. Mark is having problems with anger and frequently disrupts the class with his impulsiveness and frequent outbursts.

All of the above children are living in transitional housing and share many common problems, including homelessness, lack of medical care, disruption in educational pursuits, dysfunctional family life, and uncertainly about their future. The first question that arises is, can anything be done for children who spend so little time at any one place?

School nurses and school personnel are in a good position to work with these youngsters, since the school may provide the most consistent place in a world of constant change and inconsistencies.

Scope of Problem

One of the Healthy People 2000 goals is to increase the span of healthy life for Americans and reduce the health disparities among the poor and to achieve access to preventive services.[1]

Approximately 2 to 3 million people are homeless in any given night. A growing number of homeless people are single women and children. One study[2] reported that children represent 20% of the homeless population and 63% of the homeless family members. "The homeless children of today will be the unhealthy, unemployable, destitute and homeless adults of tomorrow."[2] Children and their families are the largest and fastest growing segment of the homeless population.[3]

Homelessness among single mothers and their children is related to poverty and not the result of mental illness.[3] The average homeless family includes 2 to 3 children, most younger than 5 years of age.[4]

Healthcare for these children and their families becomes secondary to survival. Primary to their existence is the need to use their resources and energies to obtain the basic needs of food and shelter. Additionally, many of these families do not appreciate or understand the need for preventive health services. Healthcare becomes crisis oriented with many homeless families relying on emergency departments for care. This is not only costly, but emergency care facilities rarely have the capacity for follow-up care.

School nurses, because of their experience and knowledge, are in a pivotal position to collaborate with teachers and other staff members in identifying physical and psychosocial problems interfering with developmental and academic progression. However, it is imperative for nurses and others to assess their own attitude and resources toward working with this population. Relief organizations report that public support and sympathy for homeless individuals and families is declining.[5,6] Since these children may be at a given school for only a limited time, the question of investing time and energy does arise. Identifying those services relevant to the needs of homeless children will make a difference in their lives.

A less than adequate physical and psychological environment exposes homeless children to an increased risk for lasting physical and mental health problems. Problems span the physical, psychosocial, spiritual, and developmental dimensions, including growth disorders, plus a higher incidence of acute and chronic health diseases.

Pathophysiology

The delivery of health services to this segment of the population requires specific knowledge of the multidimensional health problems facing children, plus the barriers they encounter in accessing and receiving adequate health services.

Therefore, to understand the etiology of health problems identified in homeless children, the school nurse must consider the many unhealthy behaviors and consequences of living in an unstable environment. Health problems affecting the child include the following:[7]

Physical Problems

• Higher incidence of acute and chronic

health problems, especially infections and communicable diseases.

- Increased risk for nutritional deficiencies leading to anemia and growth disorders. Meal times in transitional living quarters are often very regulated and extra food may not be allowed in the rooms, making it difficult to meet the nutritional needs of children.
- Exposure to sexual abuse, violence, physical abuse, criminal behavior, and substance abuse. Continual exposure predisposes these youngsters to physical, mental health, and behavior problems.
- Preventive healthcare is pursued less frequently than in children from more stable environments, particularly notable is the lack of immunizations.
- Healthcare received in an emergency facility is more likely to be fragmented and oriented to solving only acute problems. Compliance and follow-up care are poor in this population.
- Children are often criticized for their hygiene. Facilities to wash clothes or practice hand washing or other hygienic activities are not available.
- Dental healthcare practices are often non existent.

Developmental Problems

A study by Riley[8] stated that 61% of children under age 5 had at least one developmental lag and 44% had two or more lags. The purpose of this study was to examine the health status and utilization of health services of families living in shelters. Findings from this study and others demonstrated the need for delivery of health services to this group; 60% of the children over 5 required medical and psychiatric evaluation and 55% were performing below average in school.

Each transitional home the child lives in brings with it new restrictions and policies plus very limited living space or play area to accomplish the normal developmental tasks of childhood, such as learning interactive and social skills.

Psychosocial Problems

Research suggests that children who live in poverty are more likely to experience difficulty in school, become teen parents, and as adults earn less and be unemployed more.[9]

Problems related to mental health include negative attention-seeking behavior, aggressiveness, and learning difficulties. To solve many of these problems requires a safe and long-term place where trust can be established. Psychosocial problems common to this population include:

- Disruptions in relationships, losses of friends and possessions
- Lack of consistent routines in performance of daily activities
- Parental depression
- Lack of a male role model (especially in female-headed households)
- Exposure to family violence and abuse
- Exposure to substance and sexual abuse
- Continual exposure to other families and children with problems

As a result the environmental effects of homelessness on children often lead to:

- Depression and withdrawal
- Decreased self-esteem
- Aggressive behavior
- Poor impulse control
- Poor attention span
- Poor task persistence, often due to frequent absences from school and changes of schools, all of which result in developmental lags and learning difficulties

Additionally, homeless children must return to an unhealthy environment after school is dismissed, further exposing them to the many problems associated with meeting academic expectations. Studying and completing homework assignments may not be possible because of over-crowding or lack of parental ability to assist the child with school assignments.

Barriers to Care

Access to healthcare is a very real problem. Many women and their children do not have adequate transportation to a medical facility or, if they are able to take a bus, all the children must accompany her for lack of care. Additionally, many clinics are very busy, which means long waiting periods for patients once they do get there. Homeless children and their families lack the resources to obtain health insurance beyond short-term state/government health coupons. Other barriers may include fear of rejection by health personnel, language barriers, and the inability to navigate the bureaucracy of many health facilities.[7]

Role of the School Nurse

In developing a nursing care plan for the child facing homelessness, the school nurse needs to consider the following:

- School nurses are in a unique position to assist homeless children and their families for many reasons. They are resourceful and aware of available services and how to access them while being mindful of the economic plight of the families.
- School nurses can provide a broad range of services including physical assessments, sensory assessments, and case management and serve as an advocate for the child.
- School nurses, although unable to provide for all of the needs of the homeless child, are able to work collaboratively with agencies and other healthcare providers to offer a wide spectrum of services.
- School nurses may be the only medical personnel with whom homeless youngsters have contact.

The length of time a school nurse may have with a homeless child is limited; however, the use of the nursing process will assist in planning and implementing appropriate health promotion, disease prevention, and health maintenance strategies. Nurses in partnership with school personnel, community agencies, parents, and students can play a key role in improving the health of homeless children.

In planning intervention(s) related to a child's health needs, the school nurse must be cognizant of the child's environment. For example, if the child has lice and is excluded from school, the nurse needs to ask: 1) If the child's family can afford the medication, 2) What facilities are there for bathing and washing clothes, 3) Are clean clothes available, and 4) Is it possible for the child and his and her family to carry out all of the instructions to get rid of the lice?

INDIVIDUALIZED HEALTHCARE PLAN

Assessment

History

- Family composition—identify younger children who are not in school but may need services
- Length of time child has been homeless—has the child ever had a stable environment?
- Average length of stay in each shelter—what relationships has the child been able to establish?

- Number of times moved
- Source of healthcare and when last seen
- Medical history—past, present, acute and chronic infectious diseases
- History of injury/abuse
- Health promotion—immunizations
- Use of prescribed medications, over-the-counter medications and/or prescribed treatments
- What resources have the family successfully used in the past?
- Knowledge of resources available to the child and family in their current setting
- Review of academic achievements/disruptions
- Financial resources available
- Family goals/hopes/needs

Assessment

- Physical
  - Overall appearance and build
  - Height, weight—is child undernourished, alert, interactive?
  - Hygiene (availability of bathing facilities)
  - Obvious injuries or health problems
  - Dental problems
  - Vision and hearing results
  - Systems review: any problems noted with each system
- Developmental
  - Assess developmental level for strengths, and lags in social, motor, and language skills. (There are various standardized tools depending on the child's age. The Denver Developmental Screening Tool [DDST] is one tool appropriate for children under 5.)
- Psychosocial Assessment
  - The need to recognize and appropriately refer children with mental health concerns is imperative. The school nurse may wish to team up with counselors or other mental health professionals to make a combined comprehensive assessment. Assessment should focus on those problems associated with homelessness, such as:
    - Depression
    - Helplessness
    - Anxiety
    - Interpersonal skills and relationships
    - Learning difficulties
    - Fears
    - Anger
    - Distrust
    - Inattentiveness

These problems interfere with the child's ability to learn and even though treatment requires time, identification of these problems is an important first step.
- Environmental Assessment
  - Facilities at the shelter
  - School environment
  - Safety issues

- Spiritual Assessment
  - Life goals, values, beliefs
  - Hopelessness
- Academic Assessment
  - School(s) the student attended in the past
  - Academic achievement
  - Current or need for special education services
  - School attendance pattern
  - Child's perception of academic needs/level

Nursing Diagnoses (N.D.)

Physical

N.D. 1 Alteration in nutrition and risk for less than body requirement or inadequate supply of food (NANDA 1.1.2.2) related to economic factors.

N.D. 2 Fatigue (NANDA 6.1.1.2.1) related to:
  - overwhelming psychological or emotional demand
  - increased energy requirements to perform, activities of daily living
  - excessive social and role demands related to constant change

N.D. 3 Altered health maintenance (NANDA 6.4.2) related to:
  - inability to seek out or maintain health (health resources)
  - lack of knowledge
  - alteration in communication skills
  - ineffective coping
  - lack of material resources
  - impairment of support systems

N.D. 4 Sleep pattern disturbance (NANDA 6.2.1) related to:
  - environmental distractions in shelter
  - overcrowding

N.D. 5 Risk for injury and risk for trauma (NANDA 1.6.1 and 1.6.1.3) related to
  - lack of safety measures
  - cognitive or emotional problems
  - unsafe environment
  - high crime neighborhood
  - exposure to abuse

Developmental

N.D. 6 Altered growth and development (NANDA 6.6) related to:
  - inability to perform self-care or self-control activities (interruption in daily schedules)
  - delay in performing self-care activities due to lack of facilities

N.D. 7 Altered family processes (NANDA 3.2.2) related to:
  - disorganization of family life
  - anger, frustration, powerlessness

N.D. 8 Risk for social isolation (NANDA 3.1.2) related to:
  - affectional deprivation
  - absence of significant others (father often absent)

N.D. 9   Risk for loneliness (NANDA 3.1.3) related to:
- physical and social isolation (lack of opportunity to form long-lasting relationships)

N.D. 10   Diversional activity deficit (NANDA 6.3.1.1) related to:
- decreased opportunity for stimulation
- lack of environmental diversional activities at the shelters

N.D. 11   Self-esteem disturbance alteration (NANDA 7.1.2) related to:
- decreased opportunity for success and accomplishment

Psychosocial

N.D. 12   Ineffective individual coping skills (NANDA 5.1.1.1) related to:
- inability to meet basic needs
- alteration in societal participation
- inability to meet role expectation
- inability to ask for help

N.D. 13   Relocation stress syndrome (NANDA 6.7) related to:
- frequent changes in environment leading to anxiety and uncertainty
- losses - friends
- decrease in support system

N.D. 14   Anxiety (NANDA 9.3.1) related to:
- uncertainty
- conflict about values/goals
- changes in environment
- changes in interaction patterns

Cognitive

N.D. 15   Knowledge deficit (educational) (NANDA 8.1.1) related to:
- interruption of education
- lack of consistent routines
- absences—frequent

N.D. 16   Impaired verbal communication (NANDA 2.1.1.1) related to:
- difficulty expressing thought
- lack of opportunity to express concerns

GOALS (Student oriented)

- Improves health-enhancing behaviors (N.D. 1-6)
- Verbalizes feelings regarding health issues and homelessness (N.D. 11-14.16)
- Develops positive coping skills/strategies (N.D. 12-14)
- Increases successful completion of educational tasks (N.D. 6,15)
- Meets nutritional needs while at school (N.D. 1)
- Accesses two available resources to help meet his/her basic needs (N.D. 1,3,5,7-10)
- Accesses school health services (nursing, counseling, etc.) to meet basic needs (N.D. 1-6,15)
- Improves self-care skills: safety measures, self assessment (N.D. 6)
- Develops beginning interest and skill in one recreation activity (N.D. 9-10)
- Establishes relationship with at least one other child: pen pal if he or she moves again (N.D. 8-10,13)

INTERVENTIONS

Physical

- Identify barriers that interfere with families seeking preventive healthcare services. (N.D. 3,7)
- Perform as many assessments as possible, including vision nutritional status, height, weight, hearing, and dental. (N.D.1-5)
- Identify and prioritize health needs from history and basic health assessment. (N.D. 1-5)
- Assess child's environment for basic needs such as running hot water, soap, clean clothes, sleeping quarters, and recreational opportunities. (N.D. 4-7)
- Develop an individual health record that child can take with him/her. (N.D. 1-5)
- Provide opportunity for child to have immunizations updated. (N.D. 3)
- Link student to medical resources for evaluation and follow-up. (N.D.3)
- Teach child basic health survival skills, CPR, first aid, and when and how to call for help. (N.D. 5)
- Encourage good hygiene through role modeling and providing basic necessities, such as tooth- brush, clean clothes, etc. (N.D. 3-6)

Psychosocial

- Develop a team of staff and teachers who are willing to develop intensive short-term relationship with homeless child. (N.D. 8,9,11,15)
- Visit the shelters to meet families and personnel to establish a link between school and shelter. (N.D. 7,8,9,15)
- Provide current information on health services available and how to contact various agencies. (N.D. 3,7,12)
- Assist school staff to construct an environment at school where the child can learn self-care and increase self-esteem. (N.D. 6,11,15)
- Assist student to identify and access services needed to meet needs. (N.D. 1-6,11-12)
- Develop a referral and follow-up system to provide continuity of care for these children. (N.D. 3, 7)
- Monitor use of services and note if child's needs are being met. (N.D. 1-5,6,8,14)
- Serve as an advocate to the child and family. (N.D. 3,7,15)
- Work with staff and teachers to provide consistency in routines and class activities. (N.D. 15)
- Encourage child to express feelings related to homelessness. (N.D. 8-11,16)
- Encourage child to identify children with whom they would like to correspond. (N.D. 8,9,13,14)
- Provide a place where child can feel safe—identify at least one consistent staff person child can come to. (N.D. 14,15)

Developmental

- Encourage social interaction with children. (N.D.9,10,11,15)
- Encourage child to participate in school extracurricular activities. (N.D. 10,15)
- Assess parents' knowledge and ability to meet child's needs. (N.D. 1-5,7,12 -14)
- Identify small goals that the child can accomplish each day to meet developmental task, for example: learning proper hand washing, toothbrushing, etc. (N.D. 6,11)

Expected Student Outcomes

The student will:
- identify physical, psychosocial, and developmental needs and describe one way to meet a need in each area. (N.D. 1-5,6-11,12-14)
- identify and articulate fears and concerns to school nurses or trusted staff member. (N.D.7,13,14,16)
- identify two resources to call when needing assistance, for example: food bank and/or clothing bank. (N.D. 1-5,6-10,12)
- demonstrate proper use of 911. (N.D. 5,7)
- state one person with whom they would like to correspond. (N.D. 8,9,13,14)
- participate in one extracurricular activity. (N.D. 10)
- display improved health practices, such as improved hygiene and nutritional practices. (N.D. 3,6,11)
- list accomplishments related to educational and developmental task. (N.D. 6,15)
- assist in maintaining an updated health record (immunizations, height and weight, vision and hearing). (N.D. 3,7)
- describe how he or she can perform self-care activities considering environmental limitations. (N.D. 1-6)
- identify ways to assess shelter environment for safety and make appropriate decisions. (N.D. 1,4,5,7,12)

The following care plan is based on an 8-year-old homeless boy and illustrates many of the complex problems these children present. Although the length of stay in any one school is limited, it is possible to plan strategic interventions with positive outcomes. Note the importance of assessing all dimensions and their affect on total health. Three goals should guide you: 1) Teach and encourage self-care, 2) Connect child to appropriate resources, and 3) Assess as much as you can. You may be the child's only connection to healthcare.

CASE STUDY

David, an 8-year-old male, enrolled in the second grade at your school. This is the seventh school he has attended in three years. He lives with his mother and two younger siblings (a 3-year old and an 8-month old). Currently the family is living in one room in a transitional housing facility. Limited history includes the following: diagnosed with asthma when five years old, no follow-up, treated in emergency room settings for flare ups. There is no record of immunizations but Mom thinks he had "some." He is often kept out of school to help Mom care for the siblings. The whereabouts of David's father are unknown. David appears thin and tired and is having difficulty with school assignments.

Individualized Healthcare Plan*
Homeless

Assessment Data	Nursing Diagnosis	Goals	Nursing Interventions	Expected Outcomes
PHYSICAL ND 1 & 2 Fatigue, pale, malnourished	Alternation in nutrition and risk for less than body requirement or inadequate supply of food (NANDA 1.1.2.2) Fatigue related to: 1. overwhelming psychological or emotional demand; 2. increased energy requirements to perform activities of daily living; and/or 3. excessive social and role demands related to constant change (NANDA 6.1.2.1)	Child will have required dietary intake for age	Arrange for school; breakfast/ lunch program. Monitor 24-hr dietary intake 1x week until weight is stabilized. Work with counselor/ social worker and transition home to obtain food for child and family. Plot height/ weight on growth grid—repeat 1x week until stabilized.	Identifies resources for obtaining food. Height/ weight will progress normal for age.

Data	Nursing Diagnosis	Goal	Intervention	Evaluation
ND3 No treatment of sensory screening—having problems reading	Altered health maintenance related to: 1. inability to seek out or maintain health resources; 2. lack or knowledge; 3. alteration in communication skills; 4. ineffective coping; and/or 5. impairment of support systems (NANDA 6.4.2)	Child will identify resources to correct sensory deficits.	Assess for vision/ hearing deficits. Refer for glasses (arrange transportation and someone to accompany child). Families often cancel appointments due to no transportation or fear of rejection.	Recognizes need for vision-hearing corrections for academic success.
Incomplete history of immunization status		Child/ Mom will identify importance of completing immunizations.	Arrange for immunizations for child and family.	Accepts need for immunizations. Assists in keeping updated immunization record.
Uncontrolled asthma		Child/ Mom will state importance of adequate treatment for asthma (see asthma care plan, Vol. I).	See teaching plan on asthma. Link child up with a child who has successfully controlled his or her asthma.	Takes responsibility for self-care.
Source of healthcare— emergency room.			Provide information to child/ mom on possible insurance plans and/or clinics available to low income families.	Identifies alternate sources of healthcare.

Individualized Healthcare Plan*
Homeless

Assessment Data	Nursing Diagnosis	Goals	Nursing Interventions	Expected Outcomes
DEVELOPMENTAL ND6 Lack of opportunity to complete developmental tasks - example: exercise or play.	Altered growth and development related to: 1. inability to perform self-care or self-control activities (interruption in daily schedule); and/or 2. delay in performing self-care activities due to lack of facilities (NANDA 6.6)	Child will have developmental testing to identify lags (social and language skills often lagging).	Work with counselor/ psychologist to determine assessment protocol.	List accomplishments related to developmental level.
ND 8 & 10 Inconsistent environmental stimulation	Risk for social isolation related to: 1. affectional deprivation; and/or 2. absence or significant others (father often absent) (NANDA 3.1.2) Diversional activity- deficit related to decreased opportunity for stimulation Lack to environmental diversional activities at the shelters (NANDA 6.3.1.1)	Child will identify one extra- curricular activity that he would like to participate in that will increase social and interactive skills.	Work with PE teacher to identify appropriate activities for child with asthma.	Takes responsibility for assessing level of exercise potential.

PSYCHOSOCIAL ND13 Homeless - transitional living Frequent moves/housing instability Interruption of long-term relationship Absent father Withdrawn	Relocation stress syndrome related to: 1. frequent changes in environment leading to anxiety and uncertainty; 2. losses - friends; and/or 3. decrease support systems (NANDA 6.7)	Child will identify permanent ties with his current school setting. Child will identify the school setting as a safe and stable place.	Provide name of a child who is willing to be a pen pal for child. Solicit a staff staff adult, male role model, who child can go to and discuss his problems/accomplishments. Have child included in class pictures (to take child's picture needs to be cleared - especially if parent on run). Arrange for child's celebration of his birthday with class (if appropriate). (Visit transitional center to determine problems child may be encountering)	Expresses interest in developing ties to school personnel.

Individualized Healthcare Plan*
Homeless

Assessment Data	Nursing Diagnosis	Goals	Nursing Interventions	Expected Outcomes
COGNITIVE Below-level academic skills	Knowledge deficit (educational) related to: 1. interruption in education; 2. lack or consistent routines; and/ or 3. absences - frequent (NANDA 8.1.1)	Child will identify one small academic success per day.	Work with teachers to save and showcase child's successes. Put successful work in booklet form for child to take with him.	Takes pride in showcasing schoolwork.
Decreased access to library books or other educational stimuli		Child will identify one life skill he would like to learn (example: CPR, calling 911, etc.)	Teach and emphasize self-care skills related to first aid, CPR, assessing own health.	Demonstrates and shows pride in self-care skills learned.

*See Appendix for student profile information to include on an IHP form.

REFERENCES

1. Uphold CR, Graham MV. Schools as centers for collaborative services for families: a vision for change. Nurs Outlook. 1993; 41:204-210.
2. Norton D, Ridenour N. Homeless women and children: the challenge of health promotion. *Nurse Pract Forum.* 1995; 6:29-33.
3. Velsore FB. Homeless children and their families. *J Pediatr Nurs.* 1993; 8:293.
4. Wiley DC, Ballard DJ. How can schools help children from homeless families? *J Sch Health.* 1993; 63:291-293.
5. Velsor-Friedrich D. Homeless children and their families: the changing picture. *J Pediatr Nurs.* 1993; 8:122-123.
6. Velsor-Friedrich B. Homeless children and their families: federal programs and alternative health care delivery systems. *J Pediatr Nurs.* 1993; 8:190-192.
7. Reimer JG, Van Cleve L, Galbraith M. Barriers to well child care for homeless children under age 13. *Public Health Nursing.* 1995; 12:1.
8. Riley-Eddins EA. Health status of sheltered homeless families: an ethic-cultural assessment. *J Multicult Nurs Health.* 1995; 1(4):16-22.
9. America's Children Publication, The Forum, Washington, DC. *Key National Indicators on the Well Being of Children and Families.* Government Document No. PR-42.8: C-43. 1997.

BIBLIOGRAPHY

Bassuk EL, Buckner JC, Weinreb LF, et al. Homelessness in female headed families: childhood and adult risk and protective factors. *Am J Public Health.* 1997; 87:241-248.

Hattan DC. Managing health problems among homeless women with children in a transitional shelter. *Image: J Nurs Sch.* 1997; 29:33-37.

Hunter JK. *Nursing and Health Care for the Homeless.* New York, NY: State University of New York Press, 1993.

North American Nursing Dignosis Association. *NANDA Nursing Diagnoses: Definitions and Classification 1999-2000.* Philadelphia, Pa: North American Nursing Diagnosis Assn, 1999. (NANDA, 1211 Locust Street, Philadelphia, PA 19107. 800-647-9002; fax 215-545-8107; e-mail: NANDA@nursecominc.com)

Northam S. Access to health promotion, protection, and disease prevention among impoverished individuals. *Public Health Nurs.* 1996; 13:353-364.

Perkins JM, Tryssenaar J, Noland MR. Health and rehabilitation needs of a shelter population.*Can J Rehabil.* 1998; 11:117-122.

Immigrant and Refugee Students: Legal, Health, and Cultural Considerations

Ann Hoxie

INTRODUCTION

When assessing immigrant and refugee students in order to develop individualized healthcare plans (IHPs), the school nurse must take into consideration cultural issues as well as legal and health issues.

Schools across the United States are changing due to the growth of immigrant and refugee populations as a result of worldwide demographic shifts. As the population grows more diverse, schools face new opportunities and new demands to participate in the promotion of healthy immigrant communities. [1] School nurses are challenged to provide effective crosscultural interactions that will benefit students and their families.

The United States accepts approximately 75,000 refugees each year from diverse regions of the world.[2] Over the past two decades more than two million refugees have resettled in the United States, predominantly from Southeast Asia as a result of the Vietnam War. Currently refugees are being resettled in the United States from countries in the former Soviet Union, the former Yugoslavia (Bosnia-Herzegovina), Somalia, Iraq, Ethiopia, Sudan, Afghanistan, Cuba, and Haiti. At times, a large group of refugees may settle in one community, presenting particular challenges to educational, health, and social services. [3] In addition, secondary migration may contribute to the growth of a specific community within a certain geographical area.

Immigration and migration are fueled by economic and political forces that make leaving home and country either a necessity or more desirable than staying. People from all over the world still choose to come to the United States just as they always have. Bringing energy and enthusiasm they come to join familsy members, to find a better life, to escape persecution, and to find employment. One of every five people under age 18 in the United States is an immigrant or has parents who are immigrants. [4] Nearly one million new arrivals enter this country each year [3] as refugees, immigrants, and foreign-born adopted children and as undocumented immigrants.

For school health staff seeking to address the needs of foreign-born students, it is essential to remember that race, ethnicity, and citizenship status are important variables to consider when assessing student health, educational needs, and adaptation. It is helpful to understand the different categories under which people qualify as immigrants and refugees, potential health conditions, and the medical examinations, which are either required or voluntary.

Legal Status

Legal status can add to the understanding of the student's background and present health status and may determine what services are available to the student and family. The manner in which a person enters this country determines his/her status. The US Department of Immigration and Naturalization Service (INS) provides the following definitions:

Alien—A person who is not a citizen or national of the United States.

Asylee—A foreign-born resident who is not a US citizen and who cannot return to his or her country of origin or last residence because of persecution or the well-founded fear of persecution because of race, religion, nationality, membership in a particular social group, or political opinion, as determined by the INS. An asylee receives this status after entering the United States.

Parolee—An alien who has been given permission to enter the United States under emergency conditions or when that alien's entry is considered to be in the public interest.

Refugee—A foreign-born resident who is not a US citizen and who cannot return to his or her country of origin or last residence because of persecution or the well-founded fear of persecution because of race, religion, nationality, membership in a particular social group, or political opinion, as determined by the INS. A refugee receives this status prior to entering the United States.

Immigrant—An individual who chooses to make a new home in this country has a passport from his/her home country and a visa issued by the United States Immigrants may petition the government to become permanent residents.

Nondocumented immigrant—An individual who enters or lives in the United States without official authorization, by entering without INS inspection, overstaying his or her visa, or violating the terms of his or her visa.

Note: refugees differ from immigrants due to a fear of persecution because of religious or political beliefs or ethnicity. Refugees enter the United States under the Refugee Act and are therefore not subject to the immigration quotas that dictate the entrance of immigrants.

Since immigrants chose to come to the United States, they have had time to prepare emotionally and to thoughtfully plan their new lives. Often they have waited for a lengthy period of time to receive approval for immigration. Most often they have family to provide support and assistance during their resettlement. Immigration law requires that they be able to support themselves. On the other hand, refugees generally do not have marketable job skills, rarely speak English, and may have experienced trauma, disruptions, and deprivations that result in physical and emotional problems. In addition, circumstances have given them no choice but to resettle. [5]

Medical-legal issues

The health status of these individuals will be strongly influenced by their background. Many refugees have had poor quality healthcare in their country of origin and in refugee camps. Crowded conditions, poor sanitation, and traumatic experiences all affect current health. Children will have had little or no preventive healthcare or dental care. Immigrants may have had better access to healthcare in their home country but may be without healthcare coverage in the United States.

Undocumented immigrants may be reluctant to seek healthcare due to concerns about their legal status and lack of healthcare coverage. Persons living in this country illegally are not entitled to healthcare and social services. Children of undocumented immigrants often do not have access to preventive care, including prenatal care, dental care, health supervision, or immunizations. Family members often have different immigration statuses, which further complicates access to care, because the entire family may be fearful of investigation and therefore delay seeking care. [6]

Eligibility for medical services is determined by legal status and varies from state to state. The Welfare Reform Act of 1996 directs states to determine eligibility for Medicaid, Temporary Assistance to Needy Families (TANF), Women, Infants and Children (WIC), and Medicaid for pregnant women and children.[7]

In addition any noncitizen may be subject to deportation as a result of being accused of a serious crime. This can lead to fear and misunderstanding among refugees and immigrants. Families may not seek help for family or emotional issues fearing accusations of child abuse or concern for other legal repercussions.

Immigrant and Refugee Medical Examinations

Refugees and/or immigrants may have completed three different medical examinations. [8] The examinations differ significantly in scope and purpose. Criteria for these examinations are found in the Immigration and Nationality Act and amended by the Immigration Act of 1990.

1. Overseas Visa Medical Examination

Both refugees and immigrants are required to pass this examination within the year prior to arrival in the United States. The purpose of this examination is to identify medical conditions that would by law prohibit the individual from entering the United States. The exam is not meant to provide healthcare to the person, but rather is structured as an exclusionary process in order to protect the US population and to exclude individuals with conditions that would present a financial burden to the United States. *This examination is mandatory for all immigrants and refugees.* The State Department arranges for refugee examinations but all other immigrants pay for their own examination. The Overseas Visa Medical Examination is performed under the oversight of the US Centers for Disease Control and Prevention, Center for Prevention Services, Division of Quarantine. The International Organization for Migration conducts the overseas examinations in Southeast Asia and the former Soviet Union under a contract with the US State Department. In other countries "panel physicians" appointed by US embassies and consulates perform the examination. The quality of the examination varies according to site, the panel physician, and the length of time the overseas examination process has been in place in a given location. The visa medical examination can be completed up to a year prior to departure, therefore, the possibility exists that a person may develop a health condition after the exam but before entrance into the United States. Exclusionary conditions are[9]:
- Communicable diseases of public health significance
  - infectious tuberculosis
  - HIV infection
  - Hansen's disease (leprosy)
  - certain sexually transmitted diseases

- Current or past physical or mental disorder with associated harmful behavior
- Substance abuse or dependence
- Other physical or emotional disorders

Refugees and immigrants pass through a US Public Health Service Quarantine Station at the port of entry into the United States. Individuals are visually inspected for observable conditions and may be denied entrance at that time.

2. Domestic Refugee Health Assessment

State refugee health programs manage the Domestic Health Assessment program and as a result variations exist in the design and implementation of the services. Questions may be directed to the state refugee health coordinator. This exam is focused on eliminating health-related barriers to successful refugee resettlement. *Immigrants do not participate in this process and, although highly encouraged, refugees are not required to undergo this examination.* The exam is meant to provide protection for the US population by identifying and treating infectious diseases. This assessment also focuses on the individual's health and, in addition to the comprehensive examination, is meant to assist the individual in securing necessary healthcare and services. Refugees are eligible for Medicaid coverage during their first months of residency in the United States and Medicaid covers the cost of this exam. The components of this examination generally include evaluation of:

- Immunization status
- Tuberculosis infection and disease
- Hepatitis B infection
- Intestinal parasite infections
- Sexually transmitted disease

- Other health problems, including pregnancy testing, dental abnormalities, vision, and hearing screening
- Referral and follow-up of identified conditions
- Linkage with primary healthcare resources

Refugees are assisted by resettlement agencies, often referred to as sponsors, which are an important source of information and assistance during the refugee's first months in the United States. An agency representative meets the family at the airport, arranges for housing, and prepares a resettlement plan that includes initial contact with governmental services and employment agencies. Resettlement agencies may be religious-based organizations, private organizations, state agencies, or ethnic organizations. Resettlement workers aided by relatives, friends, and volunteers help refugees become established. [2] Immigrants have no such formalized system of support but rely on family, friends, and ethnic organizations to provide assistance.

3. Adjustment of Status Medical Examination

The purpose of this examination is to determine if health conditions exist which require care and intervention prior to the individual being granted legal permanent resident status. *The examination is required for individuals applying for permanent resident status.* Applicants pay for this examination themselves; it is not covered by health insurance. The components of this examination include:

- Physical examination
- Immunizations
- Evaluation of tuberculosis disease and infection
- Serology for syphilis
- Serology for HIV antibody

Health Issues of Immigrants and Refugees

Table 1. Medical Problems in Refugees, Based on Country of Origin or Residence

Problems	Southeast Asia	Former Soviet Union	Former Yugoslavia	East Africa	Middle East	Haiti	Cuba
Malnutrition	X			X			X
Depression	X		X		X		
Intestinal Parasites*	X			X	X	X	
Filariasis				X		X	
Leishmaniasis				X	X		
Hepatitis B	X	X	X	X	X	X	
Tuberculosis	X	X	X	X	X	X	X
Posttraumatic stress disorder	X		X		X		
Low immunization rate		X	X	X	X	X	
Diphtheria		X					
Alcohol abuse		X					
Dental caries		X	X	X	X		
Typhoid fever				X		X	
Malaria				X	X		
Trachoma				X	X		
Syphilis	X			X			
Dengue fever				X		X	X
HIV infection				X		X	
Plague		X					
Cholera		X					
Radiation exposure		X					

HIV – human immunodeficiency virus
X – disease reported in refugees from the country or considered at risk for importation.
*Includes *Enterobius, Trichuris, Strongyloides,* and *Ascaris.*

Reprinted, with permission, from Ackerman.[3]

Immunizations

Immunization status is the first priority for new students entering a school. Foreign-born students are at risk for vaccine preventable diseases because of exposure to disease and the immunization practices unique to their native countries. [10] Many immigrant families do not have immunization records with them and will not be able to retrieve them from the home country. Some refugees arriving in the United States may not have had access to vaccines. Although most refugees do have a vaccine record, it is often incomplete when applied to local immunization laws, which vary from state to state. Records that document immunizations, which meet the recommended vaccine schedule of state school immunization laws, are acceptable. [10] Some students may believe they are current because of immunizations (such as yellow fever or cholera) received just prior to departure from the country of origin and may not be familiar with the immunizations required for school in the United States. Many countries give measles vaccine but not the combined MMR (measles, mumps, rubella) required in many US schools. Handwritten records, foreign language records, and records that report dates in an unfamiliar manner (i.e., day/month/year) can further complicate interpretation of immunization records. Required vaccines as indicated for age should be administered prior to school entrance.

Tuberculosis

Tuberculosis (TB) is the most important public health problem of refugees, [10]particularly those from Southeast Asia and other developing countries, such as many African nations, where TB is endemic. Refugees and immigrants have accounted for a substantial and increasing proportion of new cases of tuberculosis within the United States in the past decade. During the first five years of resettlement, a significant risk exists for development of tuberculosis disease.[11] Persons with clinically active TB must begin treatment in the country of origin but may resettle once they are no longer contagious. Tuberculosis treatment must continue in the United States. Screening for TB and appropriate preventive therapy are an important priority in order to protect the US population, particularly during the first five years of residence in the United States. Therefore, Mantoux skin testing is recommended for all refugees regardless of previous BCG (bacille Calmette-Guérin) vaccinations.[10] School nurses should collect and record the results of TB testing, assist students in obtaining follow-up care, and monitor the results. It is also important to recognize that significant stigma is attached to tuberculosis infection and disease among refugee and immigrant populations. Consequently, patients with the disease should be treated with sensitivity and confidentiality.

Other Health Concerns

Hepatitis B is prevalent in many areas of the world, which results in relatively high rates among refugee populations. Individuals should be tested to detect carriers and those who are nonimmune should be immunized. Malnutrition and iron deficiency anemia are common. Many refugees have dental caries. Intestinal parasites are endemic in tropical areas and occur in up to 40% of refugees. Intestinal parasites can result in malnutrition, anemia, chronic diarrhea, and growth retardation or failure to thrive. [8] Other concerns include sexually transmitted diseases, malaria, and leprosy. Although refugee and immigrant children may have been exposed to infectious diseases, most will be free of contagious conditions. [6,10]

Many refugees and some immigrants have experienced significant emotional trauma, torture, and/or have witnessed extreme violence. As a result, posttraumatic stress disorder, anxiety, withdrawal, somatic complaints, and depression can be common among individuals of all ages. These conditions occur at higher rates among refugee populations, although significant variations are noted among groups.[3, 6,7] Some research suggests that the family can buffer stresses which affect children and can be a protective factor against the development of emotional disorders. [12]

Posttraumatic stress disorder is characterized by persistent reexperience of the event through intrusive recollections, dreams, and reliving the experience. The person has persistent avoidance of thoughts associated with the event, avoids anything that triggers memories, feels detached from others, and has diminished interest in activities. Posttraumatic stress disorder can cause sleep disruptions, irritability and hypervigilance, concentration difficulties, exaggerated startle responses, and physiologic reactivity. [13,14] Children who suffer from posttraumatic stress disorder can be retraumatized by health procedures (Kathleen McCullough, BSN, oral communication, February 23, 1999). [15]

Health Issues in Internationally Adopted Children

Each year, US families adopt approximately 10,000 foreign-born children. International adoptions have been primarily from Asian countries (Korea, Philippines, India) and Central and South America. In recent years however, increasing numbers of adoptions are occurring from Eastern Europe and the Caribbean. Internationally adopted children are required to have an overseas visa medical examination in the country of origin in order to receive an immigrant visa. This examination is for the purposes discussed earlier and is not a comprehensive evaluation. [6,10] Health problems exhibited by these children are a reflection of the circumstances they have experienced and therefore vary widely. Many of internationally adopted children have been institutionalized, some for long periods of time, and many have experienced abandonment and deprivation. [16] Studies indicate that at least half of the children arrive in the United States with at least one health problem that requires treatment. The health reports that accompany the children vary in the amount of detail and documentation of healthcare and at times significant discrepancies exist in the preadoptive evaluations and subsequent assessments done in the United States.[16] Health concerns for these children include growth and developmental delays, undiagnosed infectious diseases including chronic hepatitis B, tuberculosis, and intestinal parasites, and incomplete immunization status. [10,16,17]

All international adoptees, after arrival in the United States, should undergo a medical examination [10] that focuses on:
- Vision and hearing assessments
- Developmental testing
- Nutritional assessment
- Physical examination
    - Complete blood count
    - Identification of infectious diseases
    - Identification of congenital anomalies

Adjustment Issues for Children and Youth

New immigrants and refugees can be expected to experience culture shock as they discover the profound differences between their practices and beliefs and the values and behaviors of those among whom they now live. [18] Adjustments and adaptations and efforts to understand and navigate the educational, health, and social service systems all demand a great deal of energy and can lead to misunderstanding, frustration, and despair. However, the growth of healthy immigrant communities depends on recognition by mainstream society of the strengths of immigrants and refugees: dignity, resiliency, survivorship skills, ability to adapt to change, as well as the willingness of society to support the adaptation process. [1]

The stress of adapting to a new culture and the losses of the familiar homes, routines, languages, and cultures can cause difficulties for children in adapting to new schools and communities. Adjustment problems, school failure, and deviant behaviors that occur as immigrant and refugee children and youth struggle to assimilate put them at risk for mental health problems. The initial phase of adjustment is often characterized by silence due to inability to communicate and/or awareness of different cultural expectations. Children may appear withdrawn yet be actively observing and listening. Reacting to pressures to assimilate into the new culture may cause children to pretend they are not connected to their past, to their culture and, at times, to their families. Other children may feel and behave one way at home and another at school. Parent-child relationships are altered as the children learn English and adopt American cultural behaviors more quickly than the older generation. In addition, immigrant and refugee children find few support systems within the school and community. Language barriers contribute to difficulties in accessing and benefiting from available services. Efforts are needed to develop multilingual and multicultural programs which meet the mental health needs of immigrant and refugee youth. [6,12,14,19]

Healthy adjustment occurs through acculturation as the individual changes, accepts, and participates in mainstream culture without abandoning traditional cultural beliefs and values. When parents are supported and assisted in the parental role, children feel safer. Children also benefit when helped to appreciate and value both cultures—to make sense of both worlds. Schools can provide significant assistance by promoting the value of diversity within the student body, working against prejudice, and developing ways to assist parents to understand and navigate the educational system. [1,12,14]

Cultural Considerations

Culture is how we are raised to understand and live life. Culture can be viewed as a framework for how we live. Culture mediates—it affects and influences our perceptions, defines our choices, and affects our interactions with other people. [20]

Nowhere is the impact of culture more powerful than in health, as it affects both the students' health beliefs and behaviors and the school nurse's health beliefs and behaviors. Culture affects perceptions about illness, health, and disability. In addition to determining the student's immigration status and the resultant health and legal issues, it is also crucial for the school nurse to include an assessment of cultural beliefs, practices, and meanings when developing an IHP. The challenge to school nurses when assessing and planning for the needs of immigrant and refugee students is to provide care that conforms to each student's values, beliefs, and practices.

Transcultural Nursing

School nurses working with students of cultural backgrounds differing from that of the nurse are called upon to develop crosscultural expertise. Transcultural nursing authors and theorists provide a body of research to assist nurses. [20-23] The founder and leader of transcultural nursing, Madeline Leininger, was the first to note, in the 1950s, cultural differences between patients and nurses. Her theory of culture care diversity and universality provides the structure on which the transcultural nursing speciality is based. Leininger's Sunrise Model, [22] which depicts this theory, is based on the concept of cultural care. This theory is focused on care which is culturally congruent, that is, care which is meaningful and beneficial to the person involved. Taking into consideration the many influences and factors that may be present, she describes three modalities of nursing decisions and actions which demonstrate how to deliver culturally congruent care:

1. **Culture care preservation and/or maintenance** – the nurse and student agree to use cultural care such as folk medicine or healing rituals known to be helpful and not harmful. The cultural ways are preserved.
2. **Culture care accommodation and/or negotiation** - the nurse accommodates the cultural patterns or habits of the student into the plan of care. For example, extended families are encouraged to participate in decision making.
3. **Culture care repatterning or restructuring** – together the nurse and student design different patterns for the health and well being of the student. With respect for the student's cultural beliefs, the school nurse helps the student to understand and benefit from the American healthcare system, develop self-care skills, or practice preventive health measures. [18,22,24]

Cultural Assessment

Cultural assessment skills are learned. An assessment of student and family values, beliefs, and health practices can be conducted separately using one of the cultural assessment tools which are available [20,21,23] or by incorporating a cultural perspective into the usual health history. Use open-ended questions such as "Tell me about the problem," "What do you think is causing this," "What does your mother say is happening to you," "What does your family do at home for this problem?" [24,25] Expect to discover differences in health beliefs and practices when working with a culturally diverse population.[24]

Remember that the plan is for the student. If there are elements of the family's actions or choices that the school nurse assesses as harmful in light of current professional practice, problem solve a solution, involve cultural liaisons or mediators, or help the family to restructure their understanding. Continue to evaluate and reassess. [22]

It is important and helpful to learn those beliefs, practices, and unique health problems and needs that are specific to each cultural group. Because this process can take a long time, it is often necessary to attempt to apply what is learned from one group to another while avoiding stereotypes. Certainly the competence and skills developed in assessing a student or several students of a particular culture can enhance the nurse's abilities when assessing a student from another culture.[5]

Crosscultural Competence: A Journey for School Nurses

Developing competency in interactions with students and families from other cultures is a journey—a process of acquiring understanding and skills. The skills and abilities to provide culturally competent care are important now and will become increasingly so as we move into the 21st century. Begin the journey with an acknowledgment of the profound effect culture has on health and health outcomes for all people. [26] Examine the effects your own culture has on your beliefs and practices. How are you affected by the way you were brought up, the nursing education you received, the work situations you have experienced, the professional standards that guide your practice? How and why have you changed your values and behaviors from those of your family of origin? Examine how your own cultural beliefs influence your attitudes, behaviors and expectations.

Next, seek to learn and understand the cultural beliefs, and values of students and their families that influence their attitudes, beliefs, and behaviors. If you do not speak the language of the student or family, use an interpreter. Find a cultural liaison or mediator to teach you about the culture. Look for similarities and differences between cultures. Avoid stereotypes, remembering that individuals within a culture vary significantly. Each family modifies the culture of the larger group in ways that are unique. Families will adhere to the old ways that have meaning and adopt new beliefs that work for them. Culture is fluid and is influenced and changed by experiences and environment. [21,27-29]

Move toward an acceptance of other cultural perspectives by adapting your thinking to respect and value the students' or families' beliefs, and practices. Believe that students have a right to their values, beliefs and practices. Integrate the family's beliefs with your beliefs and be willing to tolerate ambiguity. Ask questions and find answers, portray a desire to learn, remain nonjudgmental, and keep your sense of humor. Involve the student and family in making decisions about their care. Be sure to consider financial issues and access-to-care issues. Don't expect to do it alone—find resources in your school and community and build partnerships within the immigrant community and the community at large. You will be developing effective crosscultural communication and understandings, which will increase your skills. You will learn to be effective in assessing students and in planning, implementing, and evaluating the plan of care and health outcomes. [21,26,29] Do not expect to complete this journey—it will continue throughout your years of professional practice.

Assessing Family Patterns

Table 2 illustrates a continuum of the cultural characteristics of families. This can be helpful in working with families when the cultural background of the nurse differs from that of the student. These examples of cultural continua illustrate differences in behavior not only across cultures but also between specific families within cultural groups. There is no right or wrong to these behaviors. However, failure to understand such differences in approaches can cause misunderstanding, conflicts, wasted time and effort, and poor outcomes for the student. [18]

Differing perspectives on beliefs and values are not fixed positions. Age, education, friends, economic situations, life experiences, and other variables can affect an individual's beliefs and thus position on the continuum. Also, family members may be at different points along each continuum. This framework can be used to assess a student or family response to a new situation, to an expectation from school, to a medical or educational diagnosis, to a treatment plan, or to a medication regimen. The seven value sets listed can be used for evaluation and interpretation of individual perspectives, not only those of the student and family members but also those of the school nurse.

Table 2. Cultural Continuum of Family Characteristics*

Extended family and kinship networks	Small unit families with little reliance on the extended family
Interdependence	Individuality
Nurturance of young children	Independence of young children
Time is given	Time is measured
Respect for age, ritual, tradition	Emphasis on youth, future, and technology
Ownership defined in broad terms	Ownership, individual and specific
Differentiated rights and responsibilities	Equal rights and responsibilities
Harmony	Control

*Reprinted, with permission, from Lynch EW[18]

The first continuum addresses extended families versus small, independent unit families. Extended families often rely on family members for assistance but may expect help or agreement in return. By contrast, the small unit family may be more independent in decision making but have less access to family support resources. Some families value individuality and foster self-esteem. Other families value the family whole over the individual—the person's worth is determined by his or her contribution to the family.

Nurturance looks different from one family to another. Some families keep children close to them physically, for example, while others encourage early independence and value the abilities to calm and entertain oneself.

Time is a variable, which can have significantly different levels of importance among people and can cause significant conflicts. For many, the clock and calendar dictate the day's activities and schedule. For others, it may be more important to respond to the immediate needs of friends and family, as things come up, than to meet a schedule.

For some, the wisdom of the elders, and the rituals and traditions of the ancestors are basic to life. In contrast, for many Americans, the emphasis is on the future, on technology, on what is new and better. American children are often taught early about "mine," about ownership and property rights. At the other end of this continuum is the child who grows up in a culture where things are shared by a wide group of family and community members.

The sixth value set contrasts rights and responsibilities. Families define gender roles, responsibilities for childcare, and decision-making power in varying ways. Some families value traditional, established gender roles whereas others place value on equal rights and responsibilities for each parent. The final continuum is harmony/control. Some families seek harmony in their environment. Their lives may be centered on this principle and structured spiritually to attain harmony. For others, often those of mainstream US culture, a common belief is that things can be controlled, fixed, changed, and acted upon.[18]

Assessing Students with Special Needs

The challenges of being culturally competent become even more apparent when working with children with special healthcare, developmental, or educational needs. Families with children with special health or developmental needs face many challenges - families of ethnically or culturally diverse backgrounds experience even greater obstacles. [27] The family's perceptions of their child's needs vary greatly among cultures and it is necessary for school nurses to recognize and assess cultural influences on a family's response to illness, disability, or developmental delays in order to respond appropriately, make effective plans of care, intervene, and evaluate.

The possible responses of parents from diverse cultures to a child with illness or a disability are infinite. Some of these possibilities are described in this paragraph. Family members may seek advice from an elder, seek help from a cultural or spiritual healer, or use native medicines or healing practices in addition to or in place of western medicine. Family and extended family are very important in many cultures and decisions may not be made before consulting the extended family or the elders. Often the extended family is very involved in raising the children, with multiple caregivers present in the child's life. Some cultures teach that respect is shown by

avoiding eye contact, by not asking questions. Providers can misinterpret these behaviors to mean lack of understanding, agreement, or interest on the part of the family. Because some immigrants and refugees may be cautious of government services and of signing papers that they do not understand based on past experiences in their country of origin, they may refuse services for their child.

Spirituality may be very important. Families may have a strong belief in the possibility of miracles. Some Asian cultures believe that a child's illness or disability is the result of a wrongdoing by an ancestor. Many cultures explain illness or disability as a punishment or a curse, and the community may seek an explanation by attempting to discover what wrong was committed and who is to blame. Others believe that the cause or cure is within the individual. For some cultures, admitting a problem publicly causes humiliation and shame. Touching a child's head is a comforting or friendly gesture to many Americans but is disrespectful in some Asian cultures. Families may feel that a disability was meant to be and that surgical intervention, medication, or therapies are not appropriate. Some believe that surgical procedures, even minor operations such as insertion of PE tubes for chronic middle ear effusions, may release the child's spirit and that the spirit may never return. Other family issues, such as adjusting to American culture, financial insecurity, and/or feelings of anger or depression, may take precedence over the child's need. [18,21,27,28]

Perceptions, beliefs, and practices such as these can cause confusion, disbelief, dismay, frustration, and anger in western healthcare providers and education staff. In order to be effective one must embark on the cultural journey described earlier and continually try to understand the meaning of the situation for the student and family.

Considerations Related to the Nursing Process

Assessment of students from diverse cultural backgrounds requires the school nurse to strive to develop cultural competence and transcultural nursing skills. It is essential to integrate a cultural history into the nursing assessment. It is also essential to recognize that not only will students come from many cultures and subcultures but they may also be at any point along a continuum of the acculturation process from new arrival to second or third generation. An understanding of culture will be important in assessing all children (Margaret Andrews, PhD, RN, [mmandrew@naz.edu], e-mail, March 1,1999).[30]

When determining nursing diagnoses to define the student's health concern and direct the individual health plan, the school nurse must be aware of the effect that cultural biases and the perspective of western medicine may have on his/her selection of nursing diagnoses. [21-23,31] It is necessary to guard against describing a condition as impaired or altered when the behavior may be considered normal within another cultural group. [31] An understanding of culture will guide the nurse in making assessments. The culturally competent school nurse determines with the student and the family what the student expects and needs. By clarifying of perceptions of the problem and then checking the accuracy of nursing diagnoses with the student and/or family, appropriate nursing diagnoses and plans of care can be achieved. It is essential to develop, together with the student and family, a plan of care that is appropriate, and meaningful and that will be effective. The school nurse negotiates differences; individualizes the plan to fit the family patterns; and when appropriate, incorporates cultural care that is not harmful to the student. Finally, culturally competent care requires the school nurse to frequently evaluate and reassess the IHP.

Recommendations for Interventions in Working with Immigrant and Refugee Students

- Monitor nutritional status
- Monitor for infectious disease signs/ symptoms
- Be aware of the health needs of refugee or immigrant populations entering school
- Assess immunization status
- Assist student and family to complete immunization series/boosters
- Determine if the refugee health examination has been completed, obtain results
- Use interpreters and cultural mediators; develop comfortable working relationships with them
- Develop a knowledge base about students' culture, background, experiences, cultural view of medical practices, culture-specific diseases
- Screen hearing and vision initially to identify barriers to learning
- Add cultural history to data collection
- Determine status of student: refugee, immigrant, nondocumented immigrant
- Network with other school support staff including English as a Second Language teachers to address educational needs and language needs/barriers
- Monitor for signs/symptoms of depression, grief, posttraumatic stress syndrome
- Assist students to appreciate, understand, and accept both the culture of their family and American culture
- Collaborate with local public health to:
  - ❏ provide culturally appropriate care
  - ❏ follow tuberculosis concerns
  - ❏ obtain refugee screening results
  - ❏ provide translated health education materials

- Develop referral resources for:
  - ❏ health
  - ❏ medical
  - ❏ social services
  - ❏ cultural liaisons
  - ❏ mutual assistance organizations
- Assist student/family in locating and accessing healthcare resources
- Display posters, pamphlets, magazines, pictures, and artifacts from the cultures of the students in the school
- Obtain health education videos in the home languages of the students
- Learn to recognize how one's own culture influences beliefs, behaviors, practices
- Acknowledge and respect cultural differences, develop appreciation for diverse cultural health beliefs and practices
- Recognize that within cultures there is a continuum of beliefs and practices; each student is an individual within a culture
- Explain to student's family that they do not have to answer questions if they are uncomfortable; explain why you are asking some questions
- Ask who is the decision maker regarding health and education within the family
- Listen to student/family concerns, beliefs, perceptions
- Ask about student and family perception of illness and response to illness
- Ask if there are cultural or religious practices that influence health or sickness. Use simple explanations; repeat as necessary, take time
- Demonstrate skills; monitor student return demonstration of self-care practices
- Problem solve with student, family, educational staff, and healthcare provider

- Negotiate mutually acceptable solutions to health-related problems with students and families
- Become knowledgeable about the healthcare system: eligibility, application process, benefits
- Explain and assist family to utilize US healthcare system, need for appointments, medication regimens
- Accept that frustration does occur, be patient, collaborate, problem solve, work with cultural liaisons
- Assist student and staff to collaborate, problemsolve, work with cultural liaisons
- Support the hiring of multilingual and culturally diverse school staff
- Work with others to build healthy communities that support all of the population
- Participate in ethnic celebrations within the community

Use of Interpreters

❑ Determine which language which the student or family/guardian will use to best express themselves (some individuals speak several languages, or speak English socially but are not able to discuss in depth using English)

❑ Use interpreters who are proficient in the language, including specific dialect, can communicate, understand and make your message clear to the student and/or parent/guardian and who understand the educational and health issues

❑ Prior to the interview discuss with the interpreter the purpose of the interaction, including any specific terms that will be used or any forms that will need to be completed

❑ Consider the interpreter a member of the school team by establishing a working relationship

❑ Plan adequate time for the interview; interpreting takes more time

❑ If other school staff need to obtain similar information from the family, schedule a joint interview and share an outline prior to meeting

❑ Look directly at and speak to the student or parent/guardian not the interpreter

❑ Convey concern for and interest in the student and or family/guardian and the information they have to share

❑ Speak in short sentences and ask one question at a time

❑ Pause and wait for the interpreter to interpret

❑ Use simple terms; be cautious of medical or educational terminology

❑ Use words to express your meaning—gestures can be misinterpreted

❑ Speak normally, not too loudly and not too fast

❑ If you are giving instructions, do so in a step-by-step, logical sequence; pictures or other visual aids are helpful

❑ Say only what you want the student or parent to hear

❑ Encourage the interpreter to ask you for clarification; check accuracy

❑ Expect the interpreter to translate directly without adding to or changing the message and to remain impartial

❑ Listen closely to the student or parent/guardian for clues to their concerns, emotional response, understanding

❑ Realize that you may need to repeat or reword your message

(Adapted from material in Lynch EW, Hanson MJ,[18] Southwest Communication Resources,[27] Randall-Davis E,[28] and Downing B.[31])

In school settings, a sibling or another student may be asked to interpret. This arrangement poses concerns for confidentiality, misinterpretation and role confusion. The role reversal of the child (as the one who imparts information and answers for the family) can cause disruptions in family dynamics and puts significant burdens on the child.[18] In addition, parents may not wish to discuss some issues while their child is interpreting, because they may be embarrassed, reluctant for the child to share in decision making, and/or concerned about the loss of their authority as the parent.

REFERENCES

1. DeSantis L. Building healthy communities with immigrants and refugees. *J Transcultural Nurs.* 1997; 9(1): 20-30.
2. Center for Applied Linguistics. *Welcome to the United States: A Guidebook for Refugees.* Washington, DC: Refugee Service Center, Center for Applied Linguistics, 1996.
3. Ackerman LK. Health problems of refugees. *J Am Board Fam Pract.* 1997; 10(5): 337-348.
4. Chaney E, Hernandez D. *The Health and Well-Being of Children in Immigrant Families.* Committee on the Health and Adjustment of Immigrant Children and Families, Board on Children, Youth, and Families, National Research Council, Institute of Medicine. Washington, DC: National Academy Press, 1998.
5. Pickwell S. Providing health care to refugees. *Adv Pract Nurs Q.* 1996; 2(2):39-44.
6. American Academy of Pediatrics, Committee on Community Health Services. Healthcare for children of immigrant families. *Pediatrics.* 1997; 100(1): 153-156.
7. Gavagan T, Brodyaga L. Medical care for immigrants and refugees. *Am Fam Physician.* 1998; 57 (5):1061-1068.
8. Refugee Health Coordinator Network, Office of Refugee Resettlement. *Issues in Refugee Health. The Overseas Medical Examination and Domestic Health Examination.* United States Department of Health & Human Services, Washington, DC. 1994.
9. 56 *Federal Register* 25001-25004 (42 CFR) (1991).
10. American Academy of Pediatrics. *The Red Book 1997: Report of the Committee on Infectious Diseases.* Elk Grove, IL American Academy of Pediatrics, 1997.
11. Centers for Disease Control. *Tuberculosis Statistics in the United States, 1988.* Atlanta, Ga: Centers for Disease Control, 1990.
12. Guarnaccia P, Lopez S. The mental health and adjustment of immigrant and refugee children. *Child Adoles Psychiatric Clin North Am.* 1998; 7(3): 537-553.
13. American Psychiatric Association. *Diagnostic and Statistical Manual of Mental Disorders.* 4th ed. Washington, DC: American Psychiatric Association, 1994.
14. James D. Coping with a new society: the unique psychosocial problems of immigrant youth. *J School Health.* 1997; 67(3):98-102
15. McCullough K. Minneapolis, Minn: The Center for Cross-Cultural Health, February 1999.
16. Albers L, Johnson D, Hostetter M, Iverson S, Miller L. Health of children adopted from the former Soviet Union and eastern Europe. *JAMA.* 1997; 278(11): 922-924.
17. Hostetter M, Iverson S, Thomas W, Mckenzie D, Dole K, Johnson D. Medical evaluation of internationally adopted children. *N Engl J Med.* 1991; 325: 479-485.
18. Lynch EW, Hanson MJ. *Developing Cross-Cultural Competence: A Guide for Working with Young Children and Their Families.* Baltimore, Md: Paul H. Brookes Publishing Company, 1998.
19. Igoa C. *The Inner World of the Immigrant Child.* New York, NY: St. Martin's Press, 1995.
20. Lipson J, Dibble S, Minarik P. *Culture and Nursing Care.* San Francisco, Calif: University of California, San Francisco Nursing Press, 1996.
21. Andrews M, Boyle J. *Transcultural Concepts in Nursing,* 3rd ed. Philadelphia, Pa: JB Lippincott, Williams & Wilkins, 1999.
22. Leininger M. *Culture Care Diversity and Universality: A Theory of Nursing.* New York, NY: National League for Nursing Press, 1991.
23. Giger J, Dacidhizar R. *Transcultural Nursing: Assessment and Intervention.* St. Louis, Mo: Mosby-Yearbook, 1995.
24. Cooper T. Culturally appropriate care: optional or imperative. *Adv Pract Nurs Q.* 1996; 2(2):1-6.
25. Campinha-Bacote J. The quest for cultural competence in nursing care. *Nursing Forum,* 1995; 30(4): 19-25.

26. The Center for Cross-Cultural Health. *Caring Across Cultures: The Providers Guide to Cross-Cultural Health Care*. Minneapolis, Minn: The Center for Cross-Cultural Health, 1997.

27. Southwest Communication Resources. *Family Perspectives: Cultural/ Ethnic Issues Affecting Children With Special Health Care Needs. Educational Fact Packets for Health and Human Service Providers*. Bernalillo, NM: Southwest Communication Resources, 1996

28. Randall-Davis E. *Strategies for Working with Culturally Diverse Communities and Clients*. Bethesda, Md: Association for the Care of Children's Health, 1989.

29. Refugee Health Program. *Six Steps Toward Cultural Competence: How to Meet the Health Care Needs of Immigrants and Refugees*. Minneapolis, Minn: Refugee Health Program, Minnesota Department of Health, 1996.

30. Andrews M, Professor, Department of Nursing, Nazareth College of Rochester, New York. March, 1999.

31. Geissler E. Nursing Diagnoses of Culturally Diverse Patients. *Int Nurs Rev*. 1991;35(5):150-151.

32. Downing B. Guidelines for working with medical interpreters. In: *Caring Across Cultures*. Minneapolis, Minn: Center for Cross-Cultural Health, 1997.

Resources for Nurses

Web Sites:

Access to current and extensive information about immigrant and refugee populations is available on the Internet.

1. www.interaction.org/refugee/refugees.html/ (links to many other government and nonprofit agency sites)
2. Center for Cross-Cultural Health, Available at: http://www.umn.edu/ccch
3. The Center for Applied Linguistics. Available at: www.cal.org (cultural profiles and information about educational needs and services for second language students)
4. Chart of State TANF Plans. Available at: www.acf.dhhs.gov/news/welfare/stplans.htm
5. Ethnomed-University of Washington and Harborview Medical Center. Available at: @ Healthlinks.washington.edu/clinical/ethnomed (profiles of specific cultural groups with information about history, cultural practices, and beliefs.)
6. Immigration and Naturalization Services. Available at: www.ins.usdoj.gov
7. Office of Minority Health, US Dept Health and Human Services. Available at: http://www.omhrc.gov
8. School Health Culture Zone. Available at: http://courses.international.edu/bc680/nmcgahn/ (web site developed by N. McGahn, a school nurse)
9. Transcultural Nursing Society. Available at: http://www.nursingcenter.com/people/nrsorgs/

Immunization resource

Foreign vaccine product list. Available
at: http:\\www.health.state.mn.us\divs\dpc\
adps\ translte.htm

Language Lines

AT&T Language Line
1 Lower Ragsdale Drive
Monterey, CA 93940
1-800-874-9426
140 languages

Pacific Interpreters, Inc.
1020 SW Taylor, Suite 280
Portland, OR 97205
1-800-870-1069
email @pacinterp
65 languages

Agencies and Organizations

American Refugee Committee (ARC) International Headquarters USA, 2344 Nicollet
Ave. So., Suite 350, Minneapolis, MN 55404. e-mail: pr@archq.org

Bureau of Population, Refugees, and Migration, US Department of State, 2401 E Street,
NW, Suite L-505, SA-1, Washington, DC 20522-0105. www.state.gov/www/global/
prm/index.html

Center for Victims of Torture, 717 East River Road, Minneapolis, MN 55455

Center for Applied Linguistics. 1118 22nd Street NW, Washington, DC 20037. (202) 429-
9292. http://www.cal.org/RSC

Immunization Action Coalition, 1573 Selby Av., Suite 234, St. Paul, MN 55104. (651)
647-9131. www.imunize.org

National Insitutes of Health (NIH). www.nih.gov/

Office of Global Health, Centers for Disease Control and Prevention, 1600 Clifton Rd.,
NE, Atlanta,GA 30333.

Office of Minority Health Resource Center. P.O. Box 37337, Washington, DC 20013-
7337. (800) 444-6472.

Refugee Service Center, Center for Applied Linguistics. 1118 22nd Street NW, Washington, DC 20037. (202) 429-9292.

Transcultural Nursing Society, Madonna University, College of Nursing, 36600
Schoolcraft Drive, Livonia, MI 48150. (888) 432-5470.

World Health Organization. Headquarters Office in Geneva (HQ). Avenue Appia 20,
1211 Geneva 27, Switzerland. info@who.ch

BIBLIOGRAPHY

American Academy of Nursing. AAN Expert Panel Report: culturally competent health care. *Nursing Outlook.* 1992; 40: 277-283.

Binkin N, Zuber P,Wells C, Tipple M, Castro K. Overseas screening for tuberculosis in immigrants refugees to the United States: current status. *Clinical Infectious Dis.* 1996; 23:1226-32.

Cookson S, et al. Immigrant and refugee health. *Emerging Infectious Dis.* 1998; 4(3):427-8

Fadiman A. *The Spirit Catches You and You Fall Down: A Hmong Child, Her American Doctors, and the Collision of Two Cultures.* New York, NY: Farrar, Straus, and Giroux, 1997.

Ingstad B, Whyte S. *Disability and Culture.* Berkeley: University of California Press, 1995.

Jackson LE. Understanding, eliciting, and negotiating client multicultural health beliefs. *Nurse Practitioner.* 1993;18:30-43.

Kavanagh K, Kennedy P. *Promoting Cultural Diversity: Strategies for Health Care Professionals.* Newbury Park, Calif:SAGE Publications, 1992.

Kleinman A. Patients and healers in the context of culture. Berkeley: University of California Press, 1980.

Kosarchyn C. School nurses' perceptions of the health needs of Hispanic elementary school children. *J School Nurs.* 1993; 9 (1) : 37-43.

Leininger M. Issues, questions, and concerns related to the nursing diagnosis cultural movement from a transcultural nursing perspective. *Journal of Transcultural Nursing* 1990; 2(1): 23-31.

Leininger M. Future trends in transcultural nursing in the 21st century. *Int Nursing Rev.* 1997; 44(1): 19-23.

Roessler G. Transcultural nursing certification. *J Transcultural Nurs.* 1990; 1:59

Sack W. Multiple forms of stress in refugee and immigrant children. *Child Adolesc Psychiatric Clin North Am.* 1998 ; 7(1) 153-67.

Suro R. *Strangers Among Us: How Latino Immigration is Transforming America.* New York, NY: Albert A. Knopf, 1998.

Urrutia-Rojas X, Aday L. A framework for community assessment: designing and conducting a survey in a Hispanic immigrant and refugee community. *LA Public Health Nurs.* 1991;8(1):20-6

Vincent L. Families and early intervention: diversity and competence. *J Early Intervention.* 1992; 16 (2): 166-172.

Wenger A. Cultural meaning of symptoms. *Holistic Nursing Practice.* 1993; 7(2): 22-35.

Wong J. Cultural changes in healthcare. Postgrad Med. 1998; 103(6): 38.

10 | IHP: Anaphylaxis— Severe Allergic Reaction

Mariann Smith

INTRODUCTION

Allergies in the school-aged population are very common — so common, infact that school personnel sometimes tend to trivialize or ignore them.[1] However, severe allergic reactions or anaphylaxis can occur after insect stings or food intake in susceptible students while at school. These reactions can be life threatening. The cutaneous, gastrointestinal, respiratory, and cardiovascular systems are often affected. Prompt treatment is necessary. All school personnel need to be familiar with early recognition, prompt treatment, and prevention measures.

Food allergy, in general, is more prevalent than insect allergy. Studies estimate that between 0.3 % and 8% of the school-aged population has a food allergy; however, the vast majority are mild in nature.[1] The foods most likely to cause allergic reactions are peanuts, nuts, eggs, milk, wheat, and fish.[2] Food allergies are not always obvious because some foods and spices used as an ingredient can be "hidden" and cause problems to certain individuals even in very small amounts. Insects that can cause allergic reaction are from the *Hymenoptera* species and include honey bees, wasps, yellow jackets, and hornets. Fire ants also have been known to cause severe reactions.

Pathophysiology

Anaphylaxis is an exaggerated, life-threatening hypersensitivity reaction to a previously encountered allergen. This reaction triggers an incomplete humoral response that allows the allergen to combine with immunoglobulin (Ig)E and causes the release of histamine.[3] The reaction may be relatively mild (hives and itching) to severe (vascular collapse, bronchospasm, and shock). Severity of past reactions does not necessarily predict how severe subsequent reactions will be; however, there is often a cumulative effect in that each additional encounter with the allergen may result in more severe symptoms.

Anaphylaxis can occur within seconds to minutes from the time of exposure to the sensitizing factor. Occasionally, the student may have a recurrence of symptoms one to two hours after the initial symptoms have improved. This "biphasic" anaphylaxis is difficult to predict; therefore, it is important to continue to monitor the student after the initial reaction.[1]

Management

Managing the student who has the potential for an anaphylactic crisis involves eliminating the known allergen from the school environment as well as planning for the treatment of any allergic reactions. In the case of food allergies, school personnel need to know the trigger food(s). Teachers need to plan alternative projects involving cooking as well as inform room mothers so appropriate party treats can be provided. The food service department also needs to know the trigger food(s) so appropriate lunch and/or breakfast alternatives can be provided. If the trigger allergen is an insect, school grounds need to be monitored and appropriate pest control maintained.

Treating an allergic reaction involves educating school personnel on symptoms of the allergic reaction and appropriate treatment protocol. School personnel need to know that anaphylaxis is a medical emergency. The IHP needs to specify treatment protocol as well as who is responsible for carrying out the plan. A source of epinephrine (usually Epi-pen) and antihistamines (if ordered) should be readily available. If emergency medical personnel are called, school personnel will need to inform them about exposure to the specific allergen and treatment measures taken at school.

INDIVIDUALIZED HEALTHCARE PLAN

Assessment

History

- Student's known allergies
- Student's reactions to known allergies
- Symptoms of reactions from mild to severe
- Number of past serious reactions
- Past treatment of reactions from mild to severe; effectiveness of t[r]
- Family knowledge base
- Any other health concerns/illnesses

Current Status and Management

- Healthcare provider involved in assessment and management
- Assistance needed to implement management plan (e.g., parent, teacher, nurse)
- Knowledge about allergy reactions from mild to severe
- Knowledge about early warning signs of allergy reaction
- Involvement of school food service department
- Involvement of school transportation services if appropriate
- Monitor/treat environment (if needed)
- Current medications for treatment

Self-care

- Student's ability to avoid allergens (triggers)
- Student's level of knowledge of symptoms and treatment
- Student's ability to alert others to possible reactions and to assist with treatment
- Student's ability to self-medicate
- Student's ability/responsibility to carry medication with him/her (bus, field trips, family activities)

- Student's perception of dangers of a severe reaction
- Compliance with IHP

Psychosocial Status

- Parent's perception of dangers of severe reaction
- Involvement with support systems
- Student's fear of an anaphylactic episode occurring
- Student's feelings regarding outcome of reactions and treatment
- Peer reactions to anaphylactic episode and treatment
- Feelings of being different and needing food alternatives, etc.
- Age/developmental level

Academic Issues

- Past attendance concerns
- Regular vs. special education
- Past patterns of academic performance
- Possible need for 504 plan
- School staff perceptions — information the student and parent feel teachers need to know
- Past experiences with school food services (positive and negative)

Nursing Diagnoses (N.D.)

N.D. 1 (Risk for) ineffective breathing pattern (NANDA 1.5.1.3) related to:
  - brochospasm
  - inflammation of airways

N.D. 2 (Risk for) impaired gas exchange (NANDA 1.5.1.1) related to
  - brochospasm
  - inflammation of airways

N.D. 3 (Risk for) altered health maintenance (NANDA 1.5.1.1) related to:
  - ability to self-medicate or seek help from others

N.D. 4 Knowledge deficit: (NANDA 1.5.1.1) related to:
  - allergens
  - symptoms of allergic reactions

N.D. 5 Powerlessness (NANDA 7.3.2) related to:
  - uncertainty of an allergic reaction/outcome in the school environment

Goals

The student will:
- prevent allergic reactions from occurring (N.D. 4,5)
- increase knowledge of trigger allergens (N.D.4)
- list symptoms of allergic reaction (N.D.1,2,4)
- participate in development of an IHPand an Emergency Care Plan (ECP) (N.D.1-5)
- participate in school activities, with modifications as necessary (N.D.1-5)
- develop self-medication skills (N.D.4,5)

School Staff will:
- demonstrate beginning awareness of significance of severe allergic reactions, symptoms, and treatment (N.D.1,2,4)
- demonstrate knowledge of trigger allergen(s) and appropriate alternatives (N.D.4)

Nursing Interventions

Inservice school staff about allergic reaction/anaphylaxis (N.D. 1,2,4)
- student's known food or insect allergen(s)
- symptoms of mild to severe allergic reactions, including anaphylaxis
- importance of early warning signs and prompt treatment (emergency care plan)
- specific guidelines for treatment (from mild to severe)—emergency care plan
- documentation of episode
- field trip modifications that may be needed, medication must be taken along on all field trips, if food will be eaten
- extracurricular activities (e.g., dances, carnivals), modifications that may be needed
- need to continually monitor school environment for potential allergens
- inform bus drivers of student with known anaphylactic episodes

Encourage student to wear medical alert bracelet or necklace at all times (N.D. 1,2) (Assist parents in obtaining one, if needed)

Work with cafeteria personnel (N.D. 1.2.5)
- how to determine if a potential allergen is in a food
- cross-contamination with allergen and how to avoid it
- establishing a safe environment for student with food allergies

Collaborate with local emergency medical services (N.D. 1,2)
- EMS staff; paramedics
- additional doses of epinephrine with EMS response team
- nearest emergency room, hospital that will be used

Develop and implement a severe allergy healthcare plan. (N.D. 1-5)
- include student, parents/guardians, appropriate school personnel, and healthcare provider
- coordinate school plan with home plan
- obtain parent and healthcare provider approval of plan, including orders for medications (antihistamines and/or epinephrine)
- develop an ECP with copies given to teachers, including a copy in substitute teacher's information
- make modifications to IHP as needed
- identify person(s) who have access to and know where medication(s) are stored

Monitor medications (N.D. 1,2,3)
- epinephrine and/or antihistamines supplied by parent and stored in health office
- check medications frequently for correct dosage per medication order
- expiration date—request new supply of medication if expired and/or used

Provide necessary health education for student to participate in self-care (depending on the student's cognitive and/or physical ability). (N.D. 3,5)
- review sources of allergen(s)

- review treatment methods, including how/when to report allergic symptoms to school personnel
- teach proper technique of self-administration of epinephrine

Expected Student Outcomes

The student will:
- participate in all school activities with modifications made when necessary (N.D.3,4)
- list his/her symptoms of an allergic reaction (from mild to severe) (N.D.1,2,4)
- list trigger foods which can cause potential severe reaction (N.D.4)
- describe steps to take if an allergic reaction occurs (N.D.3,4)
- inform his/her teacher when treatment for an allergic reaction is necessary (N.D.3,5)
- demonstrate proper technique of self-medication (N.D.3,5)
- (along with parents) keep school personnel informed of any changes in medical status (N.D.4)
- wear allergy alert bracelet/necklace (N.D.3,4,5)
- help develop ECP, date_____

CASE STUDY

Manda is an 8-year-old third grade student at Place Elementary School. Two weeks ago, Manda and her parents were eating at a new Chinese restaurant when she suddenly started to wheeze, cough, and become cyanotic. Facial swelling occurred immediately, and hives developed on her neck and trunk. An ambulance was called, and Manda was transported to the hospital where she was treated for an anaphylactic reaction. Manda was kept overnight for observation. It was determined that she had suffered an extreme allergic reaction to the peanut oil used in cooking the food at the restaurant. Manda was dismissed with an order to keep an Epi-pen Jr. kit with her at all times.

Manda is usually very eager for school to start; however, this year she is apprehensive. She does not want a "shot" at school, and she is afraid that she will not know which foods might contain peanuts. She is also afraid that her classmates will be mad at her if peanut products are banned from the classroom and the lunchroom. The doctor has not determined if peanuts must be ingested before a reaction occurs or if Manda will have a reaction simply because she is in an area where peanuts are present.

Individualized Healthcare Plan*
Anaphylaxis

Assessment Data	Nursing Diagnosis	Goals	Nursing Interventions	Expected Outcomes
ND1 Student had severe allergic reaction to peanuts; hospitalized overnight for observation. Doctor's order for Epi-pen Jr. at school	Risk for ineffective breathing related to bronchospasm and inflammation of airways. (NANDA 1.5.1.3) Risk of impaired gas exchange related to bronchospasm and inflammation of airways (NANDA 1.5.1.1)	Student will have an IHP and ECP in place to include student, staff, and parental roles in preventing and managing an anaphylatic reaction.	Educate school staff on early signs of potential anaphylatic reaction and appropriate steps to take for treatment.	School staff are informed of potential for an anaphylatic reaction, the signs of a reaction, and what to do if a reaction occurs. Student will identify allergic reactions and treat immediately.
ND4 Hesitant to eat school breakfast and lunch. Able to recognize peanuts but not when an ingredient mixed in food dishes.	Knowledge deficit re: foods that contain peanut as an ingredient and to symptoms of a severe allergic reaction. (NANDA 1.5.1.1)	Student will increase knowledge about foods containing peanuts. Student will tell school personnel when his or her symptoms indicate an allergic reaction.	In-service staff regarding anaphylaxis potential and treatment. Notify food service of need for alternative food choices. Request classroom teacher to alert room mothers about food allergy and need for alternative party treats.	Student will increase knowledge of foods that contain peanut ingredients and will avoid these foods. Staff personnel will check with school nurse or food service department with any questions about ingredients in foods.

Nursing Diagnosis	Goals	Interventions	Expected Outcomes
ND3 Student fearful of another reaction at school Risk for altered health maintenance (NANDA 6.4.2) and feelings of powerless regarding uncertainty of allergic reaction outcome at school (NANDA 7.3.2)	Student will have an IHP and ECP. Student will participate in school activities with minimal disruptions.	Establish trusting, opening communication with student to provide health counseling sessions on foods containing peanut ingredients and on symptoms and treatment of allergic reaction.	Student will describe his symptoms of an allergic reaction.
Student not yet ready to self-medicate	Student will increase self-care skills regarding self-administration of medication.	Monitor and continue to educate regarding foods containing peanuts and need for alternative food choices. Educate student in proper technique of self-medication. Require return demonstration from student. Assist student to identify possible persons in school that can assist if anaphylactic episode occurs.	Student will identify school personnel responsible for helping carry out IHP and ECP. Student will participate in all school activities with modifications as needed. Student will demonstrate proper self-administration of epinephrine (Epi-pen).

*See Appendix for student profile information to include on an IHP form.

EMERGENCY CARE PLAN

School: _____

Phone: _____

FAX #: _____

Date: _____

Pupil's Name: _____   Physician's Name: _____

I.D.#: _____   Address: _____

Birthdate: _____   Phone: _____

Address: _____   FAX#: _____

Phone: _____   Hospital: _____

Parent's:

    Mother: _____   Day Phone: _____

    Father: _____   Day Phone: _____

Parent Designee: _____   Day Phone: _____

Medical Condition: Severe allergic reaction to peanuts and peanut products

Location of medication and other supplies: Epi-pen Jr. is kept in labeled drawer in locked medication cabinet in Health Room. Personnel listed below have access to key.

Persons authorized to administer treatment:

    School nurse: _____

    Nurse Designee: _____

Signs of emergency: Hives, itching, swelling, difficulty breathing, cyanosis

Treatment for Severe Allergic Reaction:

1. Administer epinephrine injection or assist student with self-administration.
2. Call 911, informing emergency personnel of severe allergic reaction to peanuts and that epinephrine injection has been given.
3. Call parent or parent designee.
4. Call student's physician to inform of emergency situation.
5. Record administration or self-administration of medication in student's health record (include date, time, source of exposure, treatment, if EMS was called, and signature).
6. Emergency personnel to transport to (hospital reference) or nearest emergency room.

REFERENCES

1. Wynn S, Anaphylaxis at school. *J School Nurs,*1993; 9(3): 4-11.
2. Mudd KE, Noone SA, Management of severe food allergy. *J School Nurs,* 1995;11(3): 30-32.
3. Anderson KE, Anderson, LE. Glanze, WD. *Mosby's Medical, Nursing, and Allied Health Dictionary,* St. Louis, MO: Mosby-Year Book, 1998.

BIBLIOGRAPHY

Anderson KE, Anderson LE, Glanze WD. *Mosby's Medical, Nursing, and Allied Health Dictionary,* St. Louis, MO: Mosby-Year Book, 1998.

Butler RE, ed. Parent pointer: warning to women against eating peanuts when pregnant or nursing, *Asthma, Strategies for Taking Control,* 1998; November-December

Committee on School Health, American Academy of Pediatrics. *School Health: A Guide for Health Professionals,* Elk Grove Village, Ill: American Academy of Pediatrics, 1987.

Kemper DW, *Healthwise Handbook: A Self-care Manual For You,* Boise, Idaho: Healthwise, 1991.

Lewis KD, Thompson HB. *Manual of School Health,* Menlo Park, Calif: Addison-Wesley Publishing Company, 1986.

Manz CJ. Food-induced anaphylaxis in children. *J Emerg Nurs,* 1994;20(5): 420-421.

Mudd KE, Noone SA, Management of severe food allergy in the school setting. *J School Nurs,* 1995;11(3): 30-32.

North American Nursing Diagnosis Association. *NANDA Nursing Diagnoses: Definitions & Classification 1999-2000.* Philadelphia, Pa: North American Nursing Diagnosis Assn, 1999. (NANDA, 1211 Locust Street, Philadelphia, PA 19107. 800-647-9002; fax 215-545-8107; e-mail: NANDA@nursecominc.com)

Wichita Public Schools Department of Health Services. *Emergency Care Guidelines,* Wichita, Kan: Wichita Public Schools, 1994.

Wold SJ. *School Nursing: A Framework for Practice,* North Branch, Minn: Sunrise River Press, 1981.

Wynn SR, Anaphylaxis at school. *J School Nurs,* 1993; 9(1): 5-11.

Wynn S, *Anaphylaxis: The Extreme Allergic Emergency*, Port Washington, NY: Center Laboratories, 1998.

11 | IHP: Burns

Patricia S. Latona

INTRODUCTION

Estimates indicate that one percent of the population incur a burn injury (approximately two million people) every year.[1] Eight out of ten burn deaths occur in the victim's home.[2] Burns in children are the second leading cause of death, second only to moving vehicular accidents.[1]

Approximately 40 percent of all burns which require hospitalization affect young children and adolescents. With a decreasing mortality rate, more will survive to return to their schools and communities.[3]

Treatment of a major burn injury is very intense and complicated. Hospitalization is determined by the age of the victim, the depth and size of the burn, the location of the burn, the cause of the burn, and the presence of associated injuries. Recovery time varies from several weeks in a minor burn to several years in a major burn.

Pathophysiology

Anatomy of the Skin

The skin is the largest organ of the body and at some point it interfaces with all major systems of the body. Therefore, the pathology of a major burn injury presents a multitude of complicated medical problems and issues.

The skin is basically divided into three layers. The outer layer is the epidermis, which is composed of epithelial cells.

These cells re-epithelialize. The middle layer is the dermis. Within the dermis are some epithelial cells, hair follicles, sebaceous glands, sweat glands, melanin cells, blood vessels, nerve fibers, and lymphatic vessels. Beneath the dermis is the hypodermis. The hypodermis contains fat, smooth muscle, and areolar tissue.

Causes of Burns

Burn treatment and management depend on the cause of the burn. Most burns are caused by thermal, chemical, and electrical injuries. Radiant heat injuries and tar injuries are seen less frequently.

Thermal burns are caused by dry heat (flame) or moist heat (hot liquid). The degree of injury is directly related to time of exposure and temperature. Thermal burns comprise 70% of all injuries. There are marked changes in the vascular and metabolic responses of the body.[1]

Electrical injuries comprise 6% of all burns. These injuries vary with the type of circuit, voltage, amperage, resistance of the body, pathway of current through the body, and the duration of contact with the current. Lightning injuries comprise 3% of all burn injuries. Lightning kills more people every year in the United States than any other natural disaster.[1]

Electrical injuries have an entrance

wound as well as an exit wound. Frequently, an electrical injury also has a thermal injury at the exit point. This occurs because the victim's clothing ignites. Loss of consciousness often occurs, and cardiopulmonary resuscitation at the scene is frequently required. Treatment and follow-up continue for several years post injury. Electrical injuries require massive fluid recuscitation, cardiac assessment, complicated multisystem stabilization, and possible amputation.[1]

A chemical injury is caused by the thermal energy produced when a chemical reacts with the body's tissue. These burns are progressive, and tissue damage continues until the agent has been neutralized.[1]

Burn Wound Description

The description of burn wounds includes their size and depth. Size is estimated using a modified Lund and Browder Chart. The extent of the burn is expressed as a percentage of total body surface area (TBSA).[4]

Burn depth is classified as superficial, partial thickness, or full thickness. Previous classification referred to the depth as first, second, or third degree burns (sometimes fourth). Superficial (first-degree) burns are usually of minor signficance. The skin remains intact. There is usually erythema and significant pain.

Partial thickness (second-degree) burns involve the first layer of skin (epidermis) and part of the second layer of skin (dermis). They appear red or mottled, contain blisters, and are wet and weeping. They are extremely painful. They usually heal within two to three weeks with a variable amount of scarring.[4]

Full thickness (third-degree) burns involve injury to the deep dermis and the hypodermis. They appear dark and are covered with eschar (dead skin tissue). Healing involves separation of eschar, debridement of the wound, and wound clo-

sure through skin grafting and other surgical interventions. This process can take months and can result in considerable scarring.[4]

Management

Destruction of the skin by a major burn injury causes numerous physiologic and hemodynamic changes throughout each of the body's systems. Some of the changes occur immediately, whereas others occur as the burn wound progresses.

Burn wound physiology and care have been divided into three phases of burn management. The first phase is the emergent phase (shock phase), the second phase is the acute phase (fluid remobilization phase), and the third phase is the rehabilitation phase (recovery phase).

During the emergent phase there is massive edema formation and a decrease in blood volume. Increased capillary permeability combined with an increase in hydrostatic pressure cause loss of water, protein, and electrolytes from the circulating volume into the interstitial spaces. Adequate fluid volume replacement is necessary to maintain vital organ function. This phase lasts anywhere from 36 to 48 hours.[4]

During the acute phase, fluid shifts from the interstitial space back into the cardiovascular space. When this occurs, there is massive diuresis. Management of the burn wound and prevention of complications such as infection and respiratory, circulatory, gastrointestinal, and central nervous system problems become imperative during this phase. Wound closure and prevention of complications are the goals during this phase.[1]

The final and most important phase is the rehabilitative phase. It begins once wound coverage has been completed. During this phase, final preparations for reentry into the burn victim's community are made. The phase includes: use of pressure bandages and splints, occupational therapy, physical therapy, and psychological and social support for dealing with issues and concerns regarding the burn injury and reintegration back into the family, school, and community.[1]

School Reentry

Next to the home, school is the most important social event for a child. Preparation for school reentry begins during the acute phase of hospitalization. The process of returning to the community and resuming life outside the hospital can be frightening for the child and his or her family, especially if the injury leaves the child visibly changed and/or different from other children.[5]

It is critical for the school nurse to establish herself/himself as the school contact person for the student's school reentry program as soon after the injury has occurred as possible. The school nurse can then assist in developing a school reentry program that includes:

1. Inclusion of the student and family in the planning and implementation of the school reentry program
2. Presentation of information on burn injury and management to staff and students
3. Presentation of specific information regarding the student
4. Presentation of information regarding psychosocial issues that the student may be experiencing.[5]

The school presentation should include discussion of topics such as the cause of the injury; history of the hospitalization; scars; splints, assistive devices, pressure garments, and other appliances; activity level and tolerance limitations; how individuals can help the student transition; and emphasis on how the child may have changed on the outside, but he or she is the same on the inside. Note: Special care must be taken to explain that accidents happen and they can be prevented, versus blaming the child and his or her parents for the injury.[5]

Teachers, staff members, and the student's peers may be very anxious. This anxiety is realistic; however, it can be decreased by assisting them to learn about burns and to discuss any questions or concerns they may have that will assist them in the school reentry program. Utilizing the staff from the burn center can assist in providing accurate information and answers to questions and concerns. Some burn centers use individualized videotapes in addition to written literature. Allowing the students to view pressure garments, splints, assistive devices, and other appliances will help them understand the complexity of burn care and wound management.

Assisting the student and his or her family to access and utilize community services such as counseling and support groups is also crucial. The student's participation in structured burn camps sponsored nationwide could enhance the student's self-esteem.[5,6]

INDIVIDUALIZED HEALTHCARE PLAN

Assessment

History

Prehospitalization (previous history)
- Preexisting medical conditions
- Surgeries
- Medications
- Allergies
- Height and weight

Prehospitalization (history related to the burn injury)
- Date and time of burn
- Cause of burn
- Did the burn occur in an open space or closed space?
- Were petroleum products involved?
- Did the victim lose consciousness?
- Were there any associated injuries?

Hospitalization
- Areas of body burned and thickness of burns
- Date of admission; date of discharge
- Surgeries (how many and what for)
- Treatment
- Complications
- Medical/psychological problems during hospitalizaton
- Academics during hospitalization
- Height/weight upon discharge

Current Status and Management

- Status of burn wounds (healed areas, open areas, treatments, etc)
- School reentry coordinator
- School reentry program (objectives, activities, timeline)
- Physician(s)
- Nurse (from hospital/burn center)
- Contact for current and further questions or concerns
- Activity restrictions
- Appliances (splints, assistive devices, etc.)
- Pressure garments
- Medications
- Nutritional status (appetite/diet requirements)

Self-Care

- Self-care abilities
- Desire to do self-care
- Motivators to do self-care
- Barriers to self-care
- Areas to encourage self-care

Psychosocial Status

- Student's concerns regarding returning to school
- Family status/dynamics

Academic Issues

- Number of days absent from school
- Academic instruction while hospitalized
- Need for health services at school
- Adaptive equipment needed
- Modifications needed
- Need for special education program or a 504 Plan
- Community resources
- Activity limitations
- Special precautions (i.e., exposure to sun, cold, etc)
- Community resources

Nursing Diagnoses (N.D.)

N.D. 1   Alteration in skin integrity (NANDA 1.6.2.1) related to:
- burn injury resulting in hypertropic scarring
- photosensitivity
- diminished/absent sweat glands
- dryness
- pruritus
- temperature sensitivity

N.D. 2   Risk for infection (NANDA 1.2.1.1) related to loss of skin integrity

N.D. 3   Risk for injury (NANDA 1.6.1) related to:
- impaired tissue integrity
- psycho/physiologic stress reaction to severe trauma
- immobility

N.D. 4   Pain (NANDA 9.1.1) related to burn injury

N.D. 5   Risk for ineffective individual (NANDA 5.1.1.1)/family coping (NANDA 5.1.2.1.2) related to:
- injury/situational crisis
- hospitalization

N.D. 6   Altered nutrition, less than body requirements (NANDA 1.1.2.2) related to:
- increased metabolic needs
- decreased appetite

N.D. 7   Body image disturbance (NANDA 7.1.1) related to:
- perception of appearance
- activity limitations and restrictions

N.D. 8   Impaired physical mobility (NANDA 6.1.1.1) related to:
- impaired joint movement
- searing

N.D. 9   Activity intolerance (NANDA 6.1.1.1) related to:
- prolonged hospitalization/period of inactivity
- impaired joint movement

N.D. 10 Self-care deficit— feeding, bathing/hygiene, dressing/grooming (NANDA 6.5.1,2,3) related to impaired joint movement/scarring

Goals

The student will be able to minimize scar contracture formation. (N.D. 8, 9)
The student will increase flexibility, strength, and endurance. (N.D. 8)
The student will have increased independence and self-care skills. (N.D. 10)
The student will utilize school and community resources for support. (N.D. 5)
The student manages pain/discomfort successfully during the school day. (N.D. 4)
The student achieves and maintains good nutritional intake. (N.D. 6)
The student increases his or her physical activity tolerance. (N.D. 9)
The student utilizes assistive devices as needed. (N.D. 3, 9)
The student demonstrates improved body image. (N.D. 7)
The student increases independent mobility in the school environment. (N.D. 8)
The student increases participation in self-care activities. (N.D. 10)
The student's skin shows signs of wound healing and improved skin integrity. (N.D. 1)
The student prevents infection of burn wounds. (N.D. 2)
The student meets height and weight requirements for age. (N.D. 6)
The student's skin maintains its integrity. (N.D. 6)

Interventions

Apply prescribed lotion that contains water and lipids to newly healed skin. (Avoid creams, lanolin, fragrances, and nonessential ingredients.) (N.D. 1)
Work with environmental staff to increase humidity in the classroom(s) air. (N.D. 1)
Assist student to avoid direct sunlight for six or more months to prevent sunburn and hyperpigmentation. (N.D. 1)
Encourage student to wear a hat and long sleeves when out in sun. (N.D. 1)
Assist student to apply sunscreen to newly formed skin. (N.D. 1)
Limit outdoor activities to early morning and late afternoon. (N.D. 1)
Avoid extreme changes in temperature. (N.D. 1)
Administer antihistamines in conjunction with topical antipruritics for itching as prescribed. (N.D. 1)
Refrigerate lotions and apply them cold. (N.D. 1)
Encourage good hygiene practices. (N.D. 1)
Assist and encourage student to actively participate in self-care. (N.D. 1)
Educate family to support student in participation in self-care. (N.D. 1)
Monitor compliance with compression therapy plan. (N.D. 1)
Assist student to maintain compliance with compression therapy plan in the school setting. (N.D. 1)
Monitor skin integrity for signs and symptoms of infection. (N.D. 2)
Assist student to notify his/her parents if signs or symptoms of infection occur. (N.D. 2)
Assist student to use assistive devices and/or adapted equipment as prescribed. (N.D. 3)
Assist in proper positioning in the classroom, and elsewhere, to prevent contractures. (N.D. 3)
Assist student and family to comply with prescribed exercise program. (N.D. 3)
Monitor effectiveness of splints. (N.D. 3)
Monitor student's range of motion with occupational and physical therapy staff. (N.D. 3)
Referral to special education if needed for academic-related issues/concerns (occupational therapy, adapted physical education, physical therapy). (N.D. 3)

Assist student to learn positive strategies to reduce stress. (N.D. 3)

Assist the student to practice using the strategies when experiencing stress at school. (N.D. 3)

Monitor need for and effectiveness of pain medication. (N.D. 4)

Administer pain medication, as prescribed. (N.D. 4)

Coordinate therapy procedures, with minimal classroom disruption. (N.D. 4)

Anticipate energy requirements and plan daily schedule to maximize energy for academic activities. (N.D. 4)

Plan rest periods, modify as needed. (N.D. 4)

Promote time and guidance for self-help activities. (N.D. 4)

Assist student to identify strategies that increase comfort/decrease pain (clothing, positioning, movement, etc.). (N.D. 4)

Encourage patient to verbalize thoughts, feelings, and concerns with family and staff. (N.D. 5)

Encourage and/or assist teacher to discuss academic and other issues with student and family. (N.D. 5)

Encourage student to keep a journal of negative and positive reactions of others toward him or her. (N.D. 5)

Encourage student and family to participate in school and community events. (N.D. 5)

Encourage student and family to participate in rehabilitative follow-up visits. (N.D. 5)

Encourage student and family to utilize community-based services and resources for counseling and support groups. (N.D. 5)

Assist the student to have available high-calorie, high-protein meals and snacks and foods that the student likes, as needed. (N.D. 6)

Provide attractive meals during times that the student desires to eat. (N.D. 6)

Assist in encouraging the student to socialize with peers during meals. (N.D. 6)

Monitor height and weight as indicated/requested. (N.D. 6)

Convey positive feedback to the student with honesty and sincerity. (N.D. 7)

Promote peer interactions and cooperative activities with peers. (N.D. 7)

Assist other students to address their questions and concerns appropriately, utilizing their parents and administrators as needed. (N.D. 7)

Prepare peers regarding child's appearance. (N.D. 7)

Encourage the student and parents to discuss issues surrounding body image. (N.D. 7)

Encourage the student to participate in support groups and activities with other children with burn injuries (burn camps). (N.D. 7)

Discuss activity limitations with the student's teachers. Assist them to modify activities based on the student's needs and abilities. (N.D. 3, 8, 9)

Discuss, develop, and plan for making up work when the student is unable to attend class or is absent. (Follow-up visits with healthcare providers and/or further treatment may occur during the school day.)

In-service staff regarding the student's return to school, prior to student's return. Cover the following:
- The student's burn injury
- The student's treatment and recovery
- Expectations for further health-related interventions
- Student and parents' concerns
- Teachers' concerns
- Resources available

Expected Student Outcomes

The student will:
- maintain/resolve wound healing (N.D. 1, 2)
- remain free from wound infection (N.D. 3)
- maintain/increase skin integrity (N.D. 1)
- demonstrate (a specific positive strategy) that reduces stress (N.D. 3)
- report freedom from pain during the school day (N.D. 4)
- request and appropriately utilize medication for pain/discomfort during the school day (N.D. 4)
- use nonmedication strategies to decrease discomfort/pain (N.D. 4)
- family will identify and describe the student's needs (N.D. 5)
- family will participate in the school and community reentry planning and implementation (N.D. 5)
- maintain nutritional intake to meet caloric needs   (N.D. 6)
- maintain and gain weight (N.D. 6)
- participate in activities with family, peers, and community (N.D. 5, 7)
- participate in planning and implementation for school reentry (N.D.5-10)
- refrigerate lotions and apply cold (N.D. 1)
- encourage good hygiene practices (N.D. 1)
- assist and encourage student to actively participate in self-care (N.D. 1)
- educate family to support student in participation in self-care (N.D. 1)
- monitor compliance with compression therapy plan (N.D. 1)
- assist student to maintain compliance with compression (N.D. 8)
- increase activity tolerance (specific criteria: ie half day attendance to full-day school attendance) (N.D. 9)
- participate in classroom/school activities with peers (N.D. 7)
- describe him/herself in positive terms (N.D. 7)
- describe his/her abilities and areas where he/she feels assistance is needed (N.D. 7, 10)
- increase participation/independence in self-care skills (specific skills) (N.D. 10)
- demonstrate independence in: (specific self skill) (N.D. 10)
- eliminate possible sources of infection (N.D. 2)
- achieve functioning to level of ability (N.D. 8)
- participate in follow-up care (N.D. 5)

BURN INJURY DISCHARGE INSTRUCTIONS TO SCHOOL

STUDENT'S NAME: _____

STUDENT'S SCHOOL: _____

History of Burn

      Date_____

      Cause_____

      Open Space Fire/Closed Space Fire_____

      Loss of consciousness_____

      Percent of body burn_____

Hospitalization Dates_____

Physical Abilities_____

Physical Limitations/Restrictions_____

Student may attend school____Part Time____Full Time_____Home School_____

Student requires a tutor_____Yes_____No

Medications_____
_____

Treatments_____
_____

Diet_____Nutritional Needs_____

Special Equipment Needs/Appliances_____
_____

Pressure Garments_____

Skin Care_____
_____

Student may participate in P.E._____Yes_____No

P.E. Limitations_____

Student may participate in contact sports_____Yes_____No

Physical Therapy Needs_____
_____

Occupational Therapy Needs_____
_____

_____

Authorized Signature

Date: _____

Telephone Number: _____

Adapted from North Carolina Jaycee Burn Center Discharge Report to School [7]

CASE STUDY

Medical Status

Samantha is an 8-year-old girl who sustained a 25 percent burn when she was playing with a lighter. She has partial and full thickness burns of her face, neck, chest, and right arm and hand. She was hospitalized at a university hospital burn center for four weeks. She had three skin graft surgeries.

Discharge Status

- No pending medical problems upon discharge
- Weight loss 12 pounds from preburn weight
- Limited ROM of right hand, wrist, elbow, and arm
- Extreme pruritus
- Splint to neck to prevent contracture
- Pressure garment to chest and right arm

Nutrition: Regular diet with supplement between meals at 10 a.m., 2 p.m., and 8 p.m. Snacks encouraged.

Activity: Full activity, however, she hesitates to participate.

Skin: Graft sites completely healed. Partial thickness burn areas healed. Frequent complaints of pruritus.

Activities of daily living: Due to right hand involvement, she needs assistance in all activities, including eating.

Academic: In-hospital educational program. Teacher-coordinated academics with student's school. Student academic progress has been good.

Psychosocial: Patient and family very anxious about student's reentry to school and community. Mother wants student to be home-schooled until she is completely healed.

Individualized Healthcare Plan*
Burns

Assessment Data	Nursing Diagnosis	Goals	Nursing Interventions	Expected Outcomes
ND1 Recent burn injury 25 percent burn (partial and full thickness) to face, neck, chest, and right arm and hand	Impaired in skin integrity related to burn injury resulting in hypertrophic scarring, photosensitivity, diminished/absent sweat glands, dryness, pruritus, and temperature sensitivity (NANDA 1.6.2.1.2.1)	The student's skin shows signs of wound healing, and improved skin integrity. The student prevents infection of burn wounds.	Apply prescribed refrigerated lotion to skin. Assist student to limit outdoor activities to early morning and late afternoon. Assist student to apply sunscreen to newly formed skin.	Student will maintain/ resolve wound healing. Student will maintain/ increase skin integrity.
Hospitalized 4 weeks. Three skin graft surgeries. Graft sites completely healed. Extreme pruritus. Pressure garment to be worn to cover chest and right arm.			Encourage student to wear a hat and long sleeves when out in the sun. Administer antihistamines in conjunction with topical antipruritics for itching as prescribed. Monitor compliance with compression therapy plan.	

ND6 12-pound weight loss from preburn to now. Regular diet with supplement at 10am, 2pm, and 8 pm.	Altered nutrition, less than body requirements, due to increased metabolic needs and decreased appetite (NANDA 1.1.2.2)	The student achieves and maintains good nutritional intake. The student meets height and weight requirements for age.	Assist the student to have available high-calorie, high-protein meals and snacks and foods that the student likes, as needed. Provide attractive meals during times that the student desires to eat. Assist in encouraging the student to socialize with peers during meals. Monitor height and weight as indicated/requested.	Student will maintain nutritional intake to meet caloric needs. Student will maintain/gain weight.
ND8 Student hesitates to participate in activities. Burn to right hand necessitates assistance in all activities, including eating.	Impaired physical mobility due to impaired joint movement and searing (NANDA 6.1.1.1)	The student will be able to minimize scar contracture formation. The student will increase flexibility, strength, and endurance. The student participates in classroom activities with modifications made as needed.	Discuss activity limitations with the student's teachers. Assist them to modify activities based on the student's needs and abilities. Refer to special education or 504 if necessary.	Student will utilize assistive devices to accomplish academic/self-care tasks at school. Student will achieve functioning to level of ability.

Individualized Healthcare Plan*
Burns (continued)

Assessment Data	Nursing Diagnosis	Goals	Nursing Interventions	Expected Outcomes
ND5 Student and family very anxious about student's re-entry to school and community. Mother wants student to be home schooled.	Potential for ineffective patient/family coping related to injury/ situational crisis, hospitalization (NANDA 5.1.1.1 & 5.1.2.1.2)	The student will utilize school and community resources for support.	Encourage student to verbalize thoughts, feelings, and concerns with family and staff. Encourage and/or assist teacher to discuss academic and other issues with student and family. Student will participate	in planning and implementation for school re-entry. Student will participate in activities with family, peers, and community.
No activity limitations per discharge plan. Student has made good progress.		Family participates in planning and implementing Samantha's return to school.	Encourage and facilitate family involvement in planning and implementing Samantha's return to school: *Timeline; *Modifications; *Health needs; *Nutritional needs; *Parent concerns; Teacher concerns; Feedback to parents(daily at first then	move to weekly) Family will identify and describe student's needs. Family will participate in the school and community re-entry planning and implementation.
			Encourage student and family to participate in school and community events. Encourage student and family to participate in rehabilitative follow-up visits.	

*See Appendix for student profile information to include on an IHP form.

REFERENCES

1. Hoeman SP, ed. *Rehabilitation: Nursing Process and Application*. St. Louis, Mo: C.V. Mosby, 1996:647-659.
2. National Fire Protection Association. *A Step by Step Guide: Planning the 1998 Fire Prevention Week Campaign in Your Community*. Quincy, Mass: Natl Fire Protection Assn, 1998.
3. Staley M, Anderson L, Greenhalgh D, Warden G. Return to school as an outcome measure following a burn injury. *J Burn Care Rehab*; 1999; 20(1):91-94.
4. Wong DL, Hockenbery-Eaton M, Wilson D, Winkelstein ML, Ahmann E, Divito-Thomas PA, eds. *Whaley & Wong's Nursing Care of Infants and Children*. 6th ed. St. Louis, Mo: Mosby, 1999:1336-62.
5. Blakeney P. School reintegration. *J Burn Care Rehab*. 1995;16(4):180-187.
6. Biggs KS, Heinrich PA, Jekel JF, Cuono CB. The burn camp experience: variables that influence the enhancement of self-esteem. *J Burn Care Rehab*. 1997;18(1):92-98.
7. Rosenstein DL. A school reentry program for burned children. Part I: Development and implementation of a school reentry program. *J Burn Care Rehab*. 1987; 8(4):319-324.

BIBLIOGRAPHY

Abdullah A, Blakeney P, Hunt R, et al. Visible scars and self-esteem in pediatric patients with burns. *J Burn Care Rehab*. 1994; 15:164-168.

Achauer BM, ed. *Management of the Burned Patient*. East Norwalk, Conn: Appleton & Lange, 1987.

Biggs KS, Heinrich PA, Jekel JF, Cuono CB. The burn camp experience: variables that influence the enhancement of self-esteem. *J Burn Care Rehab*,1997; 18(1):92-98.

Bishop B, Filinsky V. School reentry for the patient with burn injuries: video and/or on-site intervention. *J Burn Care Rehab*, 1995; 16(4): 455-457.

Blakeney P, Moore P, Meyer W, et al. Efficacy of school reentry programs. *J Burn Care Rehab*, 1995; 16(4): 469-472.

Blakeney P. School reintegration. *J Burn Care Rehab*, 1995; 16(4):180-187.

Boswick JA. *The Art and Science of Burn Care*. Rockville, Md: Aspen, 1987.

Cahners S, Dumont J, O'Connor M, McLoughlin E. *The Burned Child's Return to School*. Boston, Mass: Shriners Burns Institute, 1976.

Carpenito LJ. *Handbook of Nursing Diagnosis*. 7th ed, Philadelphia, Pa: Lippincott, JB 1993.

Carr-Collins JA. Pressure techniques for the prevention of hypertrophic scar. *Clin Plast Surg*. 1992; 19(3):733-743.

Clochesy JM. *Critical Care Nursing*. Philadelphia, Pa: WB. Saunders, 1993.

Doctor, ME. Burn camps and community aspects of burn care. *J Burn Care Rehab*, 1992; 13(1): 68-76.

Hoeman SP, et al, eds. *Rehabilitation Nursing Process and Application*. St. Louis, Mo: CV Mosby, 1996.

Leman CJ. Splints and accessories following burn reconstruction. *Clin Plast Surg*, 1992; 19(3):721-731.

National Fire Protection Association. *A Step by Step Guide: Planning the 1998 Fire Prevention Week Campaign in Your Community*. Quincy, Mass: Natl Fire Protection Assn, 1998.

North American Nursing Diagnosis Association. *NANDA Nursing Diagnoses: Definitions & Classification 1999-2000*. Philadelphia, Pa: North American Nursing Diagnosis Assn, 1999. (NANDA, 1211 Locust Street, Philadelphia, PA 19107. 800-647-9002; fax 215-545-8107; e-mail: NANDA@nursecominc.com)

Poh-Fitzpatrick MB. Skin care of the healed burn patient. *Clin Plast Surg*, 1992; 19(3): 745-751.

Rosenstein DL. A school reentry program for burned children. Part I: Development and implementation of a school reentry program. *J Burn Care Rehab*, 1987; 8(4):319-324.

Staley M, Anderson L, Greenhalgh D, Warden G. Return to school as an outcome measure following a burn injury. *J Burn Care Rehab*, 1999; 20(1):91-94.

Wong DL. *Nursing Care of Infants and Children*.6th ed. St. Louis, Mo: CV Mosby, 1999.

IHP: Duchenne Muscular Dystrophy

Judy F. Harrigan

INTRODUCTION

Muscular dystrophies are the largest and most important group of muscle diseases affecting children. The term *muscular dystrophy* refers to a group of inherited diseases marked by progressive weakness and degeneration of the skeletal muscles. The muscular dystrophies constitute the largest group of muscle diseases that affect children. In all forms of muscular dystrophy there is insidious loss of strength, but in each there is a difference in muscle groups affected, age of onset, rate of progression, and inheritance patterns. The etiology of the muscular dystrophies is unknown, although it is probable that the basic defect is caused by a metabolic disturbance which is unrelated to the nervous system. Recent theory supports the belief that the muscle itself is the site of the primary defect.

Pathophysiology

Duchenne (pseudohypertrophic) muscular dystrophy (DMD) is the most common and severe form of muscular dystrophy affecting children and is characterized by progressive, symmetric weakness and wasting of skeletal muscles, with increasing disability and deformity. Duchenne muscular dystrophy is X-linked and therefore affects males almost exclusively with an incidence of approximately 1:3500 male births. Major complications of DMD include contractures, muscle atrophy, respiratory infections, obesity, and cardiopulmonary problems.

Although there is laboratory evidence that the disease is present from birth and there may be an early history of motor delay, the onset of muscle weakness is generally not exhibited until the child is between three and five years of age. The child generally achieves early developmental milestones such as raising his head while lying prone, rolling, and sitting upright. The disability becomes apparent when the child begins to stand and walk. At this point he may be described as clumsy with a slightly waddling gait, frequently falling and exhibiting a characteristic method of rising from a sitting position on the floor by "walking" his hands up his legs (Gower sign). Unless there is suspicion of DMD related to family history, these signs may be attributed to the normal clumsiness of a developing child. The diagnosis may not be made until the late preschool years when the child's inability to physically keep up with his peers becomes significant.

The boy with DMD often seems to be particularly well developed muscularly because of the hypertrophied muscles characteristic of the disease. The name pseudohypertrophy is applied to DMD because muscles, especially in the calves and upper arms, become enlarged from fatty infiltrates. Leg pain, lordosis, progressive muscle weakness, and more frequent falls become problematic as the child enters school. Stair climbing, running, and jumping become difficult or impossible for the child with DMD. Mild mental retardation may be associated with muscular dystrophy. Anxiety and depression are also common, first, as the child begins to realize that he is not able to keep up with peers, and later when he becomes confined to a wheelchair.

Significant muscle atrophy, contractures, and deformities involving many joints occur in later stages of the disease. Ambulation usually becomes impossible by the time the child approaches his second decade of life. A progressive kyphoscoliosis develops, interfering with an already weakened respiratory system. In its terminal stages, the disease process involves the facial, oropharyngeal, and respiratory muscles with death resulting from pneumonia and respiratory failure.

Management

There is no effective treatment for DMD; at the present time it is an incurable disease. Maintaining function of muscles for as long as possible is the primary goal of treatment. Passive stretching of heel cords and the application of nighttime splints may impede foot and ankle deformities. Maintenance of function often includes surgery to release contractures, bracing, and assistance with activities of daily living. Despite best preventive efforts, most patients eventually become confined to a wheelchair, and contractures accelerate to include knee, hip, and arm joints. Stretching exercises should include these joints. As kyphoscoliosis begins to develop, a body jacket or wheelchair insert may be used to impede progression. Progression of scoliosis is often related to failure to comply with the body jacket regimen. Patients must use the brace in order for it to be effective. Ancillary assistive devices may benefit the child who has difficulty performing activities of daily living. Consultation with physical and occupational therapists will be helpful in determining aids that will enable the child to participate as much as possible in all aspects of his life.[1]

INDIVIDUALIZED HEALTHCARE PLAN

Assessment

History

- When the diagnosis was made
- Degree and pattern of progression of physical disability related to DMD
- Past hospitalizations, surgeries, medications—respiratory complications, tendon release, scoliosis, tracheostomy
- Previous physical, occupational, and respiratory therapy
- Assistive devices (braces, splints, feeding equipment, computers, etc.) that have been used previously
- Other illnesses and/or complications related to DMD
- Family genogram—including history of others with muscular dystrophy
- Family history in relation to management of cares, stresses, finances, and the demands of having a physically disabled child with a terminal illness

Current Status and Management

- Severity of the student's DMD
- Prognosis
- Compliance with DMD plan of care
- Effectiveness of DMD plan of care
- Growth pattern—current height and weight
- Daily nutritional pattern
- Daily activity schedule—including DMD management measures
- Bowel elimination pattern
- Respiratory status—past and present
- Description and general knowledge about DMD—student and family
- Involvement of support persons/systems
- Heathcare providers involved in management of DMD and routine health maintenance

Self-care

- Knowledge about DMD—student, family, and school personnel
- Knowledge about skin care, use of assistive devices, respiratory health, prevention of constipation, etc.—student, family, and school personnel
- Student's participation in development and implementation of DMD plan of care
- Assistive devices needed for daily activities
- Ability to manage activities of daily living
- Motivation to do self-care
- Barriers to self-care
- Experience with self-care at home

Psychosocial Status

- Current developmental stage of the student
- Current developmental stage of the family
- Communication skills—student and family
- Student's self-concept
- Student's feelings about having DMD
- Student's fears, anxieties, and concerns
- Student's perception of his health and DMD
- Student's perception of his abilities and disabilities
- Family's perception of student's health and DMD
- Decision-making skills and problem-solving skills
- Coping skills—student and family
- Student's locus of control—health, school, family, and activities of daily living
- Ability to interact with peers and adults
- Support systems—student and family
- Family values

Academic Issues

- Level of cognitive functioning—learning problems, fine motor problems
- Academic, developmental, and social strengths and weaknesses

- Patterns of academic performance—grades, failures, retentions, changes in academic performance
- Need for special education services (IDEA or ADA) to adequately educate the student
- Past school attendance patterns—absences related to DMD
- Student's perceptions about school—his own strengths and weaknesses
- Teacher's perception of student's academic performance and classroom adjustment
- Comparison of student's behavior, social skills, and academic performance to peers
- Participation in regular school activities
- Participation in regular exercise program—school-related or non-school-related

Nursing Diagnoses (N.D.)

N.D. 1   Impaired physical mobility (NANDA 6.1.1.1) related to:
- muscle weakness
- contractures

N.D. 2   Alteration in self-care feeding, bathing/hygiene, dressing/grooming, toileting (NANDA 6.5.1, 2,3, & 4) related to:
- mobility limitations
- muscle weakness
- contractures

N.D. 3   Body image disturbance, self-esteem (NANDA 7.1.1 & 2) related to:
- physical limitations
- grieving
- embarrassment
- feelings of being different/physical changes
- loss of control
- intimacy concerns
- perception of stigma

N.D. 4   Risk for physical injury (NANDA 1.6.1) related to:
- poor balance and coordination
- falls

N.D. 5   Risk for respiratory infection (NANDA 1.2.1.1) related to ineffective airway clearing

N.D. 6   Constipation (NANDA 1.3.1.1) related to immobility

N.D. 7   Risk for impaired skin integrity (NANDA 1.6.2.1.2.2) related to:
- pressure from braces and wheelchair
- immobility

N.D. 8   Anticipatory grieving (NANDA 9.2.1.2) and/or hopelessness (NANDA 7.3.1) related to:
- deteriorating physical condition
- terminal prognosis

N.D. 9   Risk for altered nutrition: more than body requirements (NANDA 1.1.2.1) related to immobility

N.D. 10   Altered family processes (NANDA 3.2.2) related to having a child with a disability

N.D. 11   Alteration in student role (NANDA 3.2.1) related to cognitive delays

Goals

Student will develop minimal deformities and/or deformities currently present will not progress. (N.D. 1)

Student will maintain maximum independence in school and classroom and activities of daily living. (N.D. 2)

Student will maintain and/or improve self-management skills. (N.D. 2)

Student and family will be actively involved in making decisions about the management of the condition. (N.D. 2, 3)

Family will encourage and allow student to maintain independence and make decisions. (N.D. 2, 3)

Student will maintain positive self-image and self-esteem. (N.D. 3)

Student will maintain mobility throughout the school using a wheelchair and/or other assistive devices. (N.D. 1)

Student will be safe in the school environment and remain free from physical injury. (N.D. 4)

Student will be free of respiratory infections. (N.D. 5)

Student will have regular, soft bowel movements. (N.D. 6)

Skin will be free from breakdown. (N.D. 7)

Student and family will be able to express feelings of optimism about the present. (N.D. 8)

Student and family will exhibit peace and comfort with the terminal prognosis. (N.D. 8)

Student will develop relationships with similar age peers. (N.D. 8)

Student will maintain appropriate weight for height. (N.D. 9)

Student will choose low-fat, healthy foods in appropriate portions. (N.D. 9)

Student will maintain an optimal level of exercise, with modifications as necessary. (N.D. 9)

Student will achieve academic success appropriate to chronological age and cognitive abilities. (N.D. 10)

Interventions

Monitor student's ability to perform self-management skills and collaborate with occupational therapy (OT)/physical therapy (PT) staff to instruct him in methods to improve ability and maximize potential. (N.D. 1, 2)

Collaborate with OT/PT staff for use of appropriate assistive devices to increase independence in self-care and classroom activities and monitor use in the classroom. (N.D. 1, 2)

Assist in making arrangements for appropriate transportation to and from school. (N.D. 1)

Instruct classroom staff in performance of stretching exercises, application of braces, and transfer to and from wheelchair and provide supervision of these activities. (N.D. 1, 4)

Work with family to increase appropriate use of braces at home. (N.D. 1)

Collaborate with social worker to assist family to obtain assistive devices for use at home. (N.D. 1)

Arrange for assistance as necessary for daily school activities. (N.D. 1)

Monitor student's ability to perform self-management skills and instruct him in methods to improve skills and maximize potential. (N.D. 2)

Maintain regular communication with student and family about healthcare plan. (N.D. 2)

Encourage student to share feelings about his condition, its management requirements, limits, the stigma it imposes, and the prognosis. (N.D. 3)

Encourage student to identify his own strengths and weaknesses. (N.D. 3)

Assist student in developing strategies to handle teasing and discrimination. (N.D. 3)

Encourage continued and age-appropriate peer relationships. (N.D.3)

Refer student and family to support groups, counseling, family therapy, and/or clergy as indicated. (N.D. 3, 8, 10)

Assess school environment for accessibility and facilitate installation of equipment such as ramps, railings, etc. to allow safe access. (N. D. 4)

Collaborate with school staff and emergency personnel to establish an evacuation plan in case of fire or other emergency. (N.D. 4)

Monitor student's health and that of peers to assure that exposure to infectious diseases is minimized. (N.D. 5)

Assist student to cough and clear airway effectively. (N.D. 5)

Assist student to maintain adequate hydration to thin secretions. (N.D. 5)

Instruct school staff in proper technique for airway clearance and the need for adequate hydration. (N.D. 5)

Arrange for space and time for toileting at school. (N.D. 6)

Collaborate with family, classroom, and cafeteria staff to provide appropriate foods and fluids to decrease constipation. (N.D. 6)

Assist student and family to observe for signs of early skin breakdown. (N.D. 7)

Instruct student, family, and classroom staff in management of skin care and detection of early skin breakdown. (N.D. 7)

Reinforce student's positive abilities, interactions, etc. (N.D. 8)

Listen to student and family and encourage expressions of concern, grief, fear, and anxiety. (N.D. 8)

Monitor student's growth with height and weight measurements at least twice a year. (N.D. 9)

Assist student and family in planning nutritional diet that is low in calories and fat and high in protein and fiber. (N.D. 9)

Advise school lunch program director on inclusion of appropriate food choices. (N.D. 9)

Identify family's developmental stage. (N.D. 10)

Promote wellness for student and family with teaching and support. (N.D. 10)

Refer to Committee on Special Education or 504 Committee for evaluation of academic program needs. (N.D.11)

Refer student for adaptive physical education classes. (N.D. 9)

Develop IHP that addresses student's physical and academic needs. (N.D. 11)

Participate as a member of the interdisciplinary team, which will develop an IEP. (N.D. 11)

Expected Student Outcomes

- Student will maintain mobility around the school. (N.D. 1)
- Student will perform classroom/school activities as independently as possible. (N.D. 2)
- Student will attend all classes and participate in activities with modifications as necessary. (N.D. 1)

- Student will receive assistance for activities with which he requires assistance. (N.D. 1, 2)
- A wheelchair-adapted bus will take student to and from school. (N.D. 1)
- Student will use braces and standing table for times determined in treatment plan. (N.D. 1)
- Student will participate in range-of-motion activities for ankles, knees, and hips so range of motion will increase/contractures will not progress. (N.D. 1)
- Schedule for OT/PT will not interfere with classroom schedule. (N.D. 1)
- Student will use his braces at home for increasing times as determined by tolerance of the activity. (N.D. 1)
- Student will utilize assistive devices at school and home to achieve an optimal level of independence. (N.D. 1, 2)
- Student and family will demonstrate safe and appropriate technique in toileting, transfer, medicine-taking, skin care, etc. and report early symptoms indicating problems. (N.D. 2, 4, 6, 7)
- Student and family will be involved in problem- solving and decision- making in relation to student's care, academic program, and physical environment. (N.D. 2, 3)
- Student will verbalize feelings to appropriate adults about his concerns, grief, anger, anxiety, fear, and limitations and others' reactions to his disability. (N.D. 3, 8)
- Student will verbalize positive feelings about himself and identify individual strengths. (N.D. 3)
- Student will develop answers and will use them to explain to others about his disability and limitations. (N.D. 3)
- Bathroom adaptations, ramps, elevators, evacuation plan, etc. will be in place, accessible to the student. (N.D. 4)
- Staff will demonstrate competence in providing care. (N.D. 4)
- Student will remain free of infection. (N.D. 5)
- Student's school attendance will increase. (N.D. 5)
- Student will demonstrate effective airway clearing. (N.D. 5)
- Student will drink 4 to 6 glasses of water or juice each day in school. (N.D. 5, 6)
- Staff will encourage student to use proper technique when coughing and to drink fluids during the school day (N. D. 5).
- Student will have regular bowel movements. (N.D. 6)
- Student and family will demonstrate appropriate food choices to maintain regular bowel activity. (N.D. 6)
- Student's skin will be intact. (N.D. 7)
- Student will participate in activities and functions that he enjoys and give him positive feelings. (N.D. 8)
- Family will participate in counseling, if appropriate. (N.D. 8)
- Student's weight will be appropriate for height, as plotted on growth chart. (N.D. 9)
- Student will consistently choose appropriate, nutritional foods. (N.D. 9)
- Student will actively participate in physical education and physical therapy programs and in games played in class, with modifications as necessary. (N.D. 9)
- Family members will be encouraged to play a supportive role in assisting/managing student's care. (N.D. 10)
- Student will describe his roles and responsibilities in the family and the roles and responsibilities of other family members. (N.D. 10)

- School staff will collaborate with student and family to develop an educational program that will enable the student to achieve academic success. (N.D. 11)

Evacuation Plan

Discussion must take place with local emergency personnel to plan for evacuation of physically disabled students in case of unforeseen emergencies. Emergency personnel should be encouraged to visit the school and plan, with school personnel, for egress during drills or real emergencies.

Elevators should not be used. School staff should not be expected to carry students out of the building. If a student is able to ambulate using crutches, walker, or other assistive devices, and the student is not in a ground floor level setting, the slower student should exit the building, with adult supervision, after all other students have left. If a student is unable to ambulate and must remain in a wheelchair, it may be necessary for adaptations to be made to the building. Ramps, chutes, and egress windows above ground level are possibilities that should be considered. Evacuation plans should be developed with consideration to building construction, district finances, advice from emergency personnel and the student's personal needs.

CASE STUDY

Jason is an 11-year-old boy who was diagnosed at the age of 4 years with Duchenne muscular dystrophy after his parents began to recognize symptoms of falling and progressive weakness that they had previously seen in young cousins in both the mother's and father's families. Jason did not begin to walk until he was almost 2 years old and has never been able to run or jump. He started school one year later than his peers and is described by his teachers as being immature and unable to accomplish many routine activities of daily living. Psychological tests reveal him to be mildly mentally retarded. He is reported to be highly distractible with poor academic interest and problems with short-term and rote memory. He currently attends an in-district special education class and receives speech, physical, and occupational therapy services. He has had many absences from school because of frequent respiratory infections and has been hospitalized twice in the past two years with pneumonia.

During the last year Jason has begun to rapidly lose function. He is no longer able to ambulate, and his parents have stopped using his long leg braces at home. He is developing contractures in his ankles, knees, and hips. Jason spends most of each day in his wheelchair and is becoming more proficient in maneuvering his wheelchair. His doctor has just written a prescription for him to resume use of his braces and to stand in his braces at a standing table. The physical therapist will be monitoring this process. He has gained 12 pounds in the past six months. He takes prednisone, 12.5 mg per day. His mother reports that he has problems with constipation.

The school nurse met with Jason and his mother in her office to discuss Jason's rapidly changing physical status and to develop a healthcare plan that would accommodate his needs in school. He arrived in his wheelchair, which was pushed by his mother. His mother repeatedly answered questions that were directed to Jason and assured the nurse that he was unable to accomplish dressing, bathing, and toileting without assistance. Jason was silly and immature during the meeting and did not seem to be interested in the discussion about his care plan. When asked what he likes best about school, he stated that he did not like school.

In a private discussion with the nurse, his mother expressed guilt that "We knew this ran in the family. It's our fault that he has muscular dystrophy." She also stated that she feels so bad when he has difficulty with activities of daily living that she helps him, even though she knows she should let him do things for himself.

Individualized Healthcare Plan*
Duchenne Muscular Dystrophy

Assessment Data	Nursing Diagnosis	Goals	Nursing Interventions	Expected Outcomes
ND1 Severity of student's DMD. Current level of physical activity. Current level of weakness/contractures. Assistive equipment being used.	Impaired physical mobility (NANDA 6.1.1.1) related to muscle weakness/contractures.	Student will maintain mobility throughout the school using wheelchair and other assistive devices.	Collaborate with OT/PT staff for use of appropriate assistive devices and monitor use in classroom. Work with family to increase use of braces and standing table at home. Assist in arrangements for transportation to and from school.	Assistive devices will be available at school and home and will be useful to student achieving independence. Student will be able to manage mobility in school and perform as many activities as possible.
Compliance with plan of care. Effectiveness of plan of care. Need for assistance with daily activities. Participation in regular exercise program —school-related or non-school-related.		Student will develop minimal deformities and present deformities will not progress.	Arrange for assistance prn for daily school activities. Instruct and supervise staff in performance of stretching exercises, application of braces, transfer to and from wheelchair.	Student will be able to physically attend all classes. OT/PT schedule will not interfere with classroom schedule. A wheelchair- adapted bus will take student to and from school. Student will receive assistance as needed. Student will use braces and standing table per treatment plan. Student's range of motion will increase/contractures will not progress.

ND2 Knowledge about DMD—student and family. Developmental stage—student and family. Perception of DMD, health, abilities, and disabilities—student and family.	Alteration of self-care (NANDA 6.5.1.2 and 3) related to mobility limitations, muscle weakness, contractures.	Student will maintain maximum independence in school/ classroom activities and activities of daily living. Student will maintain and /or improve self-management skills.	Monitor student's ability to perform self-management skills. Assistive devices will be available at home and school.	Student will perform as many activities as possible that are developmentally appropriate and safe. Student will request assistance as necessary.
Knowledge about skin care, use of assistive devices, etc.—student and family. Student's participation in developing and implementing plan of care.		Student and family will be actively involved in making decisions. Family will encourage and allow student to maintain independence and make decisions.	Instruct student and family in methods to improve skills and maximize potential. Maintain regular communication with student and family about healthcare plan.	Student will utilize assistive devices to increase independence at home and school.
Ability to manage activities of daily living. Motivation to do self-care. Barriers to self-care. Experience with self-care at home. Decision-making and problem solving skills—student and family.				Student and family will demonstrate safe and appropriate techniques in toileting, transfer, medicine-taking, skin-care, etc. and report early symptoms indicating problems.
				Student and family will be involved in problem-solving and decision-making in relation to student's care, academic program, and physical environment.

Individualized Healthcare Plan*
Duchenne Muscular Dystrophy (continued)

Assessment Data	Nursing Diagnosis	Goals	Nursing Interventions	Expected Outcomes
ND5 Respiratory status—past and present. Healthcare providers involved in management of DMD and routine health maintenance.	Potential for respiratory infection (NANDA 1.2.1.1) related to ineffective airway clearing.	Student will be free of respiratory infection.	Monitor student's health and that of peers to assure minimum exposure to infectious diseases. Assist student to cough and clear airway effectively.	Student will remain free of infection. Student's school attendance will increase. Student will demonstrate effective airway clearing.
Knowledge about respiratory health—student and family. School attendance patterns.			Assist student to maintain adequate hydration to keep secretions thin. Instruct school staff in proper technique for airway clearance and the need for adequate hydration.	Student will drink 4-6 glasses of water or juice each day in school. Staff will encourage student to use proper technique when coughing and to drink fluids during the school day.
ND8 Level of acceptance of DMD—student and family. Student's self-concept. Student's feelings about having DMD. Fears, anxieties, concerns—student and family.	Anticipatory grieving (NANDA 9.2.1.2) and/or hopelessness (NANDA 7.3.1) related to deteriorating physical condition and terminal prognosis.	Student and family will be able to express feelings of optimism about the present. Student and family will exhibit peace and comfort with the terminal prognosis.	Listen to student and family and encourage expressions of concerns, grief, fear, and anxiety. Reinforce student's positive abilities, interactions, etc.	Student will verbalize to appropriate adults feelings about concerns, grief, anger, anxiety, fear, and limitations and others' reactions to his disability.

Assessment	Nursing goals	Nursing interventions	Expected student outcomes
Perception of abilities and disabilities— student and family. Coping skills— student and family. Student's locus of control —health, school, family, activities of daily living.	Student will develop relationships with similar age peers.	Refer student and family to support groups, counseling, family therapy, and/or clergy as indicated. Encourage student to participate in activities where he will meet and interact with peers.	Student will participate in activities and functions that he enjoys and that give him positive feelings. Family will participate in counseling, if appropriate.
Ability to interact with peers and adults. Support systems—student and family.			

*See Appendix for student profile information to include on an IHP form.

REFERENCES

1. Brooke MH. *A Clinician's View of Neuromuscular Diseases. 2nd ed.* Baltimore, Md: Williams & Wilkins, 1986.

BIBLIOGRAPHY

Haas MK, ed. *The School Nurse's Source Book of Individualized Health Care Plans. Vol 1.* North Branch, Minn: Sunrise River Press, 1993.(Sunrise River Press, 11605 Kost Dam Road, North Branch, MN 55056. 800-895-4585; fax 651-583-2023.)

North American Nursing Diagnosis Association. *NANDA Nursing Diagnoses: Definitions & Classification 1999-2000.* Philadelphia, Pa: North American Nursing Diagnosis Assn, 1999. (NANDA, 1211 Locust Street, Philadelphia, PA 19107. 800-647-9002; fax 215-545-8107; e-mail: NANDA@nursecominc.com)

Whaley LF, Wong DL. *Nursing Care of Infants and Children. 5th ed.* St. Louis, Mo: C.V. Mosby Company, 1995.

13 | IHP: Fragile X Syndrome

Mary Jo Martin

INTRODUCTION

Fragile X syndrome knows no boundaries. It appears in children of all ethnic, racial, and socioeconomic backgrounds. Fragile X, or Martin-Bell syndrome, is a sex-linked genetic disorder and is the most common form of inherited mental retardation.[1] In recent years, more has been learned about fragile X syndrome. Adults and children with no known cause for their mental impairment are being tested and correctly diagnosed. Multidisciplinary school programs must be provided to meet the educational and health needs of these special individuals.

Pathophysiology

The fragile X syndrome is caused by an abnormal gene on the lower end of the long arm of the X chromosome. This fragile site has been determined to be caused by a gene mutation that results in excessive repeats of nucleotide in a specific deoxyribonucleic acid (DNA) segment on the chromosome.[2]

Like other sex-linked disorders, fragile X syndrome primarily affects males. Approximately four times as many males as females have the disorder. Because females have two X chromosomes and males have one X and one Y chromosome, men with the fragile X gene pass it on to all of their daughters and none of their sons. Mothers have a fifty-fifty chance of passing it on to either their son or their daughter.[3]

The physical characteristics of fragile X may be quite subtle or pronounced. Features can include a long, narrow face, large ears, high palate, mitral valve prolapse, and enlarged testicles (macroorchidism) in males. Connective tissue and muscle abnormalities along with poor muscle tone can cause motor delays, double-jointed fingers, curvature of the back, flat feet, strabismus, and slack facial features, especially in younger children.[3]

Boys are typically more severely affected than girls. While most boys have mental retardation, only one-third to one-half of girls have significant intellectual impairment. Short attention span, hyperactivity, anxiety, and unstable mood are common in both sexes. Behavior is usually socially engaging, but individuals tend to avoid direct eye contact during conversation. Hand flapping, hand biting, and fascination with spinning objects are common. Sensory skills are often poor and those with fragile X can be easily overwhelmed by crowds, noises, textures, and so on. They may not like being touched or held.[2-4, 6]

Speech and language development are often delayed. Studies have shown that the specific communication problems associated with fragile X cannot be attributed just to mental retardation. Compared to males with Down syndrome, males with fragile X have more jargon (unintelligible strings of syllables), perseveration (frequent and inappropriate repetition of words, phrases, or a specific topic), and echolalia (repetition of verbalizations of a previous speaker, which usually indicates a lack of understanding).[2]

A DNA-based blood test was developed in 1992 to diagnose fragile X syndrome. It is an accurate test and can detect both carriers and fully affected individuals. A blood sample is collected and sent to a lab that offers the test. It usually takes several weeks to receive the results.[4] Families are advised to seek genetic counseling to understand the inheritable nature of fragile X syndrome and discuss the likelihood of other family members or future offspring having the disorder. A positive diagnosis often produces grief over the loss of the normal child the parents had hoped and expected to have. Seeking support from family, friends, and professionals is essential in coping with theses intense feelings.

Currently no cure exists for fragile X syndrome, but there are treatments that have been shown to be extremely effective. Medical treatment may include the use of serotonin agents such as carbamazepine (Tegretol) or fluoxetine (Prozac) to control violent tempers and outbursts and the use of central nervous system (CNS) stimulants or clonidine (Catapres) to improve attention span and decrease hyperactivity. The use of folic acid, which affects the metabolism of CNS transmitters, is controversial.[2]

The significant sensory processing, cognitive, and regulation problems that children with fragile X have make learning in the typical classroom challenging. These challenges require early intervention or children with fragile X can experience a progressive decline in IQ.[6] The intervention of multiple professions promotes optimal learning. Health, occupational, physical, and speech therapies should be included in the child's Individual Education Program (IEP).[5]

INDIVIDUALIZED HEALTHCARE PLAN

Assessment

History

- Family (genetic) factors that predispose to fragile X syndrome
- Review of any medical (including genetic) and/or educational testing
- Age that diagnosis was made
- Developmental milestones
- Medication history
- Any other health/medical issues
- Review of any previous special education assessment or interventions
- History from family:
    Family knowledge base of fragile X syndrome
    Any other family member affected?
    Family's concerns andneeds
    Family's coping abilities

Current Status

- Results of special education assessment, including developmental (motor and cognitive), behavioral and psychological assessments
- Results of speech and language assessment
- Vision and hearing assessment
- Ability to function in school environment (interview teachers)

Self-Care

- Self-care skill level (toilet training, dressing, eating skills)
- Barriers to self-care
- Willingness and desire to participate in self-care

Psychosocial Status

- Ability to communicate with others
- Ability to interact with peers
- Sources of emotional stress
- Development of play skills
- Development of social skills (e.g., turn-taking, eye contact)
- Ability to deal with transition and tolerate change
- Reaction to different environments (home, school, community settings)
- Effective motivators of appropriate behavior (home, school)

Academic Issues

- Ability to stay on task
- Ability to follow directions
- Review Individual Education Program (IEP) or Individual Family Service Plan (IFSP)
- Consult with teacher, special education teacher, speech therapist, occupational therapist, and any others on IEP multidisciplinary team

Nursing Diagnoses (N.D.)

N.D. 1 Impaired verbal communication (NANDA 2.1.1.1) related to speech and language delays

N.D. 2 Impaired social interaction (NANDA 3.1.1) related to communication barriers, anxiety, and altered thought processes

N.D. 3 Altered thought processes (NANDA 8.3) related to:
- impaired attention span
- impaired ability to recall information
- impaired perception
- impaired judgment
- impaired decision-making skills
- impaired conceptual reasoning ability
- sensory integration difficulties

N.D. 4 (Risk for) injury (NANDA 1.6.1) related to perceptual and cognitive impairment

N.D. 5 Self-care deficit: bathing/hygiene, dressing/grooming, toileting (NANDA 6.5.2-4) related to perceptual and cognitive impairment

N.D. 6 Altered family processes (NANDA 3.2.2) related to having a child with fragile X syndrome

Goals

The student will:
- develop abilities to communicate needs (N.D. 1)
- engage in healthy social interaction (N.D. 2)
- participate in an environment that encourages the student to learn (N.D.3)
- be free from injury (N.D. 4)
- increase participation in activities of daily living within cognitive/emotional/physical limits (N.D. 5)
- develop and/or maintain effective family communication patterns (N.D. 6)
- seek and obtain community support for self and his/her family (N.D. 6)

Nursing Interventions

Teacher/School Intervention

Refer to special education team for assessment if not already involved. (N.D. 1-5)

Participate in child study team meetings to monitor student's needs in the classroom. (N.D. 1-5)

Determine differences in chronological age and mastery of developmental milestones. (N.D. 1-6)

Interact with student on appropriate cognitive level. (N.D. 1-5)

Consult with speech therapists about methods/strategies to enhance communication. (N.D. 1)

Provide alternative ways of communication when needed (signing or using pictures). (N.D. 1)

Encourage activities that involve communication with others, especially peers: describing wants and needs, making choices, explaining experiences (home, school, friends, etc.). (N.D. 1)

Encourage student interaction with peers in the classroom, lunchroom, etc. (N.D. 2)

Provide the student with a calm atmosphere when external stimuli is overwhelming. (N.D. 3)

Provide consistent approach in care: same teacher, same routine. (N.D. 3)

Prepare the child for anticipated changes, such as having a substitute teacher tomorrow. (N.D. 3)

Allow for ample rest periods, which are important for optimal cognitive/perceptual functioning. (N.D. 3)

Provide a safe physical environment including supervision in classroom, hallways, lunchroom, gym, bus, and so on, as necessary. (N.D. 4)

Encourage staff to select and provide toys and supplies appropriate to cognitive age. (N.D. 3,4)

Teach the appropriate skills necessary for self-care in the student's terms with sensitivity to developmental needs for practice, repetition, and reluctance. (N.D. 5)

Encourage continued development of self-help skills. (N.D. 5)

Encourage continued health maintenance. (N.D.)

Student/Family Interventions

Encourage family to utilize alternative methods/strategies of communication when needed. (N.D. 1)

Provide opportunities to enhance the student's confidence in performing self-care. (N.D. 5)

Establish a caring atmosphere to keep communication open. (N.D. 6)

Involve family in case management. (N.D. 6)

Encourage parents and family members to discuss their fears and feelings. (N.D. 6)

Arrange and allow respite time for family. (N.D. 6)

Refer to genetic counseling services and other community resources as needed. (N.D. 6)

Expected Student Outcomes

The student will:

- develop effective communication abilities (N.D. 1)
- communicate his/her needs (using alternative forms of communication if necessary) (N.D. 1)
- interact with peers at home, in school, and in the community (N.D. 2)
- participate in classroom activities with modifications made as necessary (N.D. 1-3)
- perform or participate in as many activities of daily living as possible (N.D. 5)
- not experience injury (N.D. 4)
- have support from family (N.D. 6)

CASE STUDY

Name: **Carl**
DOB: 2-28-93
Age: 4 years 9 months

Health History

History was obtained from Carl's mother at his IEP conference on November 26, 1997, and from a review of health records.

Carl was delivered at full term vaginally after a normal pregnancy. He experienced mild difficulties with sucking initially but weight gain progressed typically. Developmental milestones included sitting at 9 months, crawling at 11 months, and walking at 18 months. Carl continued to be nonverbal and had poor eye contact. His parents became concerned and sought help through a variety of doctors. In May 1995, genetic testing was conducted and Carl was diagnosed with fragile X syndrome. There is a family history with the mother's brother affected, a maternal aunt who has an affected child, and a maternal uncle who is also affected (all diagnoses late in life). Further testing was conducted in November 1996 and Carl was also diagnosed with autism.

Carl suffered from recurrent otitis media infections beginning in his first year and tympanostomy tubes were placed at 18 months. Currently, Carl's mom states that the tubes are in place and he has a resolving infection. Carl's immunizations are up to date.

Carl is nonverbal and often gets frustrated with his family members and peers. He cries, moans, and sometimes screams when misunderstood. He exhibits a high energy level and has trouble falling asleep. Carl's mom states that he never seems to get tired and needs constant supervision.

Carl's mother shares that he eats frequently and the family often uses food to help calm him down. He has no limits set in regard to food. He has definite likes and dislikes. He likes pretzels, red apples, canned stew, and Popsicles. He does not like Jell-O or pudding. He has poor table manners and likes to put food in and out of his mouth.

Carl cannot adequately dress himself. He wears diapers and has about five bowel movements a day. Fecal smearing has been a problem in the past. Carl likes to chew on things and will put noneatables in his mouth. He will bite when afraid or anxious.

Carl lives with his mother, father, and five siblings. An older sister was born with a cleft palate and receives special education services. A younger sister has significant delays in motor and social skills. The family recently moved into the school district from out of state.

Currently Carl attends Early Childhood Special Education classes four mornings a week. He receives one-on-one support and enjoys circle time and riding his tricycle. He exhibits poor eye contact and demonstrates no interaction with his peers. His family receives six hours of respite time a week.

Allergies: NKA

Medication: Clonidine 0.025 mg bid
              Risperidal 1 mg - 1/2 tablet at lunch, 1 tablet at bedtime

Individualized Healthcare Plan*
Fragile X Syndrome

Assessment Data	Nursing Diagnosis	Goals	Nursing Interventions	Expected Outcomes
ND1 Carl has impaired verbal communication.	Impaired verbal communication related to speech and language delays (NANDA 2.1.1.1)	Carl will learn to communicate needs using words or signs by pointing to pictures.	Consult with special ed. teachers and speech therapist about modes to enhance communications. Look directly at Carl and speak slowly. Encourage use of visual aids for reinforcement. Discuss communications strategies at team meetings.	Carl will communicate his needs effectively.
ND5 Carl is unable to toilet, dress, or bathe independently	Self-care deficit: toileting, bathing, dressing related to perceptual and cognitive impairment (NANDA 6.5.2-4)	Carl will perform activities of daily living within his developmental capabilities.	Consult with parents and staff and develop a toileting plan to be followed at home and school. Staff will teach the appropriate skills for self-care in Carl's terms with sensitivity to developmental needs. Provide opportunities to enhance Carl's confidence in performaning self-care.	Carl will demonstrate an increase in self-care skills.

		Carl will eat only at predetermined times. Carl will eat a well-balanced diet.
Carl is a compulsive eater and does not eat a well-balanced diet.	Altered nutritional status related to compulsive behavior (NANDA 1.1.2.2)	Carl will maintain an adequate nutritional diet.	Set limits as to when Carl can eat and when he cannot. Slowly introduce new food choices. Work with family to reinforce limits and choices.
ND6 Carl has poor family functioning.	Altered family process related to having a child with fragile X syndrome (NANDA 3.2.2)	Provide support to Carl and his family.	Encourage verbalization of feelings regarding student's special needs. Use a notebook to facilitate communication between parents and the numerous professionals working with him. Refer family to ECSE Parent Support Group. Refer family to community agencies and resources as needed.	Carl will give/receive support within the family systems.

REFERENCES

1. Edelson, SM. *Fragile X Syndrome.* [Online]. Available at:http://fragileX.org Accessed 4/13/98.
2. Wong DL. *Whaley and Wong's Essentials of Pediatric Nursing.* 5th ed. St. Louis, Mo: Mosby, 1997: 578-579.
3. Webb T. Fragile X syndrome. *Am Med J Genetics.* 1986;23:6-10.
4. *Fragile X Syndrome.* [Online]. Available at: http://fraxa.org Accessed 4/13/98.
5. *What is Fragile X Syndrome?* [Online]. Available at: http://home.inreach.com/flipside/ northern.htm Accessed 4/5/98.
6. Hagerman RJ, Cronister A. *Fragile X Syndrome: Diagnosis, Treatment and Research.* 2nd ed. Baltimore:The John's Hopkins University Press, 1996:383-387.

BIBLIOGRAPHY

Braden ML. *Fragile: Handle With Care (Understanding the Fragile X Syndrome).* Chapel Hill, NC: Avanta Media Corporation, 1998.

Dykens E, Hodapp R, Leckman, J. *Behavior and Development in Fragile X Syndrome.* Thousand Oaks, Calif: Sage Publications, 1994.

Hagerman R, McBogg P. *Fragile X Syndrome.* Dillon, Colo: Spectra Publishing Company, 1983.

North American Nursing Diagnosis Accociation. *NANDA Nursing Diagnoses: Definitions & Classification 1999-2000.* Philadelphia, Pa: North American Nursing Diagnosis Assn, 1999. (NANDA, 1211 Locust Street, Philadelphia, PA 19107. 800-647-9002; fax 215-545-8107; e-mail: NANDA@nursecominc.com)

Schopmeyer B, Lowe F,eds. *The Fragile X Child.* San Diego, Calif: Singular Publishing Group, 1992.

Wilson P, Stackhouse T, O'Connor R, Scharfemaker S, Hagerman R. *Issues and Strategies for Educating Children With Fragile X Syndrome.* Dillon, Colo: Spectra Publishing Company, 1994.

Wong DL. *Essentials of Pediatric Nursing.* 5th ed. St. Louis, Mo: C.V. Mosby, 1997.

ORGANIZATIONS/AGENCIES

The Arc
National Headquarters,
PO Box 1047
Arlington, TX 76004
(817) 261-6003
http://www.thearc.org

Fragile X Advocate
75 South Elliot Road, Suite 19
Chapel Hill, NC 27514
(919) 967-0322 Ext. 200

FRAXA Research Foundation
PO Box 935
West Newbury, MA 01985
http://www.fraxa.org

National Fragile X Foundation
1441 York Street, Suite 303,
Denver, CO 80206
http://www.nfxf.org

14 | IHP: Immune Thrombocytopenic Purpura

Mary A. Swanson

INTRODUCTION

Immune thrombocytopenic purpura (ITP), also called idiopathic thrombocytopenic purpura and autoimmune thrombocytopenic purpura, is usually an acute self-limited disease in children. It is classified as an autoimmune disorder in that the person produces antiplatelet autoantibodies that destroy the body's platelets.[1]

The rate of ITP cases is increasing. Each year approximately 20,000 new cases, or about 10 to 125 per million people are diagnosed.[2] Acute ITP occurs most often in children following a seasonal viral illness. The disease usually lasts for one to two months and rarely persists longer than six months. Both sexes are affected equally in acute ITP. Chronic ITP is most often seen in adults and may last for years or indefinitely. Acute ITP is considered a milder disorder with a better prognosis than the chronic form of the disorder. About 7% to 28% of children with acute disease develop chronic ITP. The mortality rate is extremely low. [1,3,4]

The school-aged and adolescent child with ITP may have activity and/or sports restrictions, extremely cautious or anxious parents, multiple laboratory tests, and treatments with severe or chronic symptoms. The child lives with the threat of a minor or major bleeding episode, but needs to experience as near to normal activity and peer relationships as possible.

Pathophysiology

In this autoimmune disorder, the person produces autoantibody (usually 7S IgG) against platelets and possibly megakaryocytes, leading to phagocytic destruction of these cells. What triggers this production of autoantibody is not entirely understood but often follows a viral illness. The thrombocytopenia induces purpura and hemorrhage if the platelet count reaches a critical level (usually <30,000/microliter). The bleeding is predominantly seen in the skin and mucous membranes. Petechia are noticed in dependent areas of the body. Common areas for bleeding are the mucous membranes of the nose, mouth, gastrointestinal tract, and uterus. Conjunctival and retinal hemorrhages can also occur, but are rare. There is often a case history of easy bruising in absence of trauma, frequent nosebleeds, gum bleeding, prolonged menses, and hematuria. The most serious, but rare complication is bleeding into the central nervous system which can be fatal and must be rapidly and vigorously treated. The risk of hemorrhage varies and probably depends on such individual factors as platelet age, antiplatelet antibody-binding to critical functional receptors, and capillary integrity. The spleen is a major site of antibody synthesis as well as phagocytic function.[5]

The criteria[5] for diagnosis of ITP includes:

- increased platelet destruction, thrombocytopenic purpura, shortened platelet survival, increased megathrombocytes (stress platelets), and sometimes decreased platelet production
- increased megakaryocytes in bone marrow
- bound antiplatelet antibody
- exclusion of other primary clinical disorders that are capable of giving all or some of the above findings (i.e., systemic lupus erythematosus, rheumatoid arthritis, Graves' disease, Hashimoto's thyroiditis, HIV-1 related immunologic thrombocytopenia, lymphoma, chronic lymphocytic leukemia, disseminated intravascular coagulation, hypersplenism, drug-induced thrombocytopenia)
- nonpalpable splenomegaly
- response to corticosteroids, splenectomy, or intravenous gammaglobulin
- history of thrombocytopenic mother giving birth to thrombocytopenic infant

Management

Numerous therapeutic modalities for ITP have been suggested and tried over the years, but none has been uniformly curative. Treatments are aimed at maintaining the platelet count at a level which enables the child to lead a normal life, usually a count above 30,000/microliter. Many children are able to recover spontaneously without treatment. This is the preferred option if they do not have an excessively low platelet count and they lack severe symptoms, such as frequent nosebleeds or heavy bruising. The parent and child need to be informed about the risk of bleeding and management of bleeding episodes, medications that impair platelet functioning, need for platelet monitoring, and treatment options. Platelet counts are monitored intermittently, and the child's

activities and lifestyle may be restricted if the platelet levels fall below 30,000 cells per microliter to reduce the risk of internal injury and bleeding.[4,6]

Medical therapies have included steroids, immunoglobulins, and immunosuppressive drugs. Steroids such as prednisone or dexamethasone have been used to impair antibody production and/or binding to platelets. These have been given in high dosages for a short time or in "pulses" over time, with good responses for acute and chronic ITP. Immunoglobins have been given intravenously over a number of days and with further single doses and may be given in combination with steroids. Intravenous gammaglobulin blocks the destruction of antibody-coated platelets by the reticuloendothelial system. Immunosuppressive drugs such as vincristine, azathioprine (Imuran), danazol, cyclophosphamide, and cyclosporine are prescribed for patients only in severe cases where other treatments have failed because of their side effects.[7-9]

Splenectomy is often performed in cases of chronic ITP or in the case of acute ITP when life-threatening bleeding occurs. A splenectomy removes the potential site for destruction of damaged platelets and a significant source of antiplatelet antibody production. In children with chronic ITP, splenectomy improves the platelet count in approximately 70% of the cases. Following a splenectomy, the child will be monitored closely for infections and treated with antibiotics prophylactically.[6,7]

If a child has extensive hemorrhage and there is evidence of imminent or existing CNS bleeding (platelet count below 10,000/microliter), emergency treatment is required. This emergency treatment may include intravenous gammaglobulin, high-dose intravenous corticosteroids, and platelet transfusions.[5,10]

INDIVIDUALIZED HEALTHCARE PLAN

Assessment

History

- When was diagnosis made?
- Symptoms experienced? (bruising, petechia, nosebleeds, menorrhagia)
- Platelet count history?

Current status and management

- Who are healthcare providers? Frequency of doctor visits?
- What is current management plan?
- Current medications? Other medications used?
- Current platelet count?
- Physical activity restrictions?
- Plan for emergency (i.e., head injury, trauma, unconsciousness)?

Self-care

- Parent knowledge of disease and treatment
- Student knowledge of disease and treatment?
- Does student wear medical alert bracelet?

Psychosocial Status

- Involvement of family/ support persons?
- Activities with friends, peers?
- Usual school and community activities?
- Usual physical activity (i.e., sports, etc.)?

Academic Issues

- Physical education limitations (i.e. contact sports)? Is physical education required?
- School attendance patterns? (Current and prior to ITP diagnosis)
- Need for 504 Plan?
- Need for an Individual Education Program (IEP)?

Nursing Diagnoses (N.D.)

N.D. 1 Risk for injury (NANDA 1.6.1) related to thrombocytopenia
N.D. 2 Risk for social isolation (NANDA 3.1.2) related to activity restrictions with peers
N.D. 3 Altered student role performance (NANDA 3.2.1) related to:
- activity restrictions
- absence from school

N.D. 4 Risk for noncompliance (NANDA 5.2.1.1) related to:
- unknowns
- unpredictability of ITP
- denial of illness
- perceived ineffectiveness of treatment

N.D. 5 Knowledge deficit about ITP and its management (NANDA 8.1.1) related to:
- lack of information
- no experience with using the information

Goals

Prevent injuries   (N.D. 1)

Maintain peer relationships and activities (N.D.2)

Participate in classroom and school activities with modifications made as needed (N.D.2,3)

Manage bleeding episodes promptly (N.D.1)

Maintain a good school attendance pattern (N.D. 3)

Comply with medical treatment measures (N.D. 4)

Increase knowledge about ITP and its management   (N.D. 5)

Develop emergency care plan for student injury or bleeding (N.D. 1)

Nursing Interventions

Develop emergency care plan with student and parents/guardians for care of injuries and bleeding episodes. (N.D.1) Include:
- specific directions for observations and bleeding, head injuries, abdominal trauma, and unconsciousness
- plan for transportation
- plan for notification of parent

Assist in modifying educational program as needed (N.D. 1,3)
- modify physical education requirements, identify alternative activities
- modify classroom assignments, especially those that may increase potential for injury
- plan for make-up work for school days absent
- homebound education if platelets are dangerously low

Monitor playground activities — set limits on activities as necessary (N.D.1)
- inform student
- inform teachers and playground supervisor

In-service teachers and staff on ITP and emergency care plan (N.D.1,3,5)

Assist physical education teachers and classroom teachers in modifying activities (N.D.3)

Discuss with student (N.D.1,2,3,4,5)
- what ITP is and how it can be managed
- how platelet counts affect his or her activity and lifestyle to reduce risk of injury
- importance of having a plan to treat injury or bleeding
- alternatives for peer activities when platelet counts are low
- Medic Alert bracelet
- use of over-the-counter medications that contain aspirin or affect platelet formation/ functioning

Monitor school attendance (N.D. 3,4)

Request note from physician to document need for activity limitations/restrictions (N.D.2,5)

Discuss possible ways to continue to be part of a sports team with student, parents, and coach (if physical activities are restricted) (N.D. 2)

Assist student to notify parents if he/she has signs/symptoms of infections (N.D.4,5)

Request parent notify the school if there is a change in status, especially if a decrease in platelet count occurs (N.D.1,3,5)

Expected Student Outcomes

The student will:
- describe symptoms that need medical attention (N.D. 1,5)
- wear a Medical Alert bracelet (N.D.1,5)
- describe risks of injury when platelet counts are decreased (N.D.4,5)
- modify his/her activities when platelet counts are low (N.D.3,4)
- maintain good school attendance pattern (N.D. 3,7)
- report his/her platelet count to the school nurse weekly and identify its implications for safety and activities (N.D. 4,5)
- participate in physical activities (regular or modified, appropriate to platelet count) (N.D. 2,3)
- participate in activities with friends and peers (appropriate to platelet counts) (N.D. 2)

CASE STUDY

Christopher T., age 15, was taken to the doctor by his parents in November when they noticed bruising on his legs and he had several lengthy nosebleeds. He was diagnosed with ITP following several laboratory blood studies and a bone marrow exam. His platelet count was initially 23,000/microliter. He was treated with corticosteroid bursts over several months with his platelet count responding to 80,000 to 120,000 initially each time, but falling again to < 30,000/microliter. His doctor recommended that he not attend school when his platelet count was below 20,000/microliter because of the potential of injury-related or spontaneous bleeding. He also advised him not to participate in gym or contact sports when his platelet levels were below 80,000/microliter. Christopher had platelet counts done one to two times per week over several months and attended school when his platelet count was above 20,000/microliter. His parents requested homework and homebound education so that he could keep up with his coursework. At the beginning of second semester, Christopher was placed on a 504 Plan to provide an alternative for his phy-ed class and continued on homebound tutoring when his platelet counts went below 20,000/microliter. It was hoped that he could spontaneously recover and return to school and his normal activities. Christopher was completing his coursework successfully at home with a tutor. His mother arranged for him to complete a daily exercise program with an athletic trainer at the family's athletic club. Christopher logged his activities and physical education skills to submit to school for the physical education requirement.

Christopher was able to attend school for part of the second semester because his platelet count continued to fluctuate between 18,000 and 123,000/microliter. His physician diagnosed chronic ITP in May and planned a splenectomy for July.

When Christopher, post splenectomy, returned to school in September, he had platelet counts between 150,000 to 200,000/microliter and no activity restrictions. He is participating in mainstream classes and is participating in his tenth grade physical education class. His physician continues to monitor his platelet count every three months and wants him to seek medical attention with signs of infection and fever.

EMERGENCY CARE PLAN

Student: Christopher T.   Birthdate: 6-2-98   Grade: 9   School: HHS

Date: 12-12-97

Parent name: Marie T.   Workphone: Homephone: 456-3333

Parent name: Dave T.   Workphone:

Emergency Contact: Bill and Sue R.   Phone: 456-7877

Healthcare Provider: Dr. G. Seal   Phone: 456-6756

Emergency plan written by: M. Swanson, LSN

Parent/Student Signature:

Health Condition: Christopher was diagnosed with immune thrombocytopenic purpura in November 1997. His platelet count has been fluctuating between 18,000 and 120,000/microliter. He has been treated with corticosteroid bursts and responds with a higher platelet count initially, but it gradually falls over two to three weeks. The physician will be monitoring his platelet count one to two times per week and plans to continue with corticosteroids until Christopher's platelets stabilize at 100,000/microliter or higher.

There is a risk for uncontrolled bleeding if Christopher has an injury (internally or externally) because he has fewer platelets that normally clot his blood. Prevention of injuries is important, but should an accident occur, it is an emergency and Christopher will need prompt medical attention for his injuries.

Signs of Emergency:	**Actions to take:**
If Christopher sustains a cut or bruise that bleeds slowly	Apply pressure to wound and escort Christopher to the nurse's office or call the nurse to come to you. Extension 8809
If Christopher has a large injury with large amount of visible bleeding	Apply pressure to wound if possible. Call 911, stay with student, and direct someone else to call the Operator (Dial 0) to obtain help from the principal and the nurse. Notify parents of emergency.
If Christopher complains of sudden headache and/or change in consciousness	Call 911, stay with student, and direct someone to call the Operator (Dial 0) to

or orientation to his environment   obtain help from the principal and nurse. Notify parents of emergency.

Christopher wears a Medic Alert bracelet. Provide the information on this plan to the para-medics.

SECTION 504 STUDENT ACCOMMODATION PLAN

NAME: Christopher T.   BIRTHDATE: 6-2-98
GRADE: 9   SCHOOL: Hamilton High School
DATE: 2-5-981.

1. **Describe the nature of the concern:**
   Christopher was diagnosed with ITP (immune thrombocytopenic purpura) in November 1997. When his platelet count is below normal, he has a higher risk for hemorrhage/bleeding with injury, trauma, or spontaneously.

2. **Describe the basis for the determination of handicap (if any):**
   Christopher cannot attend school when his platelet count is below 20,000/microliter because he is at high risk for hemorrhage/bleeding. He is on corticosteroids (treatment) which can affect his attention span and mental stability.

3. **Describe how the handicap affects a major life activity:**
   - Christopher cannot attend school when platelets are below 20,000/microliter.
   - Christopher cannot participate in gym/contact sports when platelets are below 80,000/microliter.
   - Christopher is taking corticosteroids, sometimes at high doses, which may affect his attention span and mood.

4. **Describe the reasonable accommodations that are necessary:**
   - Homebound tutoring (1 hr/week/class of school missed) will be available to Christopher as needed for absence from school related to his ITP.
   - Christopher will discuss with teachers his need for extra time for assignments/projects/tests, as needed when he misses school.
   - Christopher will provide an activity log (physical education skills)- to counselor/assistant principal for one physical education credit consideration.
   - Christopher will wear his Medic Alert bracelet and keep the school nurse informed of his platelet count and ITP status.

Review/Reassessment Date: 3/17/98

Participants	(Name and title)		
Sue T.	(parent)	Bob B.	(math teacher)
Christopher T.	(student)	Mark K.	(Spanish teacher)
Tom P	(academic counselor)	Dan H.	(science teacher)
Mary S.	(school nurse)	Paula A.	(English teacher)
Judy M.	(assistant principal)	Marla P.	(physical education teacher)

cc. Student's Cumulative File
Attachment: Information regarding Section 504 of the Rehabilitation
**   Act of 1973**

Individualized Healthcare Plan*
Immune Thrombocytopenic Purpura

Assessment Data	Nursing Diagnosis	Goals	Nursing Interventions	Expected Outcomes
ND1 Platelets fluctuate between 18,000 and 110,000/microliters	Risk for injury related to thrombocytopenia (NANDA 1.6.1)	Prevent injury. Manage bleeding episodes promptly	Modify phy-ed requirements (see 504 plan). Develop and distribute emergency care plan. Discuss ITP and emergency plan with teachers/staff.	Christopher will wear a medical alert bracelet. Christopher will describe his symptoms that need medical attention. Christopher will report his platelet count to the school nurse weekly.
ND2 Christopher can attend school if platelets > 20,000/microliters	Risk for social isolation related to activity restrictions and absence from school (NANDA 3.1.2)	Participate in school activities with modifications. Maintain peer relationships and activities. Good school attendance pattern.	Classroom assignments modified. Homebound instruction if platelets <20,000/microliter. (See 504 Plan) Encourage social activities.	Christopher will maintain a good school attendance pattern. Christopher will participate in physical activities (appropriate to platelet count.)
ND5 Christopher diagnosed with ITP in November	Knowledge deficit about ITP and its management (NANDA 8.1.1)	Increase knowledge about ITP and its management.	Discuss with Christopher: 1) ITP and management; 2) relationship of platelet count to bleeding risk; 3) alternatives for peer activities; 4) use of OTC medications	Christopher will describe activities with friends and peers (appropriate to platelet counts). Christopher will describe risks of injury when platelet count is low.

*See Appendix for student profile information to include on an IHP form.

REFERENCES

1. George JN, Raskob GE. Idiopathic thrombocytopenic purpura: a concise summary of the pathophysiology and diagnosis in children and adults. *Semin in Hematol*,1998; 35 (Suppl 1): 5-8.
2. *About ITP*. Available at: http://www.itppeople.com/ Accessed 12/29/98.
3. Levine SP. Thrombocytopenia caused by immunologic platelet destruction. In: Lee GR, Foerster J, Lukens J, et al, eds. *Wintrobe's Hematology*. 10th ed. Baltimore: Williams & Wilkins, 1999: 1583-1611.
4. Souid AK, Sadowitz PD. Acute childhood immune thrombocytopenic purpura: diagnosis and treatment. *Clin Pediatr* 1995; 34 (9):487-94.
5. Karpatkin S. Autoimmune (idiopathic) thrombocytopenic purpura. *Lancet* 1997; 349:1531-1536.
6. George JN, Woolf SA, Raskob JS, et. al. Idiopathic thrombocytopenic purpura: a practice guideline developed by explicit methods for the American Society of Hematology. *Blood* 1996; 88: 3-40.
7. Tarantino MD, Goldsmith G. Treatment of acute immune thrombocytopenic purpura. *Semin Hematol*, 1998; 35 (Suppl 1):28-35.
8. Kirchner JT. Acute and chronic immune thrombocytopenic purpura: disorders that differ in more than duration. *Postgrad Med* 1992; 92(6):112-8, 125-126.
9. Blanchette V, Freedman J, Garvey B. Management of chronic immune thrombocytopenic purpura in children and adults. *Semin Hematol*, 1998; 35 (Suppl 1):36-51.
10. Lilleyman JS. Intracranial haemorrhage in idiopathic thrombocytopenic purpura. *Arch Dis Child* 1994; 71:251-253.

BIBLIOGRAPHY

Aronis S, Platokoudi H, Mitsika A, Haidas S, Constantopoulos A. Seventeen years of experience with chronic idiopathic thrombocytopenic purpura in childhood: is therapy always better? *Pediatr Hematol Oncol* 1994;11:487-498.

Brenner B, Guilburd JN, Tatardky I, et.al. Spontaneous intracranial hemorrhage in immune thrombocytopenic purpura. *Neurosurgery* 1988; 22:761-764.

Buchanan GR. Childhood acute idiopathic thrombocytopenic purpura: how many tests and how much treatment required? *Pediatr* 1985;106 (6):928-930.

Buchanan GR. The non-treatment of childhood idiopathic thrombocytopenic purpura. *Eur Pediat* 1987; 146:107-112.

Chronic ITP Available at: http://seconde.scripps.edu/itp/Accessed 9-19-98.

Handlin RI. Disorders of the platelet and vessel wall. In: Fauci AS, Wilson JD, Braunwald E, et al, eds. *Harrison's Principles of Internal Medicine*. 14th ed. New York, NY: McGraw Hill, 1998; 730-735.

Homas A. Disorders of platelet quantity and function. In: Gellis SS, Kagen BM, eds. *Current Pediatric Therapy*. Vol. 16. Philadelphia, PA: WB Saunders Company,1999; 705-708.

Lilleyman J. Definitions and dogma in childhood idiopathic thrombocytopenic purpura. *Pediat Hematol Oncol*, 1993; 10:xi-xiv.

North American Nursing Diagnosis Association. *NANDA Nursing Diagnoses: Definitions & Classification 1999-2000*. Philadelphia, Pa: North American Nursing Diagnosis Assn, 1999. (NANDA, 1211 Locust Street, Philadelphia, PA 19107. 800-647-9002; fax 215-545-8107; e-mail: NANDA@nursecominc.com)

Radin A, Radin B. *What's it called again?* New York, NY: ITP Society of The Children's Blood Foundation,1996; 1-13.

Robb LG, Tiedeman K. Idiopathic thrombocytopenic purpura: predictors of chronic disease. *Arch Dis Childhood*, 1990; 65:502-506.

15 | IHP: Infectious Mononucleosis

Sally Zentner Schoessler

INTRODUCTION

Infectious mononucleosis is a relatively common infectious disease with fairly nonspecific symptoms. This viral infection impacts the school-age child and adolescent not as a severe illness with dramatic complications, but as a somewhat long-term infection that creates a need to modify both the student's and family's lifestyles until the course of the illness is over.

While infectious mononucleosis can occur in any child or adolescent, children in lower socioeconomic groups have a higher incidence of mononucleosis.[1] Adolescents from lower socioeconomic levels can have up to 60% to 80 % of their peers test seropositive for the virus.[1]

Due to the prolonged nature of the symptoms of the infection, mononucleosis can be a difficult illness for the student and family to cope with. The school nurse is in a unique position to assist the student and parents in coordinating efforts to address the child's physical and academic needs during recuperation, as well the family's ability to cope with the child.

Pathophysiology

The infection is caused by the Epstein-Barr virus which is a DNA virus.[2] It is spread by salivary exchange, contact with contaminated objects or, less commonly,

by blood transfusions.[3] The illness is mildly contagious and due to the most common mode of transmission being that of salivary exchange, "mono" is often referred to as "the kissing disease."

Infectious mononucleosis is often diagnosed well into the course of the illness due to the nonspecific nature of the symptoms. After an incubation period of four to six weeks[3], an initial period of the infection with symptoms of malaise, fatigue, headache, nausea, and/or abdominal pain is often mistaken for influenza or many other viral infections. As the infection progresses, the symptoms become more pronounced. The student presents with severe pharyngitis (often with enlarged tonsils and a membranous exudate), high fever, lymphadenopathy (in the neck and throughout the body), and upper abdominal pain indicative of an enlarged spleen. Occasionally, the child will experience a rash that appears most prominently on the trunk of the body.[4] The symptoms usually disappear in one to three weeks (the fatigue may persist for up to several months), but it is not known how long the child remains infectious.[5]

Blood tests are important in the diagnosis of infectious mononucleosis due to the nonspecific nature of the symptoms. Blood work should be done to check for elevated lymphocytes. The other important test to be done is the "monospot," which screens for heterophil antibodies in which an increase is seen as soon as the fourth day of infection.[5]

Infants and young children tend to experience a mild case of infectious mononucleosis or remain asymptomatic. They often experience what appears to be a mild case of tonsillitis or an upper respiratory infection with an accompanying low-grade fever due to the fact that they tend to contract the virus by hand-to-hand contact or by an encounter with a contaminated object. Adolescents and college-age students, who tend to spread the disease by intimate salivary contact, are disposed towards a more significant case of the disease since their exposure tends to be more intimate.[1]

Complications are not common but can include neurologic problems, pneumonitis, myocarditis, hemolytic anemia, thrombocytopenia, and rupturing of the spleen.[4]

Management

Treatment is very simple. The child should be limited to bed rest during the more acute phase of the illness, followed by the addition of activities based on the child's activity tolerance level. There is no need to isolate the student.[6]

Due to the viral nature of infectious mononucleosis, treatment is mainly supportive and aimed at relieving the child's symptoms. Over-the-counter analgesics can be used to relieve the pain of headache and discomfort of malaise. Penicillin is prescribed to treat the accompanying tonsillitis if B strep is present. In severe cases, prednisone is used to lessen some of the symptoms of mononucleosis.[5] Soft foods, with attention to caloric and nutritional content, should be encouraged due to the pharyngitis that the child is experiencing.[4] If spleen enlargement is present, the child should be instructed to avoid activities that may result in an injury.

INDIVIDUALIZED HEALTHCARE PLAN

Assessment

History

- What symptoms led to the diagnosis of infectious mononucleosis?
- When was the diagnosis confirmed by a healthcare provider?
- Have any friends or family members been diagnosed with infectious mononucleosis in the past 6 weeks?

Current Status and Management

- Management plan
- What treatment has been effective?
- Have complications been experienced?
    - hepatitis
    - encephalitis
    - ruptured spleen
    - pneumonia
- How are fatigue and malaise affecting activities of daily living?
- What accommodations have been made?

- Course of illness
- Activity tolerance
- Current symptoms
    - temperature
    - streptococcal infection
    - enlarged lymph nodes
    - enlarged spleen or tenderness
    - rash
    - fatigue

Self-care

- Nutrition (eating balanced diet to support regaining strength)
- Ability to self-monitor tolerance of activity?
- Ability to modify activities to accommodate limitations due to fatigue and malaise
- Ability to engage in activities of daily living

Psychosocial Status

- How is the student maintaining peer relationships throughout prolonged absence?
    - school relationships
    - church activities
    - other social/sport activities
- If active in a team or individual sport, how can student remain part of the team in a modified capacity throughout his/her recovery period?
- How does the student feel that his/her student role is altered due to illness or related symptoms?
- What are the family's coping strategies for management of symptoms and treatment?

Academic Issues

- How many days has the student been absent from school due to infectious mononucleosis? How many total days has the student been absent this school year for any reason?
- What accommodations need to be made to facilitate attendance in full or partial days of school?
- When does the healthcare provider anticipate the student may resume participation in physical education or sports activities?
- Who is available at school to assist in arranging for homework and/or help in coordinating make-up work?
- What plan is in place to make up missed work at a manageable pace to ensure academic achievement in classes?

Nursing Diagnoses (N.D.)

N.D. 1 Alteration in activity intolerance (NANDA 6.1.1.2) related to symptoms of malaise and fatigue

N.D. 2 (Risk for) alteration in student role (NANDA 3.2.1) related to prolonged absences and fatigue

N.D. 3 (Risk for) infection (NANDA 1.2.1.1) related to increased susceptibility to other infections

N.D. 4 (Risk for) ineffective individual/family coping: compromised (NANDA 5.1.2.1.2) related to prolonged illness of self/child

N.D. 5 (Risk for) altered health maintenance (NANDA 6.4.2) related to prolonged symptoms associated with infectious mononucleosis

N.D. 6 Alteration in comfort (pain) (NANDA 9.1.1) related to infection (sore throat, headache, malaise)

Goals

Student will increase school attendance pattern beginning with half days and moving to full days over first one to two weeks. (N.D. 1,2)

Student will rest as needed at school and home. (N.D. 1)

Student will contract with teachers to complete classwork missed due to prolonged absence in small, manageable amounts. (N.D. 2)

Student will participate in extracurricular activities as activity tolerance allows. (N.D. 2)

Student will participate in physical education and sports activities as directed by his/her healthcare provider and as activity tolerance allows. (N.D. 2)

Student will increase his/her knowledge of signs and symptoms of infections to promote early intervention and treatment. (N.D. 3)

Student will verbalize concerns/issues experienced by family due to prolonged illness. (N.D. 4)

Family will identify and employ positive coping strategies in dealing with student's illness. (N.D. 4)

Student will assist in developing a management plan for symptoms. (N.D. 5,6)

Student will participate in management of discomfort. (N.D. 6)

Nursing Interventions

Monitor student's attendance on a daily basis. (N.D. 1)

Encourage student to recognize signs of fatigue and rest appropriately. (N.D. 1,6)

Provide student with an opportunity to rest as needed. (N.D. 1,6)

Procure note from healthcare provider regarding physical education and sports limitations. (N.D. 1)

Collaborate with physical education staff to provide modified PE program as needed. (N.D. 1)

Arrange for use of elevator if needed. (N.D. 1)

Discuss appropriate activity level with student and parents to ensure consistent approach between home and school. (N.D. 1)

Notify faculty and staff (with parent permission) as to student's health status. (N.D. 2)

Collaborate with the student and staff in setting realistic goals and modifying assignments for missed days or partial days during student's recovery period. (N.D. 2)

Discuss activity limitations with athletic department coaches. Find alternate role for student (i.e. timekeeper or statistician) during recuperation so that he/she can remain a member of his/her team. (N.D. 2)

Discuss appropriate time for student to rejoin extracurricular activities. (N.D. 2)

Observe for signs and symptoms of infections and/or potential complications. (N.D. 3)
- fever/chills
- sore throat
- rash
- swollen glands
- fatigue
- malaise
- abdominal pain

Discuss with parents which signs and symptoms should be reported to their healthcare provider. (N.D. 3)

Instruct student in strategies to avoid spread of communicable diseases (i.e., hand washing, not sharing cups or utensils, etc.). (N.D. 3)

Monitor possible exposure to communicable diseases such as: streptococcal sore throat, chickenpox, influenza, pneumonia, etc. (N.D. 3)

Discuss with parents and student how the family is coping with the student's illness. (N.D. 4,6)

Allow parent an opportunity to express personal issues or concerns in regard to the student's illness (i.e., large block of time missed at work while caring for child, lack of patience with symptoms of fatigue, impact on siblings, etc.) (N.D. 4)

Allow student an opportunity to express feelings in regard to being ill. (N.D. 4)

Discuss strategies to manage symptoms of malaise and fatigue in the school setting. (N.D. 5)

Arrange for home tutoring or an altered educational program if absenteeism becomes a long-term necessity. (N.D. 5)

Assist in accessing healthcare provider as needed for support of illness. (N.D. 5)

Discuss techniques for management of discomfort related to symptoms (lozenges for sore throat, medication as needed at school for headache, etc.) (N.D. 6)

Expected Student Outcomes

Student will attend school (half days for one week, then increasing to full days over the next two weeks). (N.D. 1,2)

Student will identify periods of fatigue and rest in health office as needed. (N.D. 1)

Student will participate in physical education activities as appropriate with modifications made as needed. (N.D. 1,2)

Student will arrange to complete missed course work with his/her teachers. (N.D. 2)

Student will collaborate with faculty and staff to modify school activities as needed. (N.D. 2)

Student will identify symptoms of infection and report any symptoms to the school nurse and parent. (N.D. 3)

Student will practice good hygiene behaviors. (N.D. 3)

Student will express feelings in regard to having an illness and the impact it has on him/her and his/her family. (N.D. 4)

The family will identify positive coping strategies that can be used to cope with child's illness. (N.D. 4,5)

Student will demonstrate positive coping strategies in dealing with issues of illness. (N.D. 5)

Student will identify and demonstrate strategies for managing discomfort from symptoms. (N.D. 6)

CASE STUDY

Ann Capen is a 16-year-old girl who was diagnosed with infectious mononucleosis 14 days ago. Prior to diagnosis, she had complained of nonspecific symptoms and stated she felt "lousy." Two days prior to her diagnosis by healthcare provider Dr. Louise Clarke, she ran a fever of 102° F (oral temperature) and presented with a sore throat, swollen glands, and upper abdominal discomfort. Her mother called the school to inform the health office of Ann's diagnosis of infectious mononucleosis.

Ann has missed 10 full days of school and is now attending half days. She has a physician's note excusing her from physical education and sports until further evaluation. She has obtained homework assignments but is having trouble completing them and managing her current homework load. She states, "It's so hard to make it through the time that I'm at school, and then I'm so exhausted that all I can do when I get home is sleep." She reports feeling overwhelmed by the amount of course work that remains incomplete. She is also the starting goalie for the varsity soccer team and reports feeling that she is letting her team down by not being able to play. She commented, "I've always defined myself as a soccer player, now I feel lost not being with the team."

During the acute phase of Ann's mononucleosis, her mother felt the need to be at home with her, as she remained febrile for more than seven days. Her mother has been feeling pressured by her employer to be at work as much as possible and feels frustrated at needing and wanting to care for Ann and also fulfilling her responsibilities at work. She feels additional stress due to the fact that Ann's younger brother, age 3, has regressed to the point that, although he had been "toilet trained" for eight months, he is soiling his underwear instead of using the toilet. Ann's mother feels that this is directly related to the amount of attention that she has needed to direct toward Ann and her illness.

Individualized Healthcare Plan*
Infectious Mononucleosis

Assessment Data	Nursing Diagnosis	Goals	Nursing Interventions	Expected Outcomes
ND1 Ann is often tired and complains of simply "feeling sick." Ann should not be participating in contact sports.	Activity intolerance due to symptoms of malaise and fatigue (NANDA 6.1.1.2)	Ann will increase school attendance pattern beginning with half days and moving to full days over first 1-2 weeks. Ann will rest as needed at school and home.	Monitor Ann's attendance daily. Encourage Ann to recognize signs of fatigue and rest appropriately. Provide Ann with an opportunity to rest PRN. Procure note from Ann's healthcare provider regarding physical education and sports limitations. Collaborate with PE staff to provide a modified PE program. Discuss appropriate activity level with student and parents to ensure consistent approach between home and school.	Ann will attend school (half days for 1 week, then increasing to full days over the next two weeks). Ann will identify periods of fatigue and rest in health office as needed. Ann will participate in physical education activities as appropriate with modifications made as needed.

ND2 Ann was absent for 10 full days of school and is now attending only half days. Ann is unable to compete although she is a member of the varsity soccer team.	(Risk for) alteration in student role due to prolonged absences and fatigue (NANDA 3.2.1)	Ann will contract with teachers to complete, in small manageable amounts, classwork missed due to prolonged absence.	Notify faculty and staff (with parent permission) as to Ann's health status. Collaborate with faculty to assist in setting realistic goals and modifying assignments for missed days or partial days during Ann's recovery period. Discuss activity limitations with athletic department coaches. Assist in finding an alternate role, such as statistician, during recuperation so that she can remain a member of her team.	Ann will arrange to complete course work over time and without compromising her recovery from illness. Ann will participate in PE when appropriate and with appropriate modifications. Ann will collaborate with faculty and staff to modify school activities as needed.
Ann is at an increased risk for infections.	Risk for infection due to increased susceptibility to infections (NANDA 1.2.1.1)	Ann will increase her knowledge of signs and symptoms of infections to promote early intervention and treatment.	Observe for signs and symptoms of infections and/or potential complications. Instruct Ann in strategies to avoid spread of communicable disease (hand washing, etc)."	Ann will identify symptoms of infection and report symptoms to the school nurse and parent.

Individualized Healthcare Plan*
Infectious Mononucleosis (continued)

Assessment Data	Nursing Diagnosis	Goals	Nursing Interventions	Expected Outcomes
			Monitor exposure in the school setting to communicable diseases such as: strep throat, chickenpox, influenza, etc.	
Ann's mother has missed many days of work to care for Ann. Ann expresses frustration with length of time that she has been ill.	Risk for ineffective individual/family coping: compromised, due to prolonged illness of self/child. (NANDA 5.1.2.1.3)	Ann will verbalize concerns/issues experienced by family due to prolonged illness.	Discuss with parents and Ann how the family is coping with Ann's illness.	Ann will express feelings in regard to having an illness and the impact that it has on her and her family.
Ann's young brother is exhibiting regression due to attention given to sister's illness.		Family will identify and employ positive coping strategies in dealing with Ann's illness.	Allow parent an opportunity to express personal issues or concerns in regard to the student's illness. Allow Ann an opportunity to express feelings in regard to being ill.	The family will identify positive coping strategies that can be used to cope with Ann's illness.

*See Appendix for student profile information to include on an IHP form.

REFERENCES

1. Behrmann RE Klingman RM. *Nelson Essentials of Pediatrics.* 2nd ed. Philadelphia, Pa: WB Saunders Company, 1994: 367.
2. *KidsHealth.* Infectious Mononucleosis. [Online]. Available at: http://www.kidshealth.org/parent/common/mononucleosis.html Accessed 1/25/99.
3. New York State Department of Health. (1997). *Infectious Mononucleosis* [Online]. Available at: http://www.foodsafety.org/ny/ny038.htm Accessed 1/25/99.
4. Wong, DL, Hockenberry-Eaton M, Wilson D, Winkelstein ML, Ahmann E, Divito-Thomas PA, eds. *Whaley and Wong's Nursing Care of Infants and Children.* 6th ed. St. Louis, Mo: Mosby, 1999: 1465, 1468.
5. NIAID - National Institutes of Health. *Infectious Mononucleosis.* [Online]. Available at: http://www.niaid.nih.gov/factsheets/Infmono.htm Accessed 1/25/99.
6. Benenson AS. *Control of Communicable Diseases Manual.* Washington, DC: American Public Health Assn, 1995: 314.

BIBLIOGRAPHY

Behrmann RE, Klingman RM. *Nelson Essentials of Pediatrics.* 2nd ed. Philadelphic, Pa: WB Saunders Company, 1994.

Benenson AS *Control of Communicable Diseases Manual.* Washington, DC: American Public Health Assn, 1995.

KidsHealth. Infectious Mononucleosis. [Online]. Available at: http://www.kidshealth.org/parent/common/mononucleosis.html Accessed 1/25/99.

New York State Department of Health. (1997). *Infectious Mononucleosis* [Online]. Available at: http://www.foodsafety.org/ny/ny038.htm Accessed 1/25/99.

NIAID - National Institute of Health. *Infectious Mononucleosis.* [Online]. Available at: http://www.niaid.nih.gov/factsheets/Infmono.htm Accessed 1/25/99.

North American Nursing Diagnosis Association. *NANDA Nursing Diagnoses: Definitions & Classification 1999-2000.* Philadelphia, Pa: North American Nursing Diagnosis Assn, 1999. (NANDA, 1211 Locust Street, Philadelphia, PA 19107. 800-647-9002; fax 215-545-8107; e-mail: NANDA@nursecominc.com)

Serving Students with Special Care Needs. Hartford, Conn: State of Connecticut Department of Education, 1992.

Wong, DL, Hockenberry-Eaton M, Wilson D, Winkelstein ML, Ahmann E, Divito-Thomas PA, eds. *Whaley and Wong's Nursing Care of Infants and Children.* 6th ed. St. Louis, Mo: Mosby, 1999.

16 | IHP: Inflammatory Bowel Disease

MaryAnn Tapper Strawhacker

INTRODUCTION

Inflammatory bowel disease (IBD) is a term used to describe two separate gastrointestinal conditions: Crohn's disease and ulcerative colitis. Because both diseases share many of the same symptoms as well as diagnostic tests and treatments, they are often referred to collectively as IBD. Inflammatory bowel disease is a chronic condition that persists throughout life with periods of exacerbation and remission. The annual incidence of IBD is about 4 to 7 cases per 100,000 children. The incidence of ulcerative colitis has remained stable over the past 20 to 30 years but the incidence of Crohn's disease is increasing. [1] The peak age of incidence is 15 to 20 years. [2] It occurs equally in male and female children. Inflammatory bowel disease is more common, however, among those who have a family history of the disease. [3]

Pathophysiology

The exact causes of IBD are not known. Research has proven that the immune system within the intestinal wall does not function properly in IBD. The link between heredity and trigger mechanisms is unknown. [4] It is now known that IBD is a medical disorder and not caused by food, stress, or anxiety. Stress can, however, exacerbate the illness. [5]

The child with IBD usually presents with abdominal pain, diarrhea, fever, fatigue, blood in the stool, and weight loss. [1] Delayed growth and sexual maturation may also be present. Although somewhat less common, IBD may also present with symptoms outside the gastrointestinal (GI) tract such as rashes, mouth sores, and joint pain, and swelling, particularly of the legs, may occur. Multiple tests are used to diagnosis IBD. After a complete medical history and physical examination, blood work is done. The child with active IBD often shows anemia due to blood loss, a high white blood cell count, and an elevated ESR, or sedimentation rate, due to inflammation. Additional blood tests may be done to check for the nutritional imbalances caused by poor absorption of nutrients. Upper and lower GI barium x-rays may be taken. The x-rays look for areas of inflammation that may be seen as a narrowing or swelling on the film. Upper and lower endoscopy is also done and biopsy of the tissue can be obtained during the procedure to look for abnormalities. All the information gathered helps the physician distinguish whether the child has Crohn's disease or ulcerative colitis. [4]

Crohn's Disease

Although many similarities exist with ulcerative colitis, Crohn's disease does have some unique features. Crohn's disease may be found in any part of the gastrointestinal tract but is most common in the lower part of the small intestine and the large intestines. All layers of the intestinal wall are involved. Diseased areas can be segmental with disease-free areas in-between. Abdominal pain is usually confined to the periumbilical region or right lower quadrant. Weight loss and malnutrition are related to anorexia as well as malabsorption. Anal and perianal skin tags, fissures, and fistulas are common. Intestinal obstruction, fistula, and abscess formation are frequent but intestinal perforation and hemorrhage are rare. [6] About 66% to 75% of the children with Crohn's disease require surgery at some point in the course of the disease. Procedures are most commonly done to remove diseased segments, relieve strictures, remove abscesses, and remove obstructions. Even though diseased segments have been removed, Crohn's disease may reoccur at the surgical site. In a small percentage of children only the colon is involved. If traditional therapies have failed, the perianal symptoms are severe, and sphincter damage has occurred, the family may decide to have a surgical illeostomy done to improve the child's quality of life. [7]

Ulcerative Colitis

Ulcerative colitis involves only the innermost lining of the colon causing inflammation and ulceration. The area of disease is continuous with no areas of healthy bowel in-between, as with Crohn's disease. Crampy urgent lower bowel pain is usually followed by frequent loose often bloody stools. During an acute episode the child often experiences tenesmus, which is the persistent urge to empty the bowel caused by inflammation.

Surgery may be required at some point in 25% to 40% of the children with the disease. Emergency surgery may be necessary for colon perforation, sudden severe episodes, and toxic megacolon (a severe colonic dilatation that may cause perforation). Starting ten years after diagnosis, those with ulcerative colitis are at an increased risk for colon cancer that continues to grow with each decade of life. Those with chronic severe symptoms who have experienced treatment failure and are at increased cancer risk may elect to have the colon and rectum removed. Should this become necessary, a variety of surgery options are available, many of which utilize the intact rectal sphincter for continence. Unlike Crohn's disease, surgical removal of the colon will cure ulcerative colitis. [7]

Management

Diet

Dietary modifications are not usually necessary with IBD. However when the ileum is severely inflamed, producing a narrow lumen, a low-fiber diet may be helpful until the inflammation improves. Overall good nutrition is important. Due to the associated anorexia and weight loss, the child should be encouraged to select preferred foods high in nutritional value. Sometimes vitamin and mineral deficiencies can occur and supplementation will be required. For children with severe disease in need of calories, the physician may order oral liquid supplements during the day or continuous drip feedings at night through a feeding tube.[4] Complete elemental diet through formula has been tried successfully in severe cases of IBD to obtain catch-up growth. [1]

Activity

Inflammatory bowel disease does not necessarily restrict activity. During acute episodes abdominal pain, fever, and diarrhea will affect tolerance and stamina. If the disease is under control, the child should be able to participate in sports. If strenuous sports cause fatigue or aggravate symptoms, such as abdominal or joint pain, some activity limitations may be needed. Those children on prolonged high-dose steroids may be more susceptible to bone fractures during contact sports. [4]

Medication

Research continues to result in the development of new drugs and improved treatment options for children diagnosed with IBD. The most common medication prescribed is sulfasalazine (a 5-ASA agent) which acts as a local anti-inflammatory agent in the colon. Side effects may include headaches, GI upset, and impaired folate absorption. Allergic reaction, leukopenia, and worsening of symptoms may also occur. A newer medication named *mesalamin* is similar to sulfasalazine in its local anti-inflammatory action, but is better tolerated and has less potential to cause allergic reactions. Rare but serious complications of *mesalamin* treatment include nephritis and blood dyscrasias. [1]

Corticosteroids are useful to control moderate to severe symptoms and during acute exacerbations. For disease limited to the distal colon, medication can be delivered in enemas or suppositories. When IBD involves the other areas of the gastrointestinal tract, oral or intravenous medication is necessary. Side effects of corticosteriods include weight gain, acne, facial hair, hypertension, mood swings, and increased risk of infection.[8] Prednisone (PDN) is the oral drug of choice and when used in combination with a 5-ASA agent is often effective in achieving a remission. Once therapeutic results are achieved, the dose of prednisone can be gradually tapered while monitoring the child's symptoms and lab values. If successful the child will be maintained on a 5-ASA agent alone. If symptoms resume or intensify, the dose of prednisone may be continued or an immunomodulatory medication may be added.

Immunomodulatory medications, including azathioprine, 6-mercaptopurine, and cyclosporine, are used to alter how the body's immune cells participate in the inflammatory process. These medications are prescribed when routine drugs have been ineffective. Immunomodulatory medications have been shown in some individuals to reduce dependence on corticosteroids and to be useful in maintaining remissions.[9] Side effects may include GI upset and lowered resistance to infection.[8]

INDIVIDUALIZED HEALTHCARE PLAN

Assessment

History

- What is the specific diagnosis and when was it made?
- Has the child ever been hospitalized or had surgical treatment for IBD?
- What has been the child's course with the disease? (Exacerbations, remissions?)
- Does the child have any other health concerns?

Current Status and Management

- What areas of the bowel are affected?
- Who are the healthcare providers involved in the child's care? (Primary care physicians, specialists, practitioners)

- What is the ordered medical treatment regimen? (Medications, dietary supplements, treatments)
- How has the child tolerated treatment? Any medication side effects?
- What supplies/ medications/ equipment will be needed during the school day?
- How would the family prefer to be notified when more supplies are needed at school?
- What is the child's nutritional status? Are supplements/ snacks required?
- What are the recommended fluid requirements?
- Does the child have any dietary restrictions?
- Does the child experience any extraintestinal symptoms?
- Has the child experienced discomfort with IBD? How is that discomfort managed at home?
- Does the child use any over-the-counter medications or herbal remedies?
- Has the family noticed any change in the child's activity level or tolerance?
- Does the child have any activity restrictions or limitations?

Self-care

- What medications/ treatments/ procedures does the child independently administer at home? With supervision?
- What self-care skills are the parents currently teaching at home?
- Has soiling been a problem? Does the child need supervision with personal hygiene during acute exacerbations?
- Does the child experience food intolerances? If so, is the child able to self-monitor offending foods?
- Is the child able to self-regulate activity level when fatigued, or is adult supervision needed?

Psychosocial Status

- What is the family / student perception of the child's overall health status?
- How has the family been coping with the child's diagnosis of IBD?
- Has the child experienced any disruption of usual activities?
- Has the diagnosis been shared with the child's peer group? What has been the response?
- Has the child expressed any concerns about peer reactions?
- Does the child participate in any extracurricular activities with peers?
- Has the child experienced any problems with teasing at school or in the community?
- Have family members noticed any changes in the way the child dresses or acts since the diagnosis?
- Is the family able to identify a support system within their extended family or community?
- What community resources is the family currently using? What resources are still needed?

Academic Issues

- What has been the past school attendance record? Any recent or past patterns of absences? Reason for absences?

- What has been the child's academic history? Have the scores/grades declined since the diagnosis?
- What modifications have been made for the student during the school day?
- What additional modifications are needed during the school day? At recess? During physical education class? During extracurricular activities?
- Does the child need unlimited or private bathroom privileges, snack breaks, rest periods, or modified class schedule?
- Does the child have a 504 Plan or an Individualized Educational Program that would address health and educational accommodations?
- What training will the school staff require to meet the student's needs?
- If necessary, what provisions have been made for pain management at school?

Nursing Diagnoses (N.D.)

N.D. 1 (Risk for) diarrhea (NANDA 1.3.1.2)

N.D. 2 Pain (NANDA 9.1.1) related to exacerbation of IBD symptoms

N.D. 3 (Risk for) altered nutrition: less than body requirements (NANDA 1.1.2.2) related to:
- inadequate intake
- impaired intestinal absorption

N.D. 4 Activity intolerance (NANDA 6.1.1.2) related to:
- joint pain
- fatigue
- anemia
- fever
- medication side effects

N.D. 5 Body image disturbance (NANDA 7.1.1) related to
- exacerbation of IBD symptoms
- weight loss
- medication side effects
- surgical interventions
- pain
- fatigue

N.D. 6 Self-esteem disturbance (NANDA 7.1.2) related to:
- exacerbation of IBD symptoms
- fatigue
- impaired body image
- altered role performance

N.D. 7 Altered role performance (NANDA 3.2.1) related to:
- absence from school/ class due to exacerbation of symptoms
- fatigue
- impaired body image

N.D. 8 Knowledge deficit (NANDA 8.1.1) related to:
- recent diagnosis of IBD
- complicated management of IBD

N.D. 9 (Risk for) noncompliance with prescribed medications (NANDA 5.2.1.1) related to:
- denial of need for medication

- perceived ineffectiveness of medication
- undesirable side effects of medication
- knowledge deficit

Goals

Student will attend school/ class and participate with modifications made as needed. (N.D. 1,2,4,7)

Student will experience an increased level of comfort, allowing active participation in school activities. (N.D. 2)

Student will be involved in planning and implementation of the IBD treatment plan in the school setting. (N.D. 6-9)

Student will demonstrate improved physical activity tolerance. (N.D. 4)

Student will progress towards adapting to living with a chronic illness. (N.D. 4-9)

Student will show improved nutritional status. (N.D. 3,5)

Student will demonstrate improved self-esteem. (N.D. 5-7)

Student will perform self-care skills with assistance as needed. (N.D. 1, 6-9)

Student will demonstrate increased knowledge of IBD. (N.D. 8,9)

Student will comply with prescribed IBD treatment plan. (N.D. 8,9)

Interventions

Student/Family Interventions

Obtain parental and student permission to share relevant medical information with school personnel. (N.D. 1-9)

In collaboration with the medical provider, develop an emergency plan and determine when 911 will be called and to which medical facility the student should be transported. (N.D. 1-3)

Provide pain management. (N.D. 2,4,6,7,9)
- observe the student for signs of discomfort
- determine the impact of discomfort on the student's school performance
- in association with the student, family, and medical team, evaluate the effectiveness of present comfort measures
- modify environmental factors that may contribute to the student's discomfort
- in association with the family, assemble a list of comfort measures and help the student to select appropriate choices based on level of discomfort

Provide nutritional counseling. (N.D. 3-5)
- discuss student's knowledge of the food pyramid in making healthy food choices
- discuss nutritional requirements
- discuss food intolerances
- discuss student's food preferences
- discuss ways to modify and/or supplement school lunches to provide adequate intake
- discuss ways to increase fluid intake during the school day

Provide nutritional therapy in collaboration with the child's medical team by monitoring intake, facilitating nutritious snacks, and ensuring availability of well-tolerated foods in the school lunch program. (N.D. 3, 9)

Provide support and encouragement to student. (N.D. 1-9)

Promote body image enhancement through: (N.D. 5-7)

- encouraging discussion of body changes since diagnosis of IBD
- monitor self-critical statements made by the student
- determine student's perceptions of body image alteration and compare with reality
- discuss with the student ways of minimizing outward signs of illness through cloting styles or cosmetics
- identify coping strategies used by the student
- monitor the student for signs of social isolation
- assist the student to separate physical appearance from feelings of self-worth
- locate support groups available to the student locally

Develop trusting, open communication with the student and encourage verbalization of feelings of anger, frustration, depression, concerns, and fears. (N.D. 1,2,4-9)

Establish a preferred mode of scheduled communication with parents/ guardians to facilitate coordination of medical treatment and to monitor the student's social and emotional adjustment. (N.D. 1-9)

Refer family to counseling resources as needed to facilitate the child's adaptation to living with a chronic illness. (N.D. 2,4-7,9)

Promote self-esteem enhancement. (N.D. 5-7)

- facilitate an environment that encourages self-esteem
- assist the student to examine negative self-perceptions and reasons for self-criticism
- assist the student in problem-solving social situations made difficult because of IBD
- encourage increased level of self-care and responsibility
- encourage student to discuss impact of peer group on feelings of self-worth
- assist student to identify strengths and reinforce examples of those strengths when observed
- convey confidence in the student's abilities

Provide the family with current resources on IBD. (N.D. 8)

Monitor student's medication /treatment compliance and assist in removing existing barriers. (N.D. 9)

Assist the teacher(s) in monitoring the student's activity tolerance and making adjustments in scheduling as needed. (N.D. 2-4, 7,8)

School /Teacher Interventions

Obtain a signed release of information to obtain pertinent medical records and to share information with the medical provider. (N.D. 1-9)

Obtain medical orders for IBD management in the school setting. (N.D. 1-4)

Facilitate self-medication administration when appropriate and in accordance with district policy. (N.D. 6-9)

Provide IBD educational materials to designated school personnel and allow time for questions. (N.D. 1-9)

Provide opportunities for student/ family/ nurse to educate classmates about IBD. (N.D. 4-9)

Refer to building student assistance team or 504 coordinator if not already involved. (N.D. 1-9)

Outline for school staff possible student medical accommodations such as: (N.D. 1-7)

- unrestricted restroom pass

- access to private restroom
- modified physical education class for joint pain and fatigue
- rest periods scheduled into the school day
- need for nutritional snacks during the school day
- access to private shower time after P.E. class or team sports if student has body image concerns
- modified work load if health deteriorates, or if hospitalization or surgery is required
- shortened school day during severe acute exacerbations
- assign seating next to classroom exit

Expected Student Outcomes

The student will:
- participate in classroom, physical education, and selected extracurricular activities with accommodations as needed. (N.D. 1-7)
- report an improved level of comfort after interventions. (N.D. 2)
- progress towards self-monitoring of comfort interventions. (N.D. 2,6)
- attend his/her school health planning meetings. (N.D. 6-9)
- make healthy selections from the school lunch menu. (N.D. 3)
- maintain current weight without further loss. (N.D. 3)
- progress toward self-monitoring of activity level and seek assistance as needed from school staff. (N.D. 4,6)
- demonstrate a reduction in self-critical comments. (N.D. 5-7)
- obtain counseling as needed. (N.D. 5-7)
- show evidence of improved personal appearance. (N.D. 5,6)
- identify and utilize existing community IBD resources as needed. (N.D. 6-8)
- demonstrate an understanding of the IBD disease process and begin to use that knowledge to make health management decisions. (N.D. 8)
- self-administer medications in compliance with prescribed orders and district policy/procedures (N.D. 6-9)
- have access to collaboratively planned IBD treatment. (N.D. 1-9)
- actively participate in making IBD management/treatment choices. (N.D. 6-9)
- comply with the medically prescribed treatment. (N.D. 9)

CASE STUDY

Nicole Birch is a 14-year-old white female recently diagnosed with IBD. She sought treatment after experiencing difficulties with low-grade fever, abdominal pain, ankle swelling, joint pain, weight loss, and anemia. She had also experienced several bouts of diarrhea that she had blamed on the "flu" and had missed several school days due to abdominal pain. Nicole has no previous family history of IBD. After the lower GI series showed two areas of acute inflammation, one in the proximal duodenum and one in the lower colon, the diagnosis of Crohn's disease was made. The gastroenterologist placed Nicole on oral prednisone (b.i.d.) and Pentasa (t.i.d.) to help control her symptoms. She was told by her physician to limit strenuous physical activity until her ankle swelling resolved. The physician also suspected that Nicole may have a milk intolerance. She is to limit her milk intake to 1 cup per day. The family is very supportive of Nicole but are unsure of what adaptations are needed in the school setting. Nicole has no other chronic health conditions and takes no other medications except calcium and iron supplements. Tylenol is ordered for menstrual discomfort.

Individualized Healthcare Plan*
Inflammatory Bowel Disease

Assessment Data	Nursing Diagnosis	Goals	Nursing Interventions	Expected Outcomes
ND3 (See Knowledge deficit IHP for additional assessment data) Weight loss of 15 lbs in the last 3 months. Current weight 100 lbs. Ht. 5'4".	Alteration in nutritional status: less than body requirements related to inadequate intake (NANDA 1.1.2.2)	Nicole will demonstrate an improved nutritional status.	1. Provide nutritional counseling.	
Milk intolerance diagnosed. Family will review school menu and send sack lunch as needed			2. Provide nutritional therapy in collaboration with Nicole's medical team by monitoring intake, facilitating nutritious snacks, and training the dietary staff to assist with Nicole's dietary needs.	Nicole will come to the lunchroom daily for her snack.
Parents request high school staff be trained in IBD symptoms and necessary accommodations and that the dietary department assist them in making menu selections			3. Contract the physician quarterly & prn for follow-up coordina-tion of hemoglobin values, weight loss/gain, treat-ments/ procedures, medication monitoring, activity tolerance, and/or compliance with prescribed treatment regime.	Nicole will show no further weight loss.

Calcium and iron supplements prescribed for home use. Nicole has complained of decreased energy and stamina. Nicole reports "not feeling hungry" and skipping meals. Hemoglobin was 8.4 g/dl on 7/9/98. Suggested daily fluid intake of 64 oz.			
ND6 (See Knowledge deficit and Alteration in nutritional status for additional assessment data) Parents report Nicole is wearing nothing but "baggy" clothes, has stopped wearing make-up, and "seems to care less about her physical appearance." They also report she refuses to wear a swim suit because she "looks like a boy."	Self-esteem disturbance related to impaired body image (NANDA 7.1.2)	Nicole will demonstrate improved self-esteem. Nicole will show evidence of improved personal appearance.	1. Provide support and encouragement to Nicole. 2. Promote body image enhancement through encouraging discussion of body changes since diagnosis.

Individualized Healthcare Plan*
Inflammatory Bowel Disease

Assessment Data	Nursing Diagnosis	Goals	Nursing Interventions	Expected Outcomes
Ankle swelling continues to be a problem along with pain, according to Nicole			3. Identify coping strategies used Nicole.	
Last spring several teachers reported observing older teens teasing Nicole about being "skinny" and looking sick			4. Develop trusting open communication with Nicole.	
Nicole refuses to discuss Crohn's disease with her peers. Mrs. Birch has notified the parents of several of her daughter's close friends. Parents think it's time Nicole's peers knew about her disease.			5. Assist Nicole in contacting the local teen support network.	
Nicole refuses to go to the school counselor. Her parents are willing to seek out a private therapist.			6. Refer the family to counseling resources located in the city.

7. Promote self-esteem enhancement by encouraging increased level of self-care and responsibility. | |

Individualized Healthcare Plan*
Inflammatory Bowel Disease

Nicole will show progress towards adapting to living with a chronic illness.	1. Involve Nicole in selecting which IBD handouts to give staff and discuss with her what content will be presented in the in-service. 2. Discuss with Nicole various social situations made difficult by IBD and assist her in problem solving those situations. 3. Encourage Nicole to share about her Crohn's disease with a few close friends. 4. Provide resources to Nicole as needed for peer sharing.	Nicole will demonstrate an understanding of the IBD disease process and will begin to use what knowledge to make health management decisions. Nicole will consider seeking counseling.

Assessment Data	Nursing Diagnosis	Goals	Nursing Interventions	Expected Outcomes
ND4 (See Knowledge deficit, Alteration in nutritional status, and Self-Esteem disturbance for additional assessment data) Nicole has dropped out of the swim team because she "can't keep up" with the practices Nicole has complained of decreased energy and stamina Hemoglobin was 8.4 g/dl on 7/9/98 Parents report Nicole sleeps an average of 12-14 hours per night yet still complains of being tired Nicole's grade point for last semester was 3.00, down from 3.25 Nicole missed 40 days last school year. She missed 8 days the previous year.	Activity intolerance related to fatigue (NANDA 6.1.1.2)	Nicole will attend class and participate with accommodations made as needed.	1. Assist the teachers in monitoring the student's activity tolerance and making adjustments in scheduling as needed. 2. Train staff in the use of Nicole's 504 plan which includes modifications in physical education and a provision for shortened school days during acute exacerbations. 3. Encourage Nicole to take frequent breaks during periods of exercise. 4. Provide Nicole with a designated quite rest area for use during acute exacerbations with IBD, causing extreme fatigue.	Nicole will progress towards self-monitoring of activity level and intervene as needed with school staff. Nicole will be able to complete the school day despite fatigue.

Individualized Healthcare Plan*
Inflammatory Bowel Disease

ND2 (See Knowledge deficit, Alteration in nutritional status, Self-esteem disturbance, and Activity intolerance for additional assessment data) Parents report Nicole has had several days this summer spent in bed due to abdominal cramping and leg pain Visible edema of the lower extremities with +2 pitting noted on 8/6/98 physical assessment Nicole expressed concern over walking and climbing stairs in the old high school building Tylenol and elevation used to relieve leg discomfort at home	Pain related to exacerbation of IBD symptoms (NANDA 9.1.1)	Nicole will experience an increased level of comfort, after intervention, allowing active participation in group activities. Nicole will attend class and participate with accommodations made as needed.	1. Observe Nicole for signs of pain and assist her in rating her degree of pain. 2. In association with the family, assemble a menu of comfort measures and assist Nicole in selecting appropriate choices based on her level of discomfort. 3. Work collaboratively with the student, parents, and the physician to determine the effectiveness of current pain management strategies.	Nicole will be able to participate in physical education class without experiencing discomfort. Nicole will progress towards self-monitoring of comfort interventions at school.

Assessment Data	Nursing Diagnosis	Goals	Nursing Interventions	Expected Outcomes
ND8 Diagnosed with IBD 4/98 History of low-grade fever, abdominal pain, and anemia Four episodes of loose stools lasting 2-3 weeks Lower GI series showed two areas of inflammation; diagnosed with Crohn's 5/98 No other chronic illnesses or conditions No hospitalizations since birth	Knowledge deficit related to recent diagnosis of IBD (NANDA 8.1.1)	Nicole will demonstrate an increased knowledge of Crohn's disease process and management.	1. Obtain a signed medical release to obtain pertinent medical records and to share information with the medical provider. 2. Obtain medical orders for IBD management in the school setting. 3. Obtain parental and student permission to share relevant medical information with staff. 4. Establish preferred mode of scheduled communication with parents to facilitate coordination of medical treatment and to monitor Nicole's tolerance of medication/treatments. 5. Provide them family/student with current IBD resources, provide overview of IBD, answer questions. 6. Instruct student in self-medication administration procedures at school.	Nicole will have access to school-based IBD treatment planned collaboratively with the parents, guardians, and medical providers. Nicole will actively participate in making IBD management choices. Nicole will be able to identify and utilize existing community IBD resources. Nicole will be able to self-administer medications in compliance with prescribed orders and district policy.

Pentasa and Tylenol are the only medications to be given at school. Nicole takes her medications independently at home Prednisone orally given at home Nicole has had problems with rectal fissures and needs topical medications during the school day which she self-administers		7. Review medication actions and side effects. Instruct Nicole to report any unusual side effects to the school nurse. 8. Review with the student 504 meeting procedures and prepare Nicole to attend her next schedules 504 meeting.	Nicole will attend her 504 review meeting scheduled for November.
Parents request high school staff be trained in IBD symptoms and necessary accommodations	High school staff will demonstrate knowledge of Crohn's disease management, including medication monitoring.	1. Provide educational materials to designated school personnel and allow time for questions. 2. Follow up with homeroom teacher one week after educational presentation to assess knowledge level. 3. In association with the medical providers and the family, develop an emergency plan to determine when 911 is to be called.	Nicole will receive support from the educational staff while undergoing treatment for IBD.

Individualized Healthcare Plan*
Inflammatory Bowel Disease

Assessment Data	Nursing Diagnosis	Goals	Nursing Interventions	Expected Outcomes
			4. Encourage the family to relay pertinent medical information to the local emergency response facility. 5. Outline for staff possible medical accommodations in the school setting. 6. In-service designated staff in the use of the student's IHP and emergency plans.	

*See Appendix for student profile information to include on an IHP form.

REFERENCES

1. Jackson PL, Vessey J. *Primary Care of the Child with a Chronic Condition.* 2nd ed. St. Louis, Mo: Mosby-Year Book, 1996:507-529.
2. Betz C, Sowden L. *Mosby's Pediatric Nursing Reference.* 3rd ed. St. Louis, Mo: Mosby-Yearbook, 1996:254-264.
3. Behrman R, et al. *Nelson Essentials of Pediatrics.* 3rd ed. Philidelphia, Pa: WB Saunders Company, 1998:444-445.
4. Crohn's & Colitis Foundation. *Crohn's Disease, Ulcerative Colitis & Your Child.* New York, NY: Crohn's & Colitis Foundation, 1995.
5. Crohn's & Colitis Foundation. *Questions & Answers About Emotional Factors.* New York, NY: Crohn's & Colitis Foundation, 1995.
6. Hay W, Groothuis J, Hayward A, Levin M. *Current Pediatric Diagnosis and Treatment.* 12th ed. Norwalk, Conn: Appleton & Lange, 1995:649-652.
7. Crohn's & Colitis Foundation. *Questions & Answers About Surgery.* New York, NY: Crohn's & Colitis Foundation, 1995.
8. National Digestive Diseases Information Clearinghouse. *Crohn's Disease.* Publication NIH 98-4225 E-text revised 9 October 1998. Available at: http://www.hiddk.nih.gov/health/digest/pubs/crohns/crohns.htm. Accessed 12/29/98.
9. Bonner G. Current medical therapy for inflammatory bowel disease. *South Med J* (online) 1996; (Jun). Available at: http://www.sma.org/smj/96jun2.htm. Accessed December 29, 1998.

BIBLIOGRAPHY

Crohn's & Colitis Foundation. *A Guide For Children & Teenagers to Crohn's Disease & Ulcerative Colitis.* New York, NY: Crohn's & Colitis Foundation, 1995.

Crohn's & Colitis Foundation. *A Teacher's Guide to Crohn's Disease & Ulcerative Colitis.* New York, NY: Crohn's & Colitis Foundation, 1995.

Crohn's & Colitis Foundation. *Questions & Answers About Ulcerative Colitis.* New York, NY: Crohn's & Colitis Foundation, 1995.

Crohn's & Colitis Foundation of Canada. *Surgery and Inflammatory Bowel Disease.* Toronto, Ontario: Crohn's & Colitis Foundation, 1998.

Johnson M, Maas M. *Nursing Outcomes Classification (NOC).* St. Louis, Mo: Mosby Yearbook, 1997

McCloskey J, Bulechek G. *Nursing Interventions Classification (NIC).* 2nd ed. St. Louis, Mo: Mosby Yearbook, 1996.

National Digestive Diseases Information Clearinghouse. Ulcerative Colitis. Publication NIH. 95-1597 E-text revised 28 April 1998. Available at: http://www.hiddk.nih.gov/health/digest/pubs/colitio/colitis.htm. Accessed December 29, 1998.

North American Nursing Diagnosis Association. *NANDA Nursing Diagnoses: Definitions & Classification 1999-2000.* Philadelphia, Pa: North American Nursing Diagnosis Assn, 1999. (NANDA, 1211 Locust Street, Philadelphia, PA 19107. 800-647-9002; fax 215-545-8107; e-mail: NANDA@nursecominc.com)

17 | IHP: Latex Allergy

Constance Cotter and Mariann Smith

INTRODUCTION

The school environment can be a source of allergens to some students. Allergic reactions to food, insect stings, chalk dust, and more, are well known in schools. An allergy less commonly known, but potentially life threatening in the school environment, is the allergy to latex.[1] Allergic reactions to latex can range from mild to severe. The school environment has many sources of latex; therefore, it is important for school personnel to be aware of procedures for identification and treatment of potentially serious allergic reactions to latex products.

Students with spina bifida and those who have undergone multiple surgical procedures and/or bladder/bowel programs are at risk for latex allergy. The Spina Bifida Association of America reports 18% to 73% of children and adolescents with spina bifida are sensitive to latex. However, any student with a history of respiratory symptoms or skin problems when in contact with rubber products should be considered at risk for latex allergy. Students with a known latex allergy should wear a medical alert bracelet or necklace indicating an allergy to latex.

The student's school environment should be examined for latex products. Examples of sources of latex in the school are erasers, paints, glue, rubber bands, lab and gym supplies, flooring, and latex gloves. A complete list of latex in the community can be found in Supplement A (Latex in the Home and Community).[2] This list includes latex-free alternatives. The IHP should include ways to minimize exposure to latex, an emergency care plan, as well as other considerations, such as service providers, field trips, and sharps disposal container (see Supplement A).

Pathophysiology

Latex is described as a raw material (milky sap) derived from the tropical rubber tree, *Hevea brasiliensis*, used to make many medical and consumer products (e.g., surgical gloves, balloons, and rubber additives). People who are repeatedly exposed to latex (e.g., through multiple surgical and treatment procedures) become sensitized to the latex antigen and are at risk for developing an allergic reaction. The antigen that triggers the allergic response is believed to be a water-soluble protein that occurs naturally in the latex. Reactions can include urticaria (hives) and swelling of mucosal tissues (tonsils, throat, tongue), shortness of breath, wheezing, itching eyes, feeling faint, nausea/vomiting, diarrhea, and abdominal cramping. More serious reactions include bronchospasm, hypotension, and anaphylaxis.

Management

Management of the student who has a latex allergy consists of two steps: 1) modifying the school environment to remove as many latex sources as possible and 2) treating any allergic reaction. The school environment constantly changes (class location, field trips, transportation, etc.); therefore school personnel should receive periodic in-services about sources of latex, latex-free alternatives, and necessary modifications to the environment. Nonlatex gloves should be used throughout the school. Barriers need to be provided between the skin and any latex product if no alternative is available (e.g., gym floors). Use of latex balloons should be discouraged. Parents should be notified about any party, dance, or other activity. where balloons will be used for decoration. Parents will then be able to decide if the student can attend the function. Health room and first aid supplies should be latex-free for the student. Additionally, Emergency Medical Service (EMS) personnel should be aware of the student with latex allergy so they will have appropriate supplies.

Treating an allergic reaction involves teaching school personnel about symptoms of the allergic reaction and appropriate management. School personnel need to know that a latex allergy can be a potential medical emergency. The Emergency Care Plan (ECP) should specify treatment protocol as well as designated responsibility. A source of epinephrine (usually Epi-pen) and antihistamines (if ordered) should be readily available. School personnel will need to inform EMS personnel (if called) that the student has a latex allergy and what treatment has already been given at school.

INDIVIDUALIZED HEALTHCARE PLAN

Assessment

History

- Student's medical diagnosis
- Student's medical and surgical history
- Number of reactions to latex
- Student's signs and symptoms of an allergic reaction (mild to severe)
- Date of the last allergic reaction
- Prescribed treatment for allergic reaction (e.g., medication)
- Previous allergic reactions other than to latex
- Student's level of knowledge and ability to alert others of possible reactions and assist with treatment
- Family knowledge base in relation to treatment (e.g., medications) and environmental sources of latex
- Restrictions to participate in regular education activities
- Healthcare provider involved in assessment and treatment
- Assistance needed to implement management plan (e.g., parent, sibling, teacher, nurse)

Current Status and Management

- Past healthcare records
- Knowledge about condition (student, parent, guardian, teacher, para, etc.)

- Knowledge about early warning signs (student, school staff)
- Physical and cognitive ability to self-administer medication (student)
- Current treatment for the allergic reactions
- School and classroom environment for potential sources of latex

Self-care

- Physical ability to self-administer medications
- Cognitive ability to self-administer medications
- Self-awareness of early signs and symptoms of an allergic reaction
- Knowledge of responsibility to inform appropriate personnel when experiencing allergic symptoms
- Physical and/or cognitive ability to explain his/her needs during an allergic reaction
- Knowledge and ability to avoid latex products

Psychosocial Status

- Effect of the latex allergy on student's daily living activities
- Student's perception of what family members and peers think and feel about student having latex allergy
- Student's affect, outlook, and general attitude toward the condition
- Student's age, developmental level, and intellectual level
- Student's ability to participate in normal activities of community, church, school clubs, or athletic activities
- Student's support system: family, friends, other

Academic Issues

- School environment: latex allergen sources
- Alternative products and procedures that will enable student to participate in education activities
- Faculty awareness and knowledge of condition and potential problems
- Adaptation of school environment so student may safely remain in the least restrictive environment with preferred classes and peers

Nursing Diagnoses (N.D.)

N.D.1. (Risk for) ineffective breathing pattern (NANDA 1.5.1.3) related to:
- bronchospasm
- inflammation of the airways

N.D.2. (Risk for) impaired gas exchange (NANDA 1.5.1.1) related to:
- bronchospasm

N.D.3. (Risk for) altered health maintenance (NANDA 6.4.2) related to:
- lack of physical and/or cognitive ability to self-medicate
- inability to alert staff of treatment needs

N.D.4. Knowledge deficit (NANDA 8.1.1) related to:
- latex sources
- signs and symptoms of an allergic reaction

N.D.5. Powerlessness (NANDA 7.3.2) related to:
- the uncertainty of an allergic reaction and its outcome in the school environment

Goals

The student will:
- demonstrate knowledge about symptoms of an allergic reaction/anaphylaxis. (N.D. 1,2,4)
- demonstrate knowledge about sources of latex and latex-free alternatives. (N.D. 4,5)
- be willing to help develop and participate in an individualized healthcare plan. (N.D. 1-4)
- demonstrate ability to participate in school activities with modifications as necessary. (N.D.3,4)

School staff will:
- demonstrate awareness of latex allergy significance, symptoms, and treatment. (N.D. 1,2,4)
- demonstrate awareness of sources of latex and latex-free alternatives. (N.D. 4,5)

Nursing Interventions

In-service school staff about allergic reaction/anaphylaxis. (N.D. 1,2,4) Discuss:
- symptoms of mild to severe allergic reactions, including anaphylaxis
- importance of early warning signs and prompt treatment (ECP)
- specific guidelines for treatment (from mild to severe)
- documentation of episode

In-service school staff about common sources of latex and latex-free alternatives. (N.D. 4)
- list items containing latex that are commonly found in the school environment.
- provide list of latex-free alternative items.
- discuss ways to minimize student's exposure to latex.
- explain classroom modifications that may be needed.
- discuss transportation modifications that may be needed.
- outline field trip modifications that may be needed.
- modifications for extra curricular activity (e.g., dances, carnivals, etc.) that may be needed.

Monitor school environment at regular intervals for new sources of latex. (N.D. 1,2,5)
- discourage use of latex balloons in school environment, especially in classrooms with students with known latex allergy (Mylar balloons should be used as an alternative).

Inform staff of students who have a latex allergy. (N.D. 1,2)
- encourge parents to have the student wear an allergy alert bracelet indicating a severe latex allergy.

Develop and implement a latex allergy ECP. (N.D. 1-5)
- list and describe measures to follow if reaction occurs
- include student, parent/guardian, appropriate school personnel, and healthcare provider and coordinate school plan with home plan
- allow for modifications to IHP as needed
- assist parents to supply (and resupply as needed) a source of epinephrine (Epi-pen, Anakit, etc.) to always be available in school

- assist parents to obtain physician authorization for use of epinephrine in school as needed

Have latex-free first aid supplies available. (N.D. 1,2,4)

- assist parents in obtaining and supplying latex-free health procedure supplies (catheters, gloves, etc.)
- supply health office with latex-free supplies (Band-Aids, gloves, etc.)

Provide necessary health education for student to participate in self-care (depending on the student's cognitive and/or physical ability). (N.D. 3,5)

- review sources of latex
- review treatment methods, including how/when to report allergic symptoms to school personnel
- teach proper technique for self-administration of epinephrine

Expected Student Outcomes

The student will:

- participate in all school activities with modifications made when necessary. (N.D.3,4)
- describe his/her symptoms of an allergic reaction (from mild to severe). (N.D.1,2,3,4)
- list common sources of latex in school environment. (N.D. 4)
- list steps to take if an allergic reaction occurs. (N.D. 3,4)
- inform his/her teacher(s) and school nurse when experiencing allergic symptoms. (N.D.3,4)
- demonstrate proper technique of self-medication. (N.D.3,5)
- (along with parents) keep school personnel informed of any changes in medical status. (N.D.1-5)
- wear latex allergy alert bracelet/necklace. (N.D.3,5)
- inform teachers of products that might cause allergic symptoms. (N.D. 1,2)
- avoid sources of potential allergens until environment is modified. (N.D. 1-2,4,5)

CASE STUDY

J.D. is a 13-year-old student at Wecare Middle School. He was born with spina bifida. He lives with his mother, father, brother, and sister. This past summer, J.D. had a serious allergic reaction to latex while hospitalized for orthopedic problems. He has had a long history of exposure to latex through numerous surgeries, treatments, bowel management programs, and intermittent catheterization procedures. Initially, his mother plans to transport him to school this year because she is unsure of the latex sources on the school bus.

J.D. is unable to walk and will spend his school day in a wheelchair. The school is easily accessible for him, but the environment needs to be examined for latex sources due to his recent diagnosis of "Severe Reaction to Latex." The bus will also need to be evaluated for sources of latex that he might be exposed to on his ride to and from school. Mom has also requested that we speak with the local EMS personnel who might be called for emergency problems with J.D. Due to a learning deficit, if J.D. would inadvertently be exposed to latex in the school (e.g. balloon bouquet, balls, etc.), he may not be able to advise school staff of his allergic symptoms and his need for medication or emergency treatment.

Individualized Healthcare Plan*
Latex Allergy

Assessment Data	Nursing Diagnosis	Goals	Nursing Interventions	Expected Outcomes
ND1 Potential allergic reaction	Risk for ineffective breathing related to: bronchospasms and inflammation of the airways (NANDA 1.5.1.3)	Prevent allergic reaction/ anaphylaxis	Educate school personnel on allergic signs and symptoms and appropriate treatment	School personnel will know signs and symptoms of allergic reaction to latex and what to do if it occurs.
ND2 Changing school environment, including personnel	Risk for impaired gas ex- change related to: bronchospasms and inflammation of the airways (NANDA 1.5.1.1)	Develop an ECP to include student, staff, and parental roles	Develop ECP with job roles and treatment specifications. Have parent accompany school nurse on tour of student's school environment to identify latex sources. Notify EMS personnel of student's latex allergy	Environment will be monitored and modified for safety with alternative procedures and supplies. Allergic reactions will be identified and treated early by student and/or school personnel.
ND4 Student has a learning deficit which will affect his ability to alert staff to symptoms and treatment needs	Knowledge deficit related to latex sources, signs, symptoms, and treatment (NANDA 8.1.1)	Increase knowledge about latex sources, allergic reactions, and self-medication.	Distribute list of latex sources and alternative products to school staff	Student will notify staff of potential allergens and avoid these sources until environment is modified.

Limited self-care ability	Risk for altered health maintenance related to lack of physical and/or cognitive ability to alert staff of treatment needs and self-medication (NANDA 6.4.2)		Provide necessary health education for student to participate in self-care and treatment protocol	Student will notify staff of allergic symptoms when experienced. Staff will provide treatment until student is able to demonstrate ability to self-medicate.
ND5 Student experiences differential treatment at school	Powerless related to the uncertainty of allergic reaction and the outcome in school environment (NANDA 7.3.2)	Participate in all school activities with minimal disruption.	Provide ongoing monitoring and education about sources of latex in school.	Student will remain in least-restrictive educational environment.
Student is concerned about his relationship with peers. Student is concerned about his ability to make his needs known and receive proper treatment. Student is concerned about the changing school environment and unknown sources of latex.			Provide alternative products, barriers, and modifications.	Student will be able to participate in all school activities with modifications, as needed.

EMERGENCY CARE PLAN

School: _____

Phone: _____

FAX #: _____

Date: _____

Pupil's Name: _____	Physician's Name: _____
I.D.#: _____	Address: _____
Birthdate: _____	Phone: _____
Address: _____	FAX#: _____
Phone: _____	Hospital: _____
Parent's:	
Mother: _____	Day Phone: _____
Father: _____	Day Phone: _____
Parent Designee: _____	Day Phone: _____

Medical Condition: Latex Allergy—severe reactions in past

Location of medication and other supplies: _____

Persons authorized to administer treatment:

      School nurse: _____

      Nurse Designee: _____

Signs of emergency: urticaria (hives), and itching, swelling of mucosal tissues (tonsils, throat, tongue), wheezing, shortness of breath, itching eyes, feeling faint, nausea/ vomiting, diarrhea, abdominal cramps

Treatment for Severe Allergic Reaction:

1. Administer epinephrine injection or assist with self administration
2. Call 911, informing EMS of severe latex allergy reaction and that epinephrine injection has been given
3. Call parent or parent designee
4. Call student's physician to inform of emergency situation
5. Record administration or self-administration of medication in student's health record (include date, time, source of exposure, treatment, if EMS was called, and signature)
6. EMS to transport to (hospital reference) or nearest emergency room

REFERENCES

1. Cotter C, Burbach C, Boyer M., Engelhardt M., Smith M, Hubka K. Latex allergy and the student with spina bifida. *J School Nurs*, 1996; 12: 14-18.
2. Spina Bifida Association of America. *Latex in the Home and Community*. Washington, DC: Spina Bifida Assn of America, 1998.

BIBLIOGRAPHY

Cotter C, Burbach C, Boyer M., Engelhardt M., Smith M, Hubka K. Latex allergy and the student with spina bifida. *J School Nurs*, 1996; 12: 14-18.

Gold J. Ask about latex. *RN* 1994; June: 32-34.

Gritter M. The latex threat. *Am J Nurs*, 1998; 98: 26-33.

Lee M, Kim K. Latex allergy: a relevant issue in the general pediatric population. *J Pediat R Health Care,* 1998; 12: 242-246.

Meeropol E, Frost J, Pugh L, Roberts J, Ogden JA. Latex allergy in children with myelodysplasia: a survey of shriner's Hospitals. *J Pediatr Orthoped*, 1993;13:1-3.

Meeropol E. *Alert: Latex Allergy in Children and Youth Assisted by Medical Technology Educational Settings. Guidelines for Care*. Baltimore; Md: Paul H. Brooks Publisher, 1997.

North American Nursing Diagnosis Association. *NANDA Nursing Diagnoses: Definitions & Classification 1999-2000*. Philadelphia, Pa: North American Nursing Diagnosis Assn, 1999. (NANDA, 1211 Locust Street, Philadelphia, PA 19107. 800-647-9002; fax 215-545-8107; e-mail: NANDA@nursecominc.com)

Spina Bifida Association of America *Latex in the Home and Community*. Washington, DC: Spina Bifida Assn of America, 1998.

Wynn SR Anaphylaxis at school. *J School Nurs*, 1993; 9: 5-11.

Young MA, Meyers M, McCulloch LD, Brown LJ. Latex allergy. *AORN J*, 1992;56: 488-501.

Young MA, Meyers M. Latex allergy: considerations for the care of pediatric patients and employee safety. *Nurs Clin North Am,* 1997; 32: 169-182.

SUPPLEMENT A

Latex in the Home and Community

Products That May Contain Latex	Latex-Safe Alternatives
Art supplies, paints	Some Elmer's, Crayola
Markers, glue	Liquitex products
Balloons	Mylar balloons
Balls: Koosh, tennis, bowling	PVC (Hedstrom)
Carpet backing, gym floor	Provide barrier-cloth or mat
Chewing gum	Wrigley
Condoms, diaphragms	Polyurethane, polymer
Crutch tips, hand grips	Cover with cloth, tape
Diapers, rubber pants	Huggies, Gold Seal, some
Incontinence pads	Attends, Drypers, others
Elastic on socks, underwear	Cloth-covered elastic
Erasers	Fabercastel art eraser
Food handling gloves	Synthetic gloves
Handles on rackets, tools	Vinyl, leather handles or cover
Kitchen cleaning gloves	PVC, cotton liners
Newsprint, ads, coupons	Provide barrier, such as gloves
Toys, such as old Barbies	1993 Barbie, Mattell dolls,
Stretch Armstrong	Kenner figures, toys by Fisher Price, Playschool, others
Rubber bands	String, Plastic bands
Water toys, swimming equipment	Plastic, PVC, nylon
Wheelchair cushions, tires	Jay, ROHO, cover seat, use gloves
Zippered plastic storage bags	Waxed paper, plain plastic bags

18 | IHP: Metachromatic Leukodystrophy

Jeanette H. Williams

INTRODUCTION

Metachromatic leukodystrophy (MLD) is a genetically determined progressive disorder that affects the central nervous system and peripheral nerves. It is derived from the Greek word leuko (white) because it affects the white matter of the nervous system and dystrophy meaning genetically determined and progressive. It also may affect other organs, including the kidneys, pancreas, adrenal glands, liver, and gallbladder.[1] There are several different forms of leukodystrophies: Alexander's disease, adrenoleukodystrophy, Canavan's disease, cerebrotendinous xanthomatosis, globoid cell, neonatal adrenoleukodystrophy, Pelizaeus-Merzbacher disease, Refsum disease, and Zellweger syndrome. Metachromatic leukodystrophy is the more commonly seen leukodystrophy.[2,3]

Metachromatic leukodystrophy is an autosomal recessive degenerative disease. Both parents must be carriers. Offspring have a 25% chance of having the disease, and a 50% chance of being carriers.

There are three different manifestations of MLD.[4]

Type I—late infantile form with symptoms appearing between age 6 months and 2 years

Type II—juvenile form with onset between ages 4 and 16 years

Type III—adult form with onset after age sixteen[5]

Only one form is seen in a family. The incidence of MLD is about 1 in 40,000[5] although a high incidence of the disease occurs in the Habbanite Jewish community with 1 incidence per 75 births.[6]

Metachromatic leukodystrophy is devastating to families. It takes a severe emotional, financial, and physical toll on them. The constant and total care required over an extended period of time is extremely hard. Families need nursing and respite care in order to cope with caring for a child with this serious illness. There is also a sense of guilt in having passed on this horrible disease to their child. Because the disease is inherited, families usually do not have any more children once a diagnosis has been made. Counseling and extended family support will help the parents to remain stable during this trying period of their lives.

Pathophysiology

Metachromatic leukodystrophy is an inherited disease that involves primarily the white matter of the brain.[7] It involves a disorder of myelin caused by a buildup of sulfatides in the central nervous system and also in various organs of the body, including the kidney, liver, and gallbladder. This accumulation of sulfatides is due to a missing enzyme or deficit in the activity of the enzyme, arylsulfatase A.[8, 9] Biochemically it is characterized by accumulation of sulfatide in certain tissues, brain, peripheral nerves, kidney, liver, gallbladder, and possibly spleen. Gastrointestinal reflux is also associated with the disorder.[10] It causes a lack of growth and severe loss of the myelin sheath (fatty covering), which acts as an insulator on nerve fibers.[11, 12] Demyelinization is diffuse and accumulation of metachromatic granules occurs in the central and peripheral nervous system as well as other organs (kidney, liver, and gallbladder). A severe loss of myelin occurs, especially in the late infantile form.[8] The early signs and symptoms may be vague and gradual in onset.[4]

In the late infantile form, the child has normal development until 6 to 18 months of age. Clinical features include blindness, loss of motor function, rigidity, and severe mental retardation. Seizures are common.[13] The child quickly regresses and becomes totally dependent. If he/she has reached the stage of crawling or walking, this ability is soon lost. Loss of the swallow reflex occurs and the child must be tube fed. Because of poor swallowing ability, aspiration frequently occurs and pneumonia and respiratory infections are common. The child will be floppy and mental development will halt. The child's arms and legs will later become spastic.[4,12] Death normally occurs within 3 to 6 years, although there have been exceptions because of outstanding parental and medical provider care.[2]

The juvenile form typically has an onset between age 4 and 10 years of age.[4] Normal development occurs from 4 to 12 years of age, with loss of developmental milestones usually by age 10. Symptoms include gait disturbances, behavioral and cognitive problems, slurred speech, seizures, urinary incontinence, and optic atrophy including blindness.[2] Death usually occurs 4 to 6 years after diagnosis.[12]

Symptoms of the adult form include normal development until around puberty, and then cognitive and behavioral abnormalities are seen. Progressive clumsiness and slowing occur. Seizures, peripheral neuropathy, urinary incontinence, nystagmus, optic atrophy, and blindness may also occur. Death usually occurs within 5 to 10 years of diagnosis.[10]

There is no cure for MLD. Therapy is generally symptomatic. Bone marrow transplants have been used experimentally in milder cases.[14,15] It has shown some promise in delaying the progression of the disease[16,17] Gene therapy[18] and immunosuppressant therapy[18, 19] are being investigated.

Management

Management of MLD is strictly supportive and treats the symptoms as they occur.

Nutritional support is necessary through gastrostomy tube feedings.

Suctioning and appropriate drugs are used to enhance breathing and to minimize respiratory difficulties.

Good infection control should be practiced in the child's environment to minimize infection, particularly respiratory infection.

Medications are used to control respiratory infections and seizures.

Counseling and extended family support are necessary to help the parents cope with the physical and emotional impacts of the disease.

Respite and nursing care should be available to families to assure that the family may continue the child's care in the home.

Occupational and physical therapy services help minimize contractures, rigidity, and loss of bone strength related to neuromuscular disease and lack of weight bearing.

Good skin care is necessary to prevent bedsores.

INDIVIDUALIZED HEALTHCARE PLAN

Assessment

History

- Age and developmental level
- At what age was the diagnosis made?
- Healthcare providers involved in the management and care of the student
- History of growth and weight gain
- Plan (past and current) medications, feeding, suctioning, skin care, family education, family counseling, and modifications in family environment
- Effectiveness of plan in helping family care for child and cope with disease process
- Availability and involvement of support persons/systems
- At what age was the gastrostomy done? How long has student required G-tube feedings? Does student receive any nutrition orally? What nutritional supplements have been used?
- Respiratory symptoms related to respiratory dysfunction
  –respiratory episodes/infection requiring emergency room visits and/or hospitalization
  –experience with respiratory episodes at school
  –medications used and effectiveness
  –how long and how often has student required suctioning?
  –past school attendance pattern, including number of days missed
  –plan for calling emergency medical team and order for resuscitation or DNR
- At what age did seizures begin?
- What types of seizures have been observed and how often do they occur?
- Has student experienced a seizure lasting longer than 5 minutes? If so, what intervention was needed?
- What medications have been used to control seizures?
- Level of family functioning
- Has the family had any counseling?

Current Status

- Developmental level of student
  –gross motor
  –fine motor
  –cognitive status—mental retardation
- Current height and weight
- Gastrostomy feedings
  –equipment and feeding formula, how much and how often
  –bowel elimination patterns
- Current respiratory status
  –rate, rhythm, depth
  –ability to cough
  –breath sounds
  –current procedures used to maintain respiratory function
  –positioning

  –suctioning
  –medications and side effects
- Current status of seizure activity
  –frequency
  –duration
  –behavior observed
  –change in level of consciousness
  -incidence of status epilepticus
  –medication used to control seizures and side effects
- Hearing and visual status

Self-care

- Is student able to participate in personal care?

Psychosocial Status

- Is the family intact?
- Parents' perception of student's health and condition
- Does the family have extended family members who help with the child's care?
- Is the family connected with a respite care agency and/or does the family have access to nursing care part of every day?
- Does the family appear to be grieving in a functional manner?

Academic Issues

- Parents, teachers, bus drivers, and related service personnel's knowledge about metachromatic leukodystrophy
- Staff knowledge regarding gastrostomy and feedings
- Will feedings be done at school?
- Cleaning of equipment after feedings
- Whom to contact if tube is dislodged
  - physician, hospital, parents
  - procedure for tube replacement
- Skin care of stoma
- Potential for exposure to infection in school setting
  - knowledge of infection control procedures on the part of school personnel
- Knowledge of early warning signs of respiratory difficulty
- Medications that may need to be given at school
- Knowledge of staff of seizure disorder
- IEP needed services (PT, OT, DAPE)
- Assistance needed for academic issues
- Assistance needed for health issues
- Transportation needs

Nursing Diagnoses (N.D.)

N.D. 1   Knowledge deficit (NANDA 8.1.1) related to mental retardation and neuromuscular limitations

N.D. 2   Risk for injury (NANDA 1.6.1) related to immobility, and perceptual and cognitive impairment

N.D. 3   Bathing/hygiene self-care deficit(NANDA 6.5.2) and dressing/grooming self-care deficit (NANDA 6.5.3) related to mental retardation and neuromuscular impairment related to disease

N.D. 4   Altered nutrition—less than body requirements (NANDA. l.l.2.2) related to inability to swallow

N.D. 5   Risk for altered growth and development (NANDA 6.6) related to inability to consume adequate nutrition

N.D. 6   Risk for diarrhea. (NANDA 1.3.1.2) related to gastrostomy feeding

N.D. 7   Risk for impaired skin integrity (NANDA 1.6.2.1.2.2) related to gastrostomy stoma

N.D. 8   Risk for aspiration (NANDA 1.6.1.4) related to increased intragastric pressure secondary to tube feeding

N.D. 9   Ineffective breathing pattern (NANDA 1.5.1.3) related to neurologicmuscular impairment

N.D. 10 Risk for ineffective airway clearance (NANDA 1.5.1.2) related to inability to clear oral secretions secondary to neurologic/muscular impairment

N.D. 11 Risk for impaired gas exchange (NANDA 1.5.1.1) related to increased mucus production and/or inability to clear oral secretions

N.D. 12 Risk for infection (NANDA 1.2.1.1) related to inability to clear secretions or aspiration and ineffective breathing pattern

N.D. 13 Risk for injury (NANDA 1.6.1) during seizure

N.D. 14 Risk for aspiration (NANDA 1.6.1.4) related to seizure activity

N.D. 15 Total incontinence (NANDA 1.3.2.1.5) related to neurologic dysfunction

N.D. 16 Impaired physical mobility (NANDA 6.1.1.1) related to decreased strength and endurance related to neuromuscular disease

N.D. 17 Risk for ineffective family coping—disabling (NANDA 5.1.2.1.1) related to terminal illness

N.D. 18 Risk for ineffective family coping—compromised (NANDA 5.1.2.1.2) related to terminal illness

N.D. 19 Dysfunctional grieving (NANDA 9.2.1.1) related to terminal illness

N.D. 20 Potential for family coping: potential for growth (NANDA 5.1.2.2)

Goals

Maintain the highest cognitive function possible. (N.D. 1)
Prevent injury in school environment (classroom, bus, etc.). (N.D. 2)
Maintain hygiene and grooming. (N.D. 3)
Maintain adequate nutrition and hydration and facilitate weight gain. (N.D.4-5)
Prevent/control diarrhea. (N.D. 6)
Maintain skin integrity at stoma site. (N.D. 7)
Prevent aspiration during feedings. (N.D. 8)
Maintain optimal pulmonary function. (N.D. 9 –12)
Prevent breathing difficulty. (N.D. 9 – 12)
Prevent respiratory infection. (N.D. 12)
Prevent injury during seizure activity. (N.D. 13)

Prevent aspiration during seizure. (N.D. 14)

Prevent skin breakdown from incontinence. (N.D. 15)

Prevent rigidity and maintain muscle strength as much as possible. (N.D. 16)

Family copes effectively with care of child and terminal illness. (N.D. 17-20)

Interventions

Encourage staff to stimulate student to maintain maximum potential and prevent/delay further losses in cognitive skills. (N.D. 1)

Provide in-service and supervise educational and support staff in the following as appropriate: (N.D. 2-16)

- positioning
- seizure care *
- diapering
- skin care
- transferring
- tube feeding*
- suctioning*
- infection control with emphasis on hand washing
- CPR training (at least 2 members of classroom staff)
- emergency care plans (ECPs) as developed

Develop plan for evacuation of student in case of emergency. Collaborate with transportation staff to develop plan to meet student's needs in possible emergency on bus. Collaborate with other staff in identifying safety issues and providing for safe environment at school. (N.D. 2)

Staff will provide assistance for (N.D. 3):

- toileting
- diapering
- dressing
- mobility
- grooming (hands, face, hair)

Tube feed as directed by physician. (N.D. 4 & 5)

Weigh monthly to ascertain maintenance of weight and appropriate gain. (N.D. 4 & 5)

Monitor stools for diarrhea, and refer if necessary. (N.D. 6)

Keep stoma site clean and dry. Observe for redness or irritation. Report any abnormalities to parents and/or physician. (N.D. 7)

Position properly and feed through G-tube at recommended rate of flow and recommended amount as prescribed by physician. (N.D. 8)

Suction as necessary to maintain airway. (N.D. 9-12)

Position student to drain secretions and prevent aspiration at all times. (N.D.8-12)

Develop ECP for incidences of breathing difficulty. (N.D. 9 – 12)

Use good infection control practices and prevent transmission of infection to student. (N.D. 12)

Obtain medical orders for all procedures (feeding, suctioning, stoma care) that will be done at school and all medications that may be given at school. (N.D. 2-12)

---

*See *The School Nurse's Source Book of Individualized Healthcare Plans, Volume I,* for in-depth information on these conditions.

Administer medications as ordered. (N.D. 9'-12)

Maintain records of any seizures, procedures done, and medications administered. (N.D. 2-13)

Protect student from injury during seizure activity. Remove all sharp objects from area of student. Loosen clothing if possible. (N.D. 13)

Position student to avoid aspiration during seizure activity. (N.D. 14)

Develop ECP for seizure lasting longer than 5 minutes. (N.D. 13-14)

Change diapers frequently, clean well, and give skin care as needed to maintain skin integrity in genital area. (N.D. 15)

Consult with OT and PT for appropriate interventions and positioning. (N.D. 16)

If DNR (Do Not Resuscitate) order exists, obtain necessary documents so that parents' wishes may be honored if possible if it becomes necessary to utilize emergency medical personnel. Consult with district administration regarding district policy with regard to DNR and inform parents of same. (N.D. 17-20)

Consult with family, encourage counseling, provide information about support groups for parents of terminal children, and encourage use of respite and/available nursing care. (N.D. 17-20)

Encourage use of extended family support. (N.D 17-20)

Encourage expression of feelings. (N.D. 17-20)

Expected Student Outcomes

Student will function at maximum cognitive potential. (N.D. 1)

Student will remain safe in educational environment. ND 2)

Student will be evacuated from building in a timely and safe manner in an emergency situation.(ND 2)

Student will maintain good hygiene and grooming. (N.D. 3)

Student will maintain adequate nutrition/hydration and physical growth as periodically measured by height and weight. (N.D. 4-5)

• Student will remain free of diarrhea. (N.D. 6)

• Stoma site will remain uninfected. (N.D. 7)

• Student will not aspirate during tube feedings. (N.D. 8)

• Student will remain free of infection. (ND 12)

• Student will have good school attendance pattern. (N.D. 12)

• Student will breathe comfortably. (N.D. 9-12)

• Student will be suctioned properly by staff when necessary. (N.D. 9-12)

• Student will not experience injury during seizure. (N.D. 13)

• Student will not aspirate during seizure. (N.D. 14).

• Skin integrity will be maintained. (N.D. 15)

• Student will maintain flexibility and maintain muscle strength as much as possible. (N.D. 16)

• Family will utilize effective coping skills to deal with their child's terminal illness and the child's care. (N.D. 17-20)

• Staff will have skills and knowledge to care for student's needs. N.D. 2-14).

• Medication is given at school as needed and documented on log. (N.D. 8-13)

• Staff follows ECP if a seizure occurs or a breathing problem develops.

CASE STUDY

Justin is a 4-year-old early childhood special education student at West Elementary. He was diagnosed with metachromatic leukodystrophy at age 18 months. He lives with his mother, father, and brother, Alex, who is 8 years old. Alex is in the second grade and doing well.

Justin was the product of a nine-month non remarkable pregnancy with no history of maternal drug use, alcohol abuse, or nicotine use. He was delivered by a normal vaginal delivery and his condition was listed as good. Justin weighed 8 pounds 11 ounces and was discharged from the hospital with his mother.

Justin was an easygoing baby as an infant and fed well. He responded to his mother's voice and touch and smiled and cooed in response to pleasurable stimuli. He cried and showed displeasure and discomfort in appropriate circumstances. He gained head control and rolled over at age expectancy.

At about 9 months of age, Justin's mother became worried because she felt he had not made any motor progress. He was not scooting or trying to crawl and was unable to sit up alone. He began coughing while feeding and became resistant to eating. He was hospitalized at 11 months with pneumonia. Soon Justin was unable to swallow well and was losing weight. A swallow study showed aspiration. Justin had stopped his verbal communication and responded slowly to pleasurable stimuli. He soon was not lifting his head and was unable to eat. He had two more episodes of pneumonia and several bronchial infections. A gastrostomy was done when Justin was 13 months old and a tube for feeding was placed. Testing was done while Justin was hospitalized and the resulting diagnosis of metachromatic leukodystrophy ensued. Justin began having generalized tonic-clonic seizures at age 2.

At age 4, Justin is totally non ambulatory and dependent on caregivers meeting his physical, psychological, and educational needs. He is NPO and is tube fed. He has grown one and one half inches and gained five pounds in the last year. Currently, he will not require tube feeding at school since he is enrolled in the half-day early childhood program. He has been free of respiratory infection for the last four months. He requires oral suctioning prn. He usually requires suctioning at least three or four times while at school. Justin's seizures are fairly well controlled with Depakote, 250 mg, tid. Justin is incontinent of bowels and urine and is diapered. Justin's mother does not have any relatives to help her since the family was transferred here two years ago. She does have many friends who help and support her to the best of their ability. Justin's father does not want to discuss Justin's condition and avoids interaction with school personnel and caregivers if possible. Alex seems well adjusted, but Mom would like to spend more time with him as she feels he is being given a minimum of attention because of the energy required to care for Justin.

Individualized Healthcare Plan*
Metachromatic Leukodystrophy

Assessment Data	Nursing Diagnosis	Goals	Nursing Interventions	Expected Outcomes
ND9 Compromised respiratory status	Ineffective breathing pattern related to neurologic/muscular impairment (NANDA 1.5.1.3)	Maintain optimal pulmonary function for student.	In-service and supervise educational and support staff including bus drivers regarding:	Student will breathe comfortably. Staff will recognize signs of respiratory distress.
ND10	Risk for ineffective airway clearance related to inability to clear oral secretions (NANDA 1.5.1.2)		1. Signs of respiratory distress; 2. Proper suctioning procedure; 3. Proper positioning for ease of breathing;	Staff will suction student properly when needed. Staff will follow ECP if breathing problems occur.
ND11	Risk for impaired gas exchange related to increased mucous production and/or inability to clear oral secretions (NANDA 1.5.1.1)		4. When emergency intervention may be necessary; 5. CPR training for at least 2 classroom staff and 1 transportation employee. Develop ECP to address what to do if breathing problems develop	Staff will be qualified to perform CPR if necessary.

ND12 Susceptibility to respiratory infections, pneumonia.	Risk for infection related to inability to clear secretions or aspiration and ineffective breathing pattern (NANDA 1.2.1.1)	Prevent respiratory infection.	In-service staff as to infection control practices, especially hand washing. Monitor frequently to assure proper infection control practices are being followed.	Student will remain free of respiratory infection and maintain good school attendance record.
ND13 Need for seizure care	Risk for injury during seizure (NANDA 1.6.1)	Prevent injury during seizure.	Develop ECP for a seizure. In-service and monitor staff as to what to expect in generalized tonic-clonic seizure and how to protect student during seizure (Move sharp objects; loosen clothing, if possible, etc.) How to position student during seizure. Note when to call for 911 (ECP). Side effects of seizure medication: When parents, nurse, physician should be notified.	Student will remain safe during seizure. Staff will be knowledgeable and able to care for student in event seizure occurs at school. Staff will follow ECP if a seizure occurs. Any side effects of medication will be recognized and parents notified.

Individualized Healthcare Plan*
Metachromatic Leukodystrophy (continued)

Assessment Data	Nursing Diagnosis	Goals	Nursing Interventions	Expected Outcomes
ND14	Risk for aspiration during seizure (NANDA 1.6.1.4)	Prevent aspiration during seizure.	Student will be positioned appropriately during seizure.	Student will not aspirate during seizure.
ND7 Skin care for Gastrostomy stoma	Risk for potential skin integrity at stoma site (NANDA 1.6.2.1.2.2)	Prevent skin breakdown and/or infection.	In-service staff in how to care for stoma.	Stoma site will remain healthy and uninfected.
ND15 Genital area	Total incontinence related to neurologic dysfunction (NANDA 1.3.2.1.5)		In-service staff in diapering, skin care and symptoms of potential skin breakdown.	Skin integrity in genital area will be maintained.
ND17 Need for family support services to deal with terminal condition. ND18 ND20	Risk for ineffective family coping: disabling (NANDA 5.1.2.1.1), compromised (NANDA 5.1.2.1.2), potential for growth (NANDA 5.1.2.2) related to terminal illness	Family will cope with terminal illness in healthy manner.	Consult with family. Inform them of support groups, respite care and available nursing care. Encourage dad, especially, to attend support group and school meetings.	Family will have access to and utilize respite and nursing care. Dad will be able to express feelings and cope with son's terminal condition.

| | | | Meet with parents on regular basis to discuss needs and get updates on student's condition. | Parents will establish trusting relationship with nurse and educational staff. |
| | | | Establish Care Team and meet biweekly to discuss and resolve problems in student's care and changes in his condition. | Staff will have current knowledge of student's health status. |

*See Appendix for student profile information to include on an IHP form.

IEP Recommendations
For an MLD Student
Based on the above IHP

Justin must be watched closely because of his seizure disorder, compromised respiratory status, and need for suctioning. One classroom staff member should be assigned primary responsibility to monitor Justin while he is at school.

At least 2 classroom staff members working with Justin should be trained in CPR.

Justin must have a trained aide on his bus or be transported in a "Care Cab" (a vehicle staffed with emergency trained personnel).

Weekly School Nursing Time Required

Weekly/biweekly conferences/phone calls with parents, physician —indirect services	=	30 minutes
Weekly observations and discussion of condition with teachers paraprofessionals, transportation personnel (as appropriate)—indirect services	=	1 hour 30 minutes
Classroom observation—indirect services	=	30 minutes
Total weekly nursing needs—indirect services	=	2 hours 30 minutes

REFERENCES

1. Ries M, Deeg RH. Polyposes of the gallbladder associated with metachromatic leukodystrophy. *Eur J Pedi*. 1993; 152:450-451.
2. Department of Pediatrics, Duke University Medical Center. *The Metachromatic Leukodystrophy (MDL) page*. Available at http:www.duke.edu./~pdrh/MDL.HTML
3. Berg BO, ed. *Neurologic Aspects of Pediatrics*. Boston Mass: Butterworth-Heinemann, 1992.
4. Thoene JG, ed. *Physicians Guide to Rare Diseases*. Montvale, NJ: Dowden Publishing Company, 1992.
5. Gieselmann V, Kreysing J, vonFigura K. Genetics of metachromatic leukodystrophy. *Gene Therapy*. 1994; 1 Suppl: 1 S87.
6. Zlotogora J, Back G, Bosenberg C, Barak Y, vonFigura K, Gieselmann V. Molecular basis of late infantile metachromatic leukodystrophy in the Habbanite Jews. *Human Mutations* 1995; 5(2):137-143.
7. Aicardi J. The inherited leukodystrophies: a clinical overview. *J Inherited Metab Dis*. 1993; 16 (4):733-43.
8. Tylki-Szymanska AT, Czartoryska B, Lugowska A. Practical suggestions in diagnosing metachromatic leukodystrophy in probands and in testing family members. *Euro Neurol*. 1998; 40 (2): 67-70.
9. Kolodny FH. Dysmyelinating and demyelinating conditions in infancy. *Curr Opin Neurol Neurosurg*. 1993; 6 (3): 379-86.
10. Malde AD, Naik LD, Pantvaidya SH, Oak SN. An unusual presentation in a patient with metachromatic leukodystrophy. *Anaesthesia*. 1997; 52 (7): 690-4.
11. McKhann GM. Metachromatic leukodystrophy: clinical and enzymatic parameters. *Neuropediatrics*. 15 Supplement (PEDBASE) MITROCHROMATIC LEUKODYSTROPHY. Available at http://icondata.com/health/pedbase/files/metachro.htm Accessed 12/31/94.
12. National Institute of Neurological Disorders and Stroke, National Institutes of Health, Bethesda, Maryland. Metachromatic leukodystrophy. Available at: ninds.nih.gov/healinfo/DISORDER/metachrom.leuk/meta.leuko.htm Accessed September 1997.
13. Balslev T, Cortez MA, Blaser SI, Haslam RH. Recurrent seizures in metachromatic leukodystrophy. *Pediatr Neurol*. 1997; 17(2): 150-4.
14. Pridjian G, Humbert J, Willis J, Shapira E. Presymptomatic late infantile metachromatic leukodystrophy treated with bone marrow transplantation. *J Pediatr*. 1994; 125 (5 Pt 1): 755-8.
15. Landrien P, Blanche S, Vanier MT, et.al. Bone marrow transplantation in metachromatic leukodystrophy caused by saposin-B deficiency: a case report with a 3-year follow-up period. *J Pediatr*. 1998; 133(1): 129-32.
16. Malm G, Kingden O, Wintarski J, et. al. Clinical outcome in four children with metachromatic leukodystrophy treated by bone marrow transplantation. *Bone Marrow Transplant*. 1996; 17(6): 1003-8.
17. Shapiro EG, Lockman LS, Balthazor M, Krivit W. Neuropsychological outcomes of several storage diseases with and without bone marrow transplantation. *J Inherited Metabol Dis*. 1995; 18(4): 413-29.
18. Ohashi T, Watabe K, Sato Y, Saito I, Barranger JA, Matalon R. Gene therapy for metachromatic leukodystrophy. *Acta Paediatr Japan*. 1996; 38(2): 193-201.
19. Nevo Y, Pestronk A, Lopate G, Carroll SL. Neuropathy of metachromatic leukodystrophy: improvement with immunomodulation. *Pediatr Neurol*. 1996; 15(3): 237-9.

BIBLIOGRAPHY

Berg BO, ed. *Neurologic Aspects of Pediatrics*. Boston, Mass: Butterworth-Heinemann, 1992.
Carpenito LJ. *Handbook of Nursing Diagnoses*. 7th ed. Philadelphia, Pa: JB Lippincott Company, 1997.

Haas MB. ed. *The School Nurse's Source Book of Individualized Healthcare Plan, Volume I.* North Branch, Minn. Sunrise River Press, 1993. (Sunrise River Press, 11605 Kost Dam Road, North Branch, MN 55056. 800-895-4585; fax 651-583-2722)

Hootman J, Carpenito LJ. *Nursing Diagnosis: Application in the School Setting.* Scarborough, Me. National Association of School Nurses, 1996.

Kim TS, Kim IO, Kim WS, et al. MR of childhood metachromatic leukodystrophy. *Am J Neuroradiol.* 1997; 18(4) 733-8.

North American Nursing Diagnosis Association. *Nursing Diagnoses: Definitions & Classification 1999-2000.* Philadelphia, Pa: North American Nursing Diagnosis Ass, 1999. (NANDA, 1211 Locust Street, Philadelphia, PA 19107. 800-647-9002; fax 215 545-8107; e-mail: NANDA@nursecominc.com)

RESOURCES

United Leukodystrophy Foundation
2304 Highland Drive
Sycamore, IL 60178
(815) 895-3211
(800) 728-5483

National Tay-Sachs & Allied Diseases Association
2001 Beacon Street, Ste. 204
Brookline, MA 02146
(617) 277-4463
(800) 906-8723

National Organization for Rare Disorders (NORD)
P.O. Box 8923
New Fairfield, CT 06812-8923
(203) 746-6518
(800) 999-6673

ARC of the United States
500 East Border Street
Suite 300
Arlington, TX 76010
(817) 261-6003

19 | IHP: Migraine Headaches

MaryAnn Tapper Strawhacker

INTRODUCTION

Estimates indicate that 26 million people suffer from migraines in the United States.[1] Of those, over eight million are children and adolescents. In this group, migraines are thought to account for over one million lost school days per year. The ratio of boys to girls is equal before puberty, but after puberty migraines are more common in girls.[2] By adulthood, 70% of all sufferers are women.[3] In about 70% to 80% of children diagnosed with migraines, a hereditary component exists.[4]

Pathophysiology

Migraines are a neurologic condition of unknown origin.[5] Most experts agree, however, that blood flow changes within the brain are a key factor in the process.[6] Dr. Michael Moskowitz and other researchers have worked to discover the complex relationship between pain and blood flow during a migraine. They have discovered that during a migraine an unknown trigger in the brain activates the pain sensors in the trigeminal system, causing protein fragments to be released. These fragments cause blood vessels to dilate, further irritating the nerve fibers. Receptors designated 5-HT, discovered on the trigeminal nerve, function to turn off inflammation and pain transmission. Serotonin, a brain neurotransmitter, binds to 5HT receptors. New treatments in the last few years have focused on these important discoveries.[7]

Symptoms

Migraines are classified into two dominant types, classic and common. Classic migraines affect 10% to 15% of children with migraines.[8] An aura, or neurologic symptoms, appearing 10 to 30 minutes before an attack is the major difference between the two types. Symptoms of an aura are varied but may include flashing lights, visual disturbances, speech difficulties, tingling, limb weakness, and abdominal pain.[6] The headache may begin during an aura or up to an hour after it clears. Pain is usually moderate to severe and throbbing. In young children, pain may be felt bilaterally whereas in older children it is usually one-sided. Pain is almost always frontal and worsened by movement or exercise.

Common migraines account for 85% of all migraines in children. The aura is absent and the throbbing headache builds slowly over minutes to hours. These headaches are frequently located in the forehead but may be one sided. Severity of the headache varies from mild to severe. Many children vomit within 30 to 60 minutes of onset. Both types may be, but are not necessarily, associated with light sensitivity, sound sensitivity, nausea, vomiting, diarrhea, increased urination, dizziness, increased thirst, and sensitivity to strong odors.[8,2] Abdominal symptoms are often most prominent in school-age children. [9]

Another less common type of migraine is headache free. The other associated symptoms are those previously listed for migraines. [6] Migraines may last from 30 minutes up to several days or more. Children may choose to seek out a quiet dark room and try to relieve symptoms with sleep. In some children this may be an effective treatment. Children will experience no symptoms between attacks.[8]

Diagnosis

Currently there are no medical tests that will diagnose migraines. Thermography, an experimental technique that displays skin temperature differences, has demonstrated unique heat patterns for those who suffer from headaches.[6] Although a potential tool, much research still remains to be done. At present, physicians must rely heavily on child and family report, in addition to ruling out all other possible causes of headache, to make the diagnosis.[2] The diagnostic process is difficult for some children, enduring many medical tests/ procedures and seeing multiple physicians. It is also common for children to be misdiagnosed or underdiagnosed, especially young children.[10]

Management

Trigger Mechanisms

The role of trigger mechanisms in the development of migraines is highly subjective and not well understood.[7,11] It is thought that, for some individuals, avoidance of identified triggers can lessen the number of attacks. A sample of commonly identified factors includes:

- Foods such as those containing tyramine (cheeses, yogurt, sour cream), nitrates and nitrites (luncheon meats, hot dogs), chocolate, red wine, aspartame, and dairy products and foods with MSG added as a preservative [7,11,12]
- Environmental changes such as climate, altitude or barometric pressure, high winds, weather patterns, and extremes of heat, light, or sound, and intense smells or vapors [13]
- Medications that dilate blood vessels [4]
- Excessive use of medications to treat headaches [4]
- Variations in routine such as not eating regularly and getting too much or too little sleep[11]

The association between female endocrine changes and migraine development is proven. During ovulation or around the time of menses is the most commonly reported time for migraine attacks to increase in susceptible individuals. The use of oral contraceptives can also increase attacks for about half of sufferers. [14]

Treatment

Treatment depends on frequency, duration, and intensity of the migraines.[2]

Mild to Moderate Pain

Prompt intervention with rest and/or simple analgesics often alleviates symptoms. Nonprescription analgesics should not be taken more than three days per week. Side effects of nonprescription analgesics may include cramps, diarrhea, dizziness, drowsiness, heartburn, nausea, vomiting, or rebound headaches. If these medications do not alleviate symptoms, other treatments are available. Biofeedback and relaxation techniques may be beneficial alone or in combination with medication.[2] Narcotic analgesic combination medications may allow for lower doses of each drug and be very effective for moderate pain control. Possible side effects include dry mouth, dizziness, drowsiness, heartburn, nausea, vomiting, stomach pain, blurred vision, and constipation.[15]

Moderate to Severe Pain

Medication management is centered on one or more of three areas: preventive, abortive, or general pain control. Preventive medications are prescribed to reduce the number of attacks in individuals who suffer more than two migraines per month or severe enough symptoms to affect the quality of life.[16]   Fewer than 20% of migraine sufferers require preventive treatment.[11]   Cyproheptadine and propranolol are the most commonly prescribed preventive medications in younger children. Children with asthma, bradycardia, or depression should not take propranolol.[2] In older children, beta-blockers, antidepressants, calcium channel blockers, serotonin antagonists, or anticonvulsants may be prescribed. These medications have a variety of drug interactions, side effects, and precautions. Most are prescribed in different dosage than the original indications for use recommendations.[11] Many have not been tested on children. For these reasons it is important to consult with the child's physician or pharmacist to obtain current drug information and parameters for medication monitoring.

Abortive medications are used to lessen the severity and/or shorten the duration of migraine symptoms. They must be used early in the attack to be effective. The most common type of abortive agents include ergotamine tartrate and dihydroergotamine (Migranal®, DHE45®). These medications should not be taken more that two days per week and doses should be taken at least five days apart. Possible side effects of ergot alkaloids include nausea, vomiting, diarrhea, dizziness, leg cramps,

rebound headaches, and chest discomfort. Triptans, which are selective serotonin agonists, have possible side effects of dizziness, drowsiness, muscle aches, nausea, vomiting, chest or throat tightness, warmth, and tingling. Specific medications in this category include sumatriptan (Imitrex®), naratriptan (Amerge®), rizatriptan (Maxalt®), and zolmitriptan (Zomig®). Isometheptene mucate (Midrin®) is a combination drug that acts to constrict inflamed blood vessels in the head, relieves pain, and helps the child relax. One of the few side effects is drowsiness.[17]

Pain control is the goal of treatment once other measures have failed. Nonprescription and prescription analgesics, nonsteroidal anti-inflammatory drugs, and antinausea drugs may all be used alone or in prescribed combinations.[11] Butorphanol tartrate (Stadol NS®), Midrin®, and Fioricet® are some of the newer medications used. Consult with the child's physician or pharmacist for medication monitoring parameters. Depending on the severity and duration of pain, emergency medical treatment may become necessary.

Psychosocial Implications

The effect of migraines on the family has not been extensively studied.[18] Often complex medical management, unpredictable attacks, time missed from school and work, and financial costs of treatment are all factors that predispose the family to stress. Stress, although not the cause, can worsen symptoms for the child.[12] Historically, migraines were thought to have psychological and not physiologic origins. Unfortunately this belief has survived, despite research to the contrary, and it still plays a role in how migraine sufferers are treated by society.[7]

INDIVIDUALIZED HEALTHCARE PLAN

Assessment

History

- Has the child had a complete medical work-up?
- When was the diagnosis made?
- Does the child have any other health concerns?
- Is there a family history of migraines?

Current Status and Management

- What are the frequency, severity, and duration of the attacks?
- If the child experiences an aura, how does it usually present?
- What are the typical signs of a migraine for the child?
- What associated symptoms does the child experience?
- Has the child or family identified any potential triggers such as foods, environmental, or hormonal ?
- Does the child have any dietary or environmental restrictions?
- Who are the healthcare providers involved in the child's care? (physicians, specialists, practitioners)
- What is the ordered medical treatment plan? (medications, biofeedback, relaxation therapy)
- How effective has the treatment been in management of attacks and symptoms?
- What tools does the child use to rate/ describe the migraine attacks?
- How does the family document treatment at home? (logs, headache diaries, pain scale ratings)
- How has the child tolerated treatment? Any medication side effects?
- Does the child use any over-the-counter medications or herbal remedies?
- What supplies/ medications/ equipment will be needed during the school day?
- How would the family prefer to be notified when medication refills are needed at school?
- What changes has the family noticed in the child's general activity level/tolerance before, during, or after an attack?
- Has the child experienced any disruption of sleep patterns?
- What are the child's dietary habits? (eats regularly, skips meals, varied intake)

Self-care

- What medications/ treatments/ procedures does the child independently administer at home? With supervision?
- What self-management skills are the parents currently teaching at home?
- Is the child able to anticipate signs and symptoms of an impending migraine?
- Will the child notify an adult when experiencing signs and symptoms of a migraine or is adult guidance needed?
- Is the child able to participate in the selection of appropriate treatments based on symptom severity?

Psychosocial Status

- What is the family/ student perception of the child's overall health status?
- How has the family been coping with the child's diagnosis of migraines?
- Has the child experienced any disruption of activities?
- Has the diagnosis been shared with the child's peer group? What has been the response?
- Has the child expressed any concerns about peer reactions?
- Does the child participate in any extracurricular activities with peers?
- Has the child experienced any problems with teasing at school or in the community?
- Is the family able to identify a support system within their extended family or community?
- What community resource(s) is the family currently using? What resources are still needed?

Academic Issues

- What has been the past school attendance record? Any recent or past patterns of absences? Reason for absences?
- What has been the child's academic history? Have the scores/grades declined since the diagnosis?
- What modifications have been made for the student during the school day?
- What additional modifications are needed during the school day?
- Does the child have a 504 Plan or an Individualized Educational Program which would address health and educational accommodations at school?
- What training will the school staff require to meet the student's needs?
- What provisions have been made for migraine management at school?

Nursing Diagnoses (N.D.)

N.D.1 Pain (NANDA. 9.1.1) related to migraine symptoms

N.D.2 Activity intolerance (NANDA. 6.1.1.2) related to:
- migraine symptoms (headache; nausea; vomiting; sensitivity to light, sound, or movement)
- medication side effects
- frequency, severity, or duration of attacks

N.D.3 Knowledge deficit (NANDA. 8.1.1) related to:
- recent diagnosis of migraines
- complicated management of migraines

N.D.4 Ineffective family management of therapeutic regimen (NANDA. 5.2.2) related to:
- multiple caregiver demands
- inability to select appropriate treatments based on symptoms
- inconsistent primary caregiver
- knowledge deficit

N.D.5 Ineffective individual management of therapeutic regimen (NANDA. 5.2.1) related to:
- denial of early warning signs of impending attack
- inadequate follow-up of relaxation and biofeedback training

- multiple changes in medications/treatments
- knowledge deficit

N.D.6   (Risk for) noncompliance with prescribed treatment (NANDA. 5.2.1.1) related to:
- denial of need for medication/ treatment
- perceived ineffectiveness of medication/ treatment
- undesirable side effects of medication
- knowledge deficit

N.D. 7   Ineffective individual coping (NANDA 5.1.1.1) related to:
- fear of future attacks
- stress imposed by migraines and their management
- altered role performance
- pain

N.D.8   Altered role performance (NANDA. 3.2.1) related to:
- absence from school/ class due to migraines
- symptoms of migraines
- management of migraines

N.D.9   Self-esteem disturbance (NANDA. 7.1.2) related to:
- frequency, severity, or duration of attacks
- ineffective coping
- altered role performance

Goals

Student will demonstrate improved physical activity tolerance. (N.D.1, 2)

Primary caregiver, in association with the physician, will develop a mutually agreeable medical treatment plan. (N.D. 1-9)

Student will attend school/ class and participate with modifications made as needed. (N.D. 1,2,4,5,8,9)

Student will experience an increased level of comfort, allowing active participation in school activities. (N.D. 1,2,4,5)

Student's caregivers will demonstrate increased knowledge of migraine management. (N.D. 3, 4)

Primary caregiver will comply with prescribed medical treatment. (N.D. 4, 6)

Student will be involved in the planning and implementation of the migraine treatment plan in the school setting. (N.D. 4-9)

Student will progress towards adapting to living with a chronic condition. (N.D. 4-9)

Student will seek treatment for migraines at first sign of an attack. (N.D. 1,3,5,6,8)

Student will demonstrate improved self-esteem. (N.D. 7,8,9)

Student will perform relaxation and biofeedback strategies with assistance as needed. (N.D. 1,4-9)

Student will demonstrate increased knowledge of migraines. (N.D. 3, 5)

Student will comply with prescribed migraine treatment plan. (N.D. 6)

Primary caregiver will demonstrate an increased knowledge of migraine management. (N.D. 3-4)

Interventions

Student/Family Interventions

Obtain a signed release of information to obtain pertinent medical records and to share information with the medical provider. (N.D. 1-9)

Obtain parental and student permission to share relevant medical information with school personnel. (N.D. 1-9)

Provide support and encouragement to student. (N.D. 1-9)

Develop trusting open communication with the student, encouraging verbalization of feelings of anger, frustration, depression, concerns, and fears. (N.D. 1,2,4-9)

Establish a preferred mode of scheduled communication with parents/ guardians to facilitate coordination of medical treatment and to monitor the student's social and emotional adjustment. (N.D. 1-9)

In collaboration with the medical provider, family, and student, develop a school migraine treatment plan based on symptoms. (N.D. 1-9)

Provide pain management. (N.D. 1-9)
* Observe the student for signs of discomfort.
* Standardize, in association with the student and family, an individual pain rating scale for school use.
* In association with the family, assemble a list of comfort measures and help the student to select appropriate choices based on level of discomfort.
* Instruct the student to use prescribed treatment before symptoms are severe.
* Reinforce learned biofeedback and relaxation therapy techniques.
* Support the family in exploring alternative treatment options.
* Locate a quiet dark place for the student to rest during acute attacks.
* Determine the impact of discomfort on the student's school performance.
* In association with the student, family, and medical team, evaluate the effectiveness of present comfort measures.
* Modify environmental factors that may contribute to the student's discomfort.
* Assist the family/ student to identify possible triggers where appropriate.
* Make referrals to support groups and outside resources as appropriate.

Reinforce or provide additional migraine education to the student/ family. (N.D. 1-5)
* Assess the student/ primary caregiver's knowledge of migraines.
* Determine the readiness and ability of caregivers/ student to learn the necessary skills.
* Review the known pathophysiologic processes with the student at a developmentally appropriate level.
* Provide current migraine resources as needed.
* Reinforce teaching with the student/ primary caregiver on an ongoing basis.

Provide medication management. (N.D. 1-6)
* Determine medication required and administer per physician's orders.
* Assess student's ability to self-medicate.
* Monitor effectiveness of medications.
* Monitor for adverse drug effects.
* Review with the student/ family appropriate use of over-the-counter as well as prescription medications.

- Review medication administration technique for nasal and parenteral routes.
- Discuss the use of herbals and alternative therapies that may interact with over-the-counter or prescription medication.
- Monitor student's medication /treatment compliance and assist in removing existing barriers.
- Provide consultation with other healthcare providers regarding results of treatment and necessary modifications.

Promote family management of therapeutic plan. (N.D. 4-6)
- Determine the student's level of dependency on the family.
- Identify the family's expectations for management.
- Assess the need for reinforcement teaching.
- Assist the primary caregiver to identify strengths and challenges with current management strategies.
- Collaborate with the primary caregiver to set goals for school management.
- Support the primary caregiver through active listening.
- Assist to resolve conflicts between the student and family that serve as barriers to treatment.

Assist the family to minimize disruption of their daily life due to migraine management. (N.D. 4-6)
- Determine the impact of the family's cultural practices and beliefs on migraine management.
- Determine, in association with the primary caregiver, the scope of family disruption.
- Assist the family to adapt prescribed treatment into their lifestyle.
- Assist the family to focus on their child's strengths and not on the migraines.
- Encourage participation in age-appropriate activities.
- Encourage the parents to set age-appropriate limits and expectations for the child.
- Encourage the parents to set consistent age-appropriate expectations for all children in the family.
- Discuss strategies for managing acute attacks in a variety of settings.
- Identify and promote the family's use of adaptive coping mechanisms.
- Assist the primary caregiver to advocate for their child in a variety of settings.
- Encourage the family to seek and maintain a social support network.
- Assist the primary caregiver to locate and utilize existing community resources as needed.
- Make referrals to outside agencies as appropriate.

Facilitate student participation in the therapeutic plan. (N.D. 5- 9)
- Determine the student's current level of participation.
- Set goals in collaboration with the student and primary caregiver.
- Explore strategies with the student to progress towards goal attainment.
- Break down treatment plan into discrete teachable components.
- Maintain consistency in student supervision through written protocol and support staff training.
- Encourage the student to participate in monitoring progress toward goal attainment.
- Provide ongoing feedback to the primary caregiver about the child's progress towards goal attainment.
- Provide positive reinforcement to the student.
- Provide the student with choices in migraine management, whenever possible.

Promote self-esteem enhancement. (N.D. 7-9)
- Facilitate an environment that encourages self-esteem.
- Assist the student to identify the impact of migraines on self-concept.
- Assist the student to examine negative self-perceptions and reasons for self-criticism.
- Monitor self-critical statements.
- Assist the student to identify self-destructive behaviors.
- Assist the student in problem-solving situations made difficult because of migraines.
- Encourage increased level of self-care and responsibility.
- Encourage student to discuss the impact of peer group on feelings of self-worth.
- Facilitate self-expression with peers.
- Monitor the student for signs of social isolation.
- Assist student to identify strengths and reinforce examples of those strengths when observed.
- Convey confidence in the student's abilities.

Refer family to counseling resources as needed to facilitate the child's adaptation to living with a chronic condition. (N.D. 1,2,4-9)

Assist the student to adapt to the stress of migraines and their management. (N.D. 7-9)
- Provide an attitude of unconditional acceptance.
- Assist the student to develop an objective appraisal of his/her migraine status.
- Assist the student to identify his/her own strengths and challenges.
- Discuss alternative responses to stress.
- Encourage constructive outlets for expression of frustration and anger.
- Facilitate the acceptance of others' limitations.
- Evaluate the student's decision-making ability.
- Teach new coping and problem-solving skills.
- Introduce the student to an adult mentor, with family approval, who successfully manages his or her own chronic condition.
- Encourage the use of spiritual resources as appropriate.

School /Teacher Interventions

Obtain medical orders for migraine management in the school setting. (N.D. 1-6)

Facilitate self-medication administration when appropriate and in accordance with district policy. (N.D. 4-9)

Provide migraine educational materials to designated school personnel and allow time for questions. (N.D. 1-9)

Assist the teacher(s) in monitoring the student's activity tolerance and making adjustments in scheduling as needed. (N.D. 1-2, 7-9)

Provide opportunities for student/ family/ nurse to educate classmates about migraines. (N.D. 1-3, 6-9)

Refer to building student assistance team or 504 coordinator if not already involved. (N.D. 1-9)

Outline for school staff possible student medical accommodations such as: (N.D. 1-7)
- quiet place to rest during an acute attack
- modified work load if attacks are severe and frequent
- shortened school day if attacks are severe and difficult to control
- mentor assigned to assist coordination of missed school work

Expected Student Outcomes

The student will:
- improve school attendance with accommodations as needed. (N.D. 1-7)
- recognize the early warning signs of an oncoming migraine. (N.D. 1,3-5,7-9)
- report an improved level of comfort after interventions. (N.D. 2)
- progress towards self-monitoring of comfort interventions. (N.D. 2,6)
- receive consistent management of migraines. (N.D. 1,4, 6)
- demonstrate an understanding of the migraine process and utilize that knowledge to make health management decisions. (N.D. 3,5,6)
- demonstrate a reduction in self-critical comments. (N.D. 5-7)
- obtain counseling as needed. (N.D. 5-7)
- utilize biofeedback and/ or relaxation therapy techniques in pain management. (N.D. 1,5,6)
- attend his/her school health planning meetings. (N.D. 6-9)
- demonstrate the use of adaptive coping skills. (N.D. 7)
- identify and utilize existing community resources as needed. (N.D. 6-8)
- demonstrate a reduction in self-destructive behavior. (N.D. 7-9)
- self-administer medications in compliance with prescribed orders and district policy/ procedures. (N.D. 5-9)
- participate in development of the migraine treatment plan. (N.D. 1-9)
- actively participate in making migraine treatment choices. (N.D. 5-9)
- comply with the medically prescribed treatment. (N.D. 6)

The primary caregiver will:
- participate in development of the migraine treatment plan. (N.D. 1,3-6)
- effectively manage the child's therapeutic regimen. (N.D. 4)
- utilize community resources to assist in the therapeutic management of migraines. (N.D. 4)
- maintain consistent treatment strategies across all settings. (N.D. 1,4, 6)

CASE STUDY

Lindsey Newell is a 16-year-old white female diagnosed five years ago with common migraines. Usual symptoms are nausea, vomiting, light/noise/movement sensitivity, and headache. No food or environmental triggers have ever been identified. Up until the last two years Lindsey was able to control her migraine pain with the use of OTC medication and the occasional use of Migranol®. In the past year, however, Lindsey has gone from one to two migraines per month to almost weekly. She has missed 36 school days this year and has been hospitalized twice for pain management. School health office visits average four to five times per week and counselor visits average one to two times per week. Lindsey's grade point average has dropped this semester and she has quit band and pep squad. Current treatment prescribed by the neurologist includes biofeedback and relaxation therapy. Medication options include Excedrin Migraine®, Naproxine®, and Imitrex®. Her parents disagree on medical treatment approach. Lindsay is an only child whose parents recently divorced. Custody is shared on an every-other-week basis. Both parents travel out of town routinely for business. Lindsey's maternal grandparents live in a nearby suburb and are actively involved in her care. Lindsey denies having any other chronic health conditions or taking any additional medications. Last month Lindsey was given an in-school suspension for possession of alcohol on school grounds.

Individualized Healthcare Plan*
Migraines

Assessment Data	Nursing Diagnosis	Goals	Nursing Interventions	Expected Outcomes
ND4 Absent 36 school days this year. Hospitalized twice for migraines 1998-1999 school year Health office visits average 4-5 times per week Counselor office visits average 1-2 times per week Lindsey's mother prefers that herbals, biofeedback, and relaxation therapy be used before traditional medications	Ineffective family management of therapeutic regimen related to inconsistent primary caregiver and multiple treatment strategies (NANDA 5.2.2)	The family will, in collaboration with their neurologist, develop a mutually agreeable migraine treatment plan.	1. Obtain a signed medical release to obtain pertinent medical records and to share information with the medical provider. 2. Obtain medical orders for migraine management in the school setting. 3. Obtain parental and student permission to share relevant medical information with staff. 4. Identify the parent's expectations for management. 5. Assist to resolve conflict between family members with regards to medication management. 6. Determine Lindsey's level of dependence of caregivers.	Management of Lindsey's migraines will be consistent across all settings.

		Lindsey will receive prescribed treatment for migraines in the school setting.
Lindsey's father prefers the use of traditional medication therapy and does not believe alternative therapies are beneficial		7. Establish preferred mode of scheduled communication with parents/ grandparents to facilitate coordination of medical treatment and to monitor Lindsey's tolerance of medication/ treatments and her social and emotional adjustment.
Three occasions this semester Naproxine supply was depleted; refills were not obtained until one week later	Primary caregivers will comply with prescribed medical treatment.	1. Collaborate with the family to set goals for school management. 2. Assist the family to adapt prescribed treatment into their lifestyle. 3. Assist the family to focus on Lindsey's strengths. 4. Encourage the family to set age-appropriate limits and expectation. 5. Assist the parents to advocate for Lindsey. 6. Collaborate with the school counselor to locate additional community counseling services.

Individualized Healthcare Plan*
Migraines (continued)

Assessment Data	Nursing Diagnosis	Goals	Nursing Interventions	Expected Outcomes
ND3 See Family management IHP for additional data. Neurologist appointment 2/19/99, management plan negotiated, orders received. Medications prescribed include Imitrex®, Naproxine®, and Excedrine Migrainal® Stadol NS® was added. Herbal supplements will be discontinued Relaxation therapy and biofeedback training will continue	Knowledge deficit related to recent therapeutic management modifications (NANDA 8.1.1)	Lindsey will demonstrate an increased knowledge of migraine management.	1. Obtain a signed medical release to obtain pertinent medical records and to share information with the medical provider. 2. Obtain medical orders for migraine management in the school setting. 3. Obtain parental and student permission to share relevant medical information with staff. 4. Establish preferred mode of scheduled communication with parents to facilitate coordination of medical treatment and to monitor Lindsey's tolerance of medication/treatment.	Lindsey will be able to utilize her knowledge of migraine management to make health decisions.

		5. Review resources obtained at pain management seminar, answer questions, and provide reinforcement as needed. 6. Instruct student in self-medication administration procedures at school. 7. Review medication actions and side effects. Instruct Lindsey to report any unusual side effects to the school nurse.	Lindsey will be able to self-administer medications in compliance with prescribed orders and district policy.
Family is scheduled for a pain management seminar at the community college next weekend		School staff will demonstrate knowledge of the migraine process and treatment implications.	
		1. Provide educational materials to designated school personnel and allow time for questions. 2. Follow up with homeroom teacher one week after educational presentation to assess knowledge level. 3. In association with the medical providers and the family, outline for staff possible modifications required during the school day.	Lindsey will receive support from the educational staff while undergoing treatment for migraines.

Individualized Healthcare Plan*
Migraines

Assessment Data	Nursing Diagnosis	Goals	Nursing Interventions	Expected Outcomes
			4. In-service designated staff in the use of the student's IHP and overall goals for therapeutic regimen.	
ND1 *See family management and knowledge deficit IHPs for additional assessment data*	Pain related to migraine symptoms (NANDA 9.1.1)	Lindsey will experience an increased level of comfort, after intervention, allowing her to stay in school	1. Work with Lindsey to standardize a pain rating scale.	Lindsey will improve her school attendance with accommodations as needed.
Lindsey has expressed confusion over which medication to select			2. Observe Lindsey for signs of pain and assist her in rating her pain on the scale.	
Lindsey has not utilized the relaxation therapy or biofeedback training she received several years ago, according to her mother			3. In association with the family and neurologist, assemble a menu of comfort measures and assist Lindsey in selecting appropriate choices based on her pain rating.	Lindsey will progress towards self-monitoring of comfort interventions at school.

Assessment Data	Nursing Diagnosis	Goal	Nursing Interventions	Expected Outcome
Lindsey does not currently utilize a pain rating scale, although she was given a copy of one at her last neurologist visit Once a migraine begins, Lindsey prefers to call her family to take her home			4. Work collaboratively with the student, parents, and the physician to determine the effectiveness of current pain management strategies. 5. Provide medication management. 6. Review the use of over-the-counter medication and possible abuse. 7. Provide reinforcement of biofeedback and relaxation strategies and assist Lindsey to apply strategies and assist Lindsey to apply strategies in the school setting.	Lindsey will be able to utilize biofeedback and relaxation therapy to assist in pain management.
ND7 *See family management knowledge deficit, and pain IHPs for additional assessment data*	Ineffective individual coping related to stress imposed by migraines and their management (NANDA 5.1.1.1)	Lindsey will progress towards adapting to living with migraines	1. Obtain a signed medical release to obtain pertinent mental health records and to share information with the mental health provider.	Lindsey will demonstrate the use of adaptive coping skills.

Individualized Healthcare Plan*
Migraines (continued)

Assessment Data	Nursing Diagnosis	Goals	Nursing Interventions	Expected Outcomes
Lindsey has stated, "I just want it to all go away…Why me?…I don't want to live my life like this….Why can't things be the way they were?"			2. Maintain trusting open communication with Lindsey that encourages verbalization of feelings of anger, frustration, depression, concerns, and fears.	
In-school suspension last month for possession of alcohol on school grounds			3. Encourage Lindsey to seek and maintain a social support network.	
Parents express concern over Lindsey's "rebellious attitude"			4. Assist Lindsey to develop an objective appraisal of her migraine status.	
Grade point has dropped from and A-B average to C-D			5. Assist Lindsey to idenify destructive behaviors.	
Currently failing in algebra			6. Assist Lindsey in problem-solving situations made difficult because of migraines.	
Dropped out of band and prep squad this semester			7. Encourage increased level of self-care and responsibility.	

Parents have taken Lindsey to see a private therapist on a weekly basis since 2/18/99	8. Facilitate self expression with peers. 9. Assist Lindsey to identify strengths and reinforce examples of those strengths when observed. 10. Discuss alternative responses to stress. 11. Encourage constructive outlets for the expression of anger and frustration. 12. Facilitate Lindsey's acceptance of her parent's limitations. 13. In collaboration with the school counselor and private therapist, teach Lindsey new coping and problem-solving skills.	Lindsey will demonstrate a reduction of self-critical comments.

*See Appendix for student profile information to include on an IHP form.

REFERENCES

1. Evans RM, Scheier R. Migraine: what is migraine headache? *American Medical Association Health Insight.* 1997. Available at: http://www.ama-assn.org/insight/spec_con/migraine/whatis.htm. Accessed January 16, 1999.
2. Evans RM, Scheier R. Migraine: children and migraines. *American Medical Association Health Insight.* 1997. Available at: http://www.ama-assn.org/insight/spec_con/migraine/children.htm. Accessed January 16, 1999.
3. National Headache Foundation. *NHF fact sheet.* 1996. Available at: http://www.headaches.org/ facts.html. Accessed January 16, 1999.
4. National Headache Foundation. *Headache topics: migraine.* 1996. Available at: http://www.headaches.org.html. Accessed January 16, 1999.
5. Coleman MJ, Burchfield TM. *Myth vs. reality: an understanding of migraine disease and tips for migraine management.* Migraine Awareness Group: A National Understanding for Migraineurs. 1998. Available at: http://www.migraines.org/myth/mythreal.htm. Accessed January 16, 1999.
6. National Institute of Neurological Disorders and Stroke. *Headache: hope through research.* E-text revised 20 May 1998. Available at: http://www.ninds.hih.gov/healinfo/DISORDER/Headache/head1.htm. Accessed January 16, 1999.
7. Underwood A, Samuels A. The new war against migraines. *Newsweek* 1999;(Jan 11):46-52.
8. American Association for the Study of Headache. *Headache types.* 1997. Available at: http://www.aash.org/pediat/aura.html. Accessed January 16,1999.
9. Troost T. *Migraine and other headaches.* E-text revised 21 January 1998. Available at: http://www.rbdc.com~troost/gt/migraine/mige.html. Accessed February 4, 1999.
10. Rogers A. When pain runs in the family. *Newsweek* 1999;(Jan 11): 52-53.
11. Evans RM, Scheier R. Migraine: how is migraine treated? *American Medical Association Health Insight.* 1997. Available at: http://www.ama-assn.org/insight/spec_con/migraine/howis.htm. Accessed January 16, 1999.
12. Nordenberg T. Heading off migraine pain. *U.S. Food and Drug Administration* (online) May-June, 1998. Available at: http:www.fda.gov/fdac/features/1998/398_pain.html. Accessed January 16, 1999.
13. National Headache Foundation. *Headache topics: environmental and physical factors.* 1996. Available at: http://www.headaches.org.html. Accessed January 16, 1999.
14. National Headache Foundation. *Headache topics: hormones and migraine.* 1996. Available at: http://www.headaches.org.html. Accessed January 16, 1999.
15. Evans RM, Scheier R. Migraine: important information about drugs for mild-to-moderate migraine and tension-type headache pain. *American Medical Association Health Insight.* 1997. Available at: http://www.ama-assn.org/insight/ spec_con/migraine/mildmig.htm. Accessed January 16, 1999.
16. Migraine Awareness Group: A National Understanding for Migraineurs. *Treatment and management: current treatment methods.* 1998. Available at: http://www.migraines.org/treatment/treatctm.htm. Accessed January 16, 1999.
17. Evans RM, Scheier R. Migraine: important information about drugs for moderate-severe migraine. *American Medical Association Health Insight.* 1997. Available at: http://www.amaassn.org/insight/ spec_con/migraine/modmig.htm. Accessed January 16, 1999.
18. Smith R. Impact of migraine on the family. *Headache.* 1998;38(6): 423-426.

BIBLIOGRAPHY

American Association for the Study of Headache. *Headache types.* 1997. Available at: http://www.aash.org/pediat/aura.html. Accessed January 16, 1999.

Behrman R, Kliegman R. *Nelson Essentials of Pediatrics.* 3rd ed. Philidelphia, Pa: WB Saunders Company, 1998:715-717.

Coleman MJ, Burchfield TM. *Myth vs. reality: an understanding of migraine disease and tips for migraine management.* Migraine Awareness Group: A National Understanding for Migraineurs. 1998. Available at: http://www.migraines.org/myth/ mythreal.htm. Accessed January 16, 1999.

Evans RM, Scheier R. Migraine: children and migraines. *American Medical Association Health Insight.* 1997. Available at: http://www.ama-assn.org/insight/spec_ con/migraine/children.htm. Accessed January 16, 1999.

Evans RM, Scheier R. Migraine: how is migraine treated? *American Medical Association Health Insight.* 1997. Available at: http://www.amaassn.org/insight/spec_ con/migraine/howis.htm. Accessed January 16, 1999.

Evans RM, Scheier R. Migraine: important information about drugs for mild-to-moderate migraine and tension-type headache pain. *American Medical Association Health Insight.* 1997. Available at: http://www.ama-assn.org/insight/spec_con/migraine/ mildmig.htm. Accessed January 16, 1999.

Evans RM, Scheier R. Migraine: important information about drugs that prevent migraine. *American Medical Association Health Insight.* 1997. Available at: http://www.ama-assn.org/insight/ spec_con/migraine/drugprev.htm. Accessed January 16, 1999.

Evans RM, Scheier R. Migraine: important information about drugs for moderate-severe migraine. *American Medical Association Health Insight.* 1997. Available at: http://www.amaassn.org/ insight/spec_con/migraine/modmig.htm. Accessed January 16, 1999.

Evans RM, Scheier R. Migraine: what is migraine headache? *American Medical Association Health Insight.* 1997. Available at: http://www.ama-assn.org/ insight/spec_con/migraine/ whatis.htm. Accessed January 16, 1999.

Hay W, Groothuis J, Hayward A, Levin M. *Current Pediatric Diagnosis and Treatment.* 12th ed. Norwalk, Conn: Appleton & Lange, 1995.

Johnson M, Maas M. *Nursing Outcomes Classification (NOC).* St. Louis, Mo: Mosby Yearbook, 1997.

National Headache Foundation. *Headache topics: migraine.* 1996. Available at: http:// www.headaches.org.html. Accessed January 16, 1999.

National Headache Foundation. *NHF fact sheet.* 1996. Available at: http://www.headaches.org/ facts.html. Accessed January 16, 1999.

National Institute of Neurological Disorders and Stroke. *Headache: hope through research.* E-text revised 20 May 1998. Available at: http://www.ninds.hih.gov/healinfo/ DISORDER/Headache/ head1.htm. Accessed January 16, 1999.

Nordenberg T. Heading off migraine pain. *U.S. Food and Drug Administration* (online), May-June, 1998. Available at: http:www.fda.gov/fdac/features/1998/398_pain. html. Accessed January 16, 1999.

North American Nursing Diagnosis Association. *NANDA Nursing Diagnoses: Definitions & Classification 1999-2000.* Philadelphia, Pa: North American Nursing Diagnosis Assn, 1999. (NANDA, 1211 Locust Street, Philadelphia, PA 19167. 800-647-9002; fax 215-545-8107; e-mail:NANDA@nursecominc.com)

McCloskey J, Bulechek G. *Nursing Interventions Classification (NIC).* 2nd ed. St. Louis, Mo: Mosby Yearbook, 1996.

Migraine Awareness Group: A National Understanding for Migraineurs. *Treatment and management: current treatment methods.* 1998. Available at: http://www.migraines.org/treatment/ treatctm.htm. Accessed January 16, 1999.

Pryse-Phillips W, et al. Guidelines for the nonpharmacologic management of migraine in clinical practice. *CMAJ.JAMC* (online) 1998; (Jul). Available at: http://www.cma.ca/cmaj/vol-159/ issue-1/0047.htm. Accessed February 4, 1999.

Rogers A. When pain runs in the family. *Newsweek* 1999;(Jan 11): 52-53.

Smith R. Impact of migraine on the family. *Headache.* 1998;38(6): 423-426.

Troost T. *Migraine and other headaches.* E-text revised 21 January 1998. Available at: http://www.rbdc.com~troost/gt/migraine/mige.html. Accessed February 4, 1999.

Underwood A, Samuels A. The new war against migraines. *Newsweek* 1999;(Jan 11):46-52.

20 | IHP: Mitochondrial Disorders

Katherine J. Saffie

INTRODUCTION

Mitochondrial disorders have only been described and spoken of within the last ten years. These disorders are mainly inherited from the mother, but both parents may cause them. Mitochondrial disorders are mainly energy disorders. The reduced production of energy at the mitochondrial level results in a multifaceted impact on the individual's health, performance, and behavior. The disorders can affect the central nervous system, the musculoskeletal system, the heart, the kidneys, and the liver. The degree of involvement will vary.

Depending upon the degree of involvement, some children might appear to be well, and others may be wheelchair bound and tremulous. The mitochondrial group of diseases generally results in death in childhood or young adulthood.[1] Some of the various mitochondrial diseases are Leigh disease, Barth syndrome, Pearson syndrome, and Alpers disease. These disorders are progressive, but the speed of progression varies from individual to individual.[1]

Pathophysiology and Management

Every cell in the body except red blood cells contains mitochondria. Mitochondria are small and complex structures within the cell. Mitochondria carry their own DNA; this is separate from the cell's DNA. Each cell contains one to hundreds of mitochondria. Mitochondria are called the "power house" of the cell, because they are required to produce the majority of energy used for growth and vital functioning of the body. Mitochondria produce this energy by changing the by-products of food we eat into adenosine triphosphate (ATP), which is energy for the body. The higher the energy need of the organ, the more dependent the organ is on proper functioning mitochondria. The organs requiring the highest energy levels are the brain, heart, skeletal muscle, kidney, liver, and bone marrow.[2]

A metabolic disease develops when a significant number of mitochondria malfunction within the cells. The cells with the abnormal mitochondria vary in number from organ to organ and cell to cell. The malfunctioning of the mitochondria causes an interruption in the Krebs' cycle. The disease also leads to an increase in the organic acids of the body, which can lead to acidosis. Lactic acid is one of the organic acids that is commonly found to be increased in mitochondrial diseases, especially in the blood and spinal fluid. Mitochondrial diseases affect the functions of the brain, heart muscles, liver, and/or bone marrow. The diseases have a wide range of body systems involved and symptoms.

Mitochondrial diseases are inherited from the maternal side of the family. The reason for this is that the mitochondria are given to the fetus from the mother's egg.[3]

Due to the very different symptoms and age of onset, diagnosing a mitochondrial disease is sometimes difficult. Even within the same family, siblings may present with different symptoms and at an older or younger age.

In addition to a complete history and physical examination, samples of blood and urine are taken for specific tests, and a brain MRI and a muscle biopsy are done to make a final diagnosis. Once a diagnosis is made, the child should be referred to a healthcare site that specializes in mitochondrial disorders.

There is no cure for mitochondrial diseases at present. Individuals with a mitochondrial disease receive treatment for the signs and symptoms, such as cardiac arrhythmias, seizure disorder, or hypoglycemia. An experimental drug, diechloroacetate, is used to lower lactic acid levels. Most doctors place the patient on a regimen of cofactors and vitamins, thinking these will help the metabolic process. Some of these medicines include co-enzyme Q, carnitine, niacin, thiamine and riboflavin. Some patients are placed on special diets, from high fat to high carbohydrate to low fructose, and these are thought to help. Genetic counseling is also necessary for the parents. Education of the child and family is essential, in reference to the disease process, treatments, and prognosis. Research toward a more effective treatment and a cure is currently being conducted.

INDIVIDUALIZED HEALTHCARE PLAN

Assessment

History

- Onset of signs and symptoms
- Diagnosis and medical testing
- Primary care physician and specialists seen
- Seizure activity and neurologic involvement
- Respiratory involvement and signs and symptoms
- Growth and development history
- Nutritional supplements or interventions used during mealtime
- Food likes and dislikes
- Toileting, any assistance needed, or diapered
- Mobility, limitations, tone and strength of extremities
- Other system involvement—cardiac, liver, gastrointestinal, or urinary
- Allergies to insects, food, or medicine
- Visual or auditory concerns or problems
- Bedtime and rising time—does the student sleep through the night, if not, why and how long is her or she awake
- Migraines, head or abdominal, and if so, any aura
- Frequent colds or viruses
- Immunization history
- Communicable disease history

- Activity likes and dislikes
- Parent or guardian's knowledge of the disease process and treatment
- Student's knowledge of the disease process and treatment (if applicable)

Current Status and Management

- Baseline neurologic assessment
- Baseline respiratory assessment
- Baseline cardiac assessment
- Baseline height and weight
- Baseline skin integrity assessment
- Mobility needs, wheelchair or walker
- Extremities: strength, range of motion, tremors, and any orthotics
- Mealtime: amount of time needed, any special utensils or dishes, any assistance needed in feeding
- Toileting: frequency, any assistance needed, incontinence
- Stools: type, any constipation or diarrhea, if so treatment
- Speech: is it understandable, does the child speak in phrases or sentences, what language is used at home, what language does the child understand
- Current medications: name, dose, schedule, and route of administration
- Dietary supplements or snacks, type, amount, and times
- Treatments needed
- Therapy schedules and routines, if applicable
- Example of current routine day
- Signs and symptoms of impending illness: temperature, crying, lethargic, headache or stomach ache
- Amount of activity or class time the child is able to tolerate before needing rest periods
- Fine motor: any assistance needed from a modified pencil to computer equipment
- Special seating, glasses, or hearing aides needed
- Determine child's best and worst time of the day
- Signs and symptoms of fatigue: may need more rest periods or naps on certain days due to constantly changing energy level, may need modified activities, may need to eliminate activity
- Access to healthcare providers and services, facilities, insurance or financial needs
- Individual supplies needed
- Who are the caretakers at home, at daycare, before or after school

Self-care

- Ability to dress self
- Ability to feed self
- Ability to toilet self or signal when toileting is necessary
- Ability to carry out personal hygiene
- Knowledge of activity limits and when rest periods are needed
- Child knowledge of the signs and symptoms to watch for that signal the onset of illness

- Ability to self-administer medications, experience at home
- Decision-making skills

Psychosocial Status

- Child's perception of his/her health status
- Does the child interact with peers, how, specific activities in school, church and community?
- What is the child's age and developmental level?
- How does the child cope with doctor's visits and/or hospitalizations?
- Does the child participate in counseling or is counseling needed? Describe
- What classes does the child enjoy?
- What are the child's motivators?
- Behavioral issues, either at school or home
- Parent's/guardian's perception of child's current health status
- Support at home for the student with homework
- Family participation in community resources for psycho social issues regarding the child and his/her health status

Academic Status

- If the child was in school previously, were any schedule modifications or changes necessary?
- Does the child have a current special education program or 504 plan?
- Were any therapies given during school, or speech, occupational, or physical therapy?
- Previous school attendance and reason for absences
- Preferential seating due to vision or hearing disabilities
- Schedule: allow for rest periods and more important classes in the morning
- Need for a modified school day: early release, late start
- Special education or 504 involvement
- Nursing care needed during school
- Assistance needed for toileting, eating, mobility, or writing
- Transportation needs: to and from school, mobility around school (stairs, long distances)
- Therapies needed during school
- Out of school educational program: homebound, hospital-based

Nursing Diagnoses (N.D.)

N.D. 1 Alteration in nutrition - less than body requirements (NANDA 1.1. 2.2) related to:
  - high energy requirements
  - decrease in ability to chew/swallow

N.D. 2 Risk for alteration in urinary functional incontinence (NANDA 1.3. 2.1) related to:
  - involvement of the kidneys

N.D. 3 Risk for decrease in cardiac output (NANDA 1.4. 2.1) related to
  - involvement of heart muscle

N.D. 4 Risk for ineffective breathing pattern (NANDA 1.5. 1.3) related to:

- involvement of the lungs
- low energy

N.D. 5   Risk for alteration in neurologic status (NANDA 1.6. 1.3) related to:
- seizure activity
- stroke-like symptoms

N.D. 6   Risk for pain (NANDA 9.1.1) related to:
- frequent migraines, head and/or abdominal

N.D. 7   Risk for injury (NANDA 1.6.1.3) related to:
- trauma
- seizure activity
- stroke-like symptoms
- fatigue
- low muscle tone and strength

N.D. 8   Altered growth and development (NANDA 6.6) related to:
- high energy need
- poor nutritional intake

N.D. 9   Risk for impaired skin integrity (NANDA 1.6.2.1.2.2) related to:
- decrease in mobility
- incontinence
- orthotics
- G-tube placement
- altered fluid and nutritional intake

N.D. 10   Risk for sensory alteration (NANDA 7.2) related to:
- visual function/vision deficit
- sensory-neural hearing loss/hearing deficit

N.D. 11   Risk for impaired verbal communication (NANDA 2.1.1.1) related to:
- speech delay
- student's understanding of class/material
- student's decreased self-confidence

N.D. 12   Alteration in learning (NANDA 8.3) related to:
- absences from school/school attendance pattern
- decreased academic achievement
- amount of incomplete work
- activity tolerance
- lack of help/support from home
- school schedule in relation to activity tolerance/fatigue

N.D. 13   Risk for impaired physical mobility (NANDA 6.1.1.1) related to:
- low muscle tone and strength
- low energy level
- decreased activity tolerance

N.D. 14   Risk for activity intolerance (NANDA 6.1.1.3) related to:
- fatigue and low energy

N.D. 15   Risk for ineffective individual coping: student and family (NANDA 5.1.1.1 and 5.1.2.1.2) related to:
- resources of the family
- student's age
- student and/or parent knowledge deficit

N.D. 16 Impaired social interactions (NANDA 3.1.1) related to:
- decreased self-esteem
- school absences/ attendance pattern
- fatigue

N.D. 17 Alteration in self care (NANDA 6.5) related to:
- disease involvement
- fatigue
- knowledge deficit regarding the disease
- knowledge deficit regarding self-care activities
- healthcare procedures, treatments
- medication administration

Goals

Student will eat a balanced diet. (N.D. 1, 8, 9)

Student will maintain a stable weight and will not lose weight. (N.D. 1, 8)

Student will maintain proper fluid intake. (N.D. 1, 2, 9)

Student will increase knowledge of the signs and symptoms of the disease to report and the causes for the signs and symptoms. (N.D. 2, 3, 4, 5, 6)

Student will avoid triggers of pain, cough, or illness. (N.D. 2, 4, 6)

Student will ask for assistance, when needed. (N.D. 2, 3, 4, 5, 6, 7)

Student will increase knowledge of what activities to avoid and why. (N.D. 6, 7)

Student will maintain good urinary and bowel elimination pattern. (N.D. 2, 9)

Student will perform regular position changes. (N.D. 9)

Student will maintain proper/prescribed use of orthotics. (N.D. 9)

Student will report any hearing or visual change. (N.D. 10)

Student will wear prescribed glasses, or hearing aides or use preferential seating as needed. (N.D. 10)

Student will communicate needs to teachers, peers, and caregivers. (N.D. 11, 16)

Student will maintain a good school attendance pattern. (N.D. 12, 16)

Student will know and communicate the need for a rest period or possible changes in schedule. (N.D.12, 17)

Student will ask for extra help, when needed. (N.D. 12, 15)

Student will follow his/her prescribed exercise program from physical therapy. (N.D. 13, 15, 17)

Student will demonstrate good decision-making skills in choosing activities—in school, after school and/or in the community—that do not exceed his/her physical limitations. (N.D. 13, 14)

Student will increase his/her knowledge about his/her disease. (N.D. 15, 16, 17)

Student will participate in the development of his/her schedule and care plan. (N.D. 15, 16, 17)

Student will comply with his/her medical management plan. (N.D. 15, 17)

Interventions

Develop an Individual Education Program (IEP) for student. (N.D. 1-17)
- Include student, parent or guardians, healthcare providers, teachers, and other staff in development process.

- Coordinate home care with school hours, incorporating necessary treatments into the school day.
- Participate in IEP assessment plan, incorporating required health-related services into the IEP.
- In-service the staff to educate them on the signs and symptoms that should be brought to the nurse's attention.
- In-service the staff regarding special measures for transportation, recess, and field trips.
- In-service the staff regarding activity restrictions and modified or alternate activities for the student.
- Provide a list of staff members trained in the care of the student.
- Provide staff with emergency phone numbers and emergency contacts.
- Assist in obtaining medical releases signed to allow information to be shared between school and healthcare provider throughout the year.
- Arrange to have parent send in required equipment and/or supplies on a regular schedule.

Obtain orders and authorization for any treatments, medication, and special diet, if necessary, from both parent and physician. (N.D. 1-10, 13)
- Daily and PRN medications
- Special dietary intake and supplements
- Nursing treatments needed throughout the school day
- Special instructions for administering medication to the student
- Specific side effects to monitor for
- Any change in medication or treatments must be obtained in writing from the doctor and parent

Monitor activity tolerance, level of fatigue, and any contributory factors. (N.D. 1, 3, 4, 5, 6, 7, 8, 12, 13, 14)
- Develop a daily schedule with student, parent, and teacher.
- Avoid long walks to and from class or to the bathroom.
- Use the elevator instead of stairs.
- Assign a hall buddy and/or staff person to stop and rest with student and to carry his/her books.
- Allow student to have a second set of books at home to avoid carrying them back and forth to school.
- Provide alternate activities for student during gym period and recess, if necessary.
- Provide a rest or nap time, if necessary.
- Modify school schedule, as needed.
- Provide a quiet, designated area for resting.
- Encourage student to voice how he/she is feeling.
- Document the occurrence of any signs of fatigue and notice if there is a pattern.
- Notify parent and healthcare provider of a change in condition.
- If student uses a wheelchair, provide a travel friend between classes, to and from the bus, and to and from lunch and recess.
- Assign a staff person for responsibility and supervision of transporting the student.
- Develop an emergency plan (fire or other emergency), whether the student is ambulatory or in a wheelchair.

Assist teachers to modify curriculum, as needed. (NANDA 10,11,12,13)
- Avoid any excess writing for assignments, both in school and for homework.

- Use multiple choice, opposed to essay, questions for testing.
- Use computer in school or photocopy student's work or have someone assist student to write out assignments.
- Provide a longer time for specific assignments.

Provide a well-balanced, nutritious diet. (N.D. 1, 8)

- Incorporate the student's likes and dislikes pertaining to food.
- Know how student is able to drink.
- Provide texture of food student is able to tolerate (grind, cut).
- Provide adaptive equipment as needed.
- Allow student ample time for eating.
- Assist the student by preparing meals for eating (open cartons, cut meat, etc.).
- Give supplements as ordered.
- Provide a snack, if needed.
- If G-tube fed, administer the prescribed formula at the set rate.
- Note any signs of abdominal distention and notify parent and physician.
- Monitor intake of fluids and solids.
- Thicken liquids, if necessary.
- Document any change in intake and notify parent and physician.
- Monitor student's need for a short rest period during meals.
- Note any signs of dysphasia and report to parent and physician.
- If student must be fed, instruct the person doing the feeding in proper feeding technique; allow ample time between bites for chewing and swallowing, train feeder in Heimlich maneuver, and require a demonstration of skill.
- Weigh student monthly and record.
- Notify parent and physician of any weight loss and change weight checks to every two weeks.
- Avoid periods of fasting.

Monitor student's output. (N.D. 2)

- Discuss with parent and/or student: urine and bowel frequency at home.
- Toilet student at regular intervals and when needed.
- Provide staff to assist with toileting, if needed.
- If needed, ask parent to send a change of clothing to school.
- If diapered, change at regular times and when needed.
- Assist parents to provide needed supplies (diapers, clothes, etc.).
- Note color, odor, and amount of urine and stool.
- Document baseline urine and stool outputs.
- Notify parent and healthcare provider of any changes or concerns regarding output; document.
- Note any edema; document and notify parent and doctor.
- Note any change in stools, diarrhea or constipation, and notify parent and physician.

Monitor student's cardiac status. (N.D. 3)

- Obtain baseline apical pulse, rate and rhythm, and blood pressure and document assessment.
- Check pulse and blood pressure weekly, notify parent and physician of any change.
- If student complains of chest pain, assess type and location of pain and monitor vital signs and notify parent.

Monitor respiratory status. (N.D. 4)

- Obtain baseline assessment of respiratory rate, rhythm, and breath sounds and document.
- Check respiratory rate and breath sounds weekly and as needed, document assessment.
- Note any change in respiratory rate, rhythm, or breath sounds, notify parent and physician.
- Administer treatments and medications as ordered.
- Reassess student after treatment.
- Document response to treatment.
- Position child for optimal air exchange.
- Refer child to physician for new onset cough or congestion.
- Keep child away from others with respiratory infections.
- Note activities that cause child to become short of breath and avoid these or shorten the time to allow for rest.
- If suctioning is ordered, suction for increased congestion to maintain a patent airway.
- Avoid any allergens that might lead to respiratory congestion.

Assist student to dress appropriately for the weather, especially cold and rainy climates. (N.D. 4)

Monitor complaints of pain. (N.D. 6, 7)

- Assess type of pain and location.
- Assess for trauma that may be causing pain.
- Provide comfort measures, especially those that have worked in the past.
- Determine if this is new-onset or chronic pain.
- Try to determine factors precipitating pain and plan to avoid factors in the future.
- Provide medication for pain, as ordered.
- Document pain, type, onset, known causes, and relief.
- Document specific regimens that help alleviate the student's pain.
- Notify parent and physician of any new or increase in pain.

Monitor seizure activity and neurologic status. (N.D. 5, 6)

- Do a baseline neurologic assessment and document.
- Communicate with parent to keep school informed of any seizure activity changes in medication, and any alteration in neurologic status.
- Maintain a seizure record.
- Reassess neurologic signs monthly and as needed.
- Notify parent and/or physician of any change in neurologic status.
- Have student wear helmet, if needed, for ambulation.
- Make any accommodations, if student has weakness or immobility of one side.
- Take seizure precautions—stairs, swimming, and climbing.
- Note any specific time of day or activity that coincides with seizures. Inform parent and physician and plan to avoid activities that precipitate seizures, in the future.

Monitor vision status. (N.D. 10, 11, 12)

- Refer any visual complaints to healthcare provider.
- Provide visual screenings yearly.
- Assign preferential classroom seating, as needed.

- If student has glasses, assist the student to wear them.
- Inform the staff of the possible involvement of the mitochondrial disease on the eye.
- Discuss special education visual impaired services with special education team, if needed.
- Offer extra help in short intervals of time. Encourage incorporating alternate methods of learning, use keyboard, tape recorder and large print books in the classroom, as needed.
- Assist the student and teacher to obtain a reading buddy to read to student, as needed.
- Speak before approaching student.

Monitor hearing status. (N.D. 10, 11, 12)
- Provide audiological screenings yearly.
- Refer student to healthcare provider, if indicated.
- Obtain records from audiologist, if seen.
- Give preferential seating in class, if needed.
- Sit student away from window, door, projectors, ventilation system, and other noise-making areas.
- If student is to wear hearing aides or an FM transmitter, assist the student to insure he or she wears the hearing device and monitor function daily.
- Speak slowly and clearly.
- Look at student when talking.

Encourage student to verbalize needs. (N.D. 11, 15, 16, 17)
- Refer student to speech therapy, as needed.
- Assist the student to feel comfortable with surroundings and staff and peers.
- Provide a place with privacy.
- Listen carefully to child.
- Observe for facial expressions and grimaces.
- Coordinate services to provide the student with consistent care providers so the child can develop a relationship.
- Maintain student confidentiality; explain to the student that some information must be shared with parents, physicians, and/or teachers and the reason for it.
- Help educate the student on the disease process and symptoms to be aware of. (N.D. 1-17)
- Assist the student to report the symptoms to his or her parents and healthcare providers.

Educate teachers and other school staff. (N.D. 1-17)
- Describe what mitochondrial disorder is.
- Explain possible symptoms involved.
- Describe common symptoms.
- Relate importance of rest periods or shortened classes.
- Explain treatment and medication schedule during the school day.
- Describe ways to minimize energy use.
- Spell out activity restrictions/modifications needed.
- State importance of listening to student and reporting any symptoms.
- Describe signs and symptoms to watch for and report to the school nurse.
- Specify actions to take if a seizure occurs.
- Illustrate alternate learning techniques in class that may be needed.

- Detail need for good communication with the home.
- Make plan for make-up work, for frequent or prolonged absences.

Assist physical education teachers or adaptive physical education teachers to understand the need to provide activities that use little energy. (N.D. 13, 14)

- Assist them to observe the student's muscle strength and tone.
- Discuss possible modifications of activities or alternate activities that use less energy but promote flexibility and muscle tone.
- Avoid any climbing or swimming due to possible seizure.
- Include child in choices of activities.
- Encourage inclusion of a few friends to do alternate activities with student.

Assist parents, teachers, and healthcare providers in understanding the social benefits of a student being in a regular education class with peers either full time or for appro priate subject matter. (N.D. 16)

- Describe class modifications that may be required.
- Provide assistance of an adult.
- Assist the parent to observe the class.

Encourage the parent to communicate with school nurse and classroom teacher regularly or with any change in student's condition or treatment. (N.D. 15)

- Discuss need for change in schedule.
- Discuss need for increased nursing care at school.
- Develop a communication notebook.
- Provide one contact for healthcare providers, for necessary information to and from them.
- Encourage parents to inform school of upcoming appointments with healthcare providers.

Educate parent on school attendance policy and appropriate absences. (N.D. 15)

- Call school when child is absent.
- Send note upon student's return.
- Notify school nurse of any illness.
- Discuss signs and symptoms or complaints to listen to and keep child home.
- Contact the teacher or school for make-up work and/or tutoring.

Assist the child in self-care activities, treatments, and medications that they can participate in. (N.D. 15, 17)

- Monitor student's ability to perform self-care skills.
- Provide privacy for administration of medications or treatments.
- Discuss with the student the purpose and benefit of the treatment and/or medication.
- Reinforce proper technique in self-care activities.
- Assist student to store and access supplies.
- Help student identify positive and negative aspects of self-care.
- Minimize or alleviate negative aspects of self-care.
- Highlight positive aspects of self-care.

Provide health education to student's peers, if they choose. (N. D. 15, 16)

- Obtain parental permission and student permission.
- Discuss information that the parent and student want shared and information they do not want shared.
- Discuss any fears with the student and/or peers.
- Help the student feel more comfortable with peers.

Assist student, counselors, and parents to plan electives and schedule, when applicable. (N.D. 15, 16, 17)
- Identify and discuss with student alternate choices, when available.
- Educate the student on alternate activities that require low energy.

Monitor attendance pattern and reasons for absences. (N.D. 12)

Monitor academic performance. (N.D. 12)
- Watch academic progress: grades, ability to participate, increase in skills and knowledge.
- Make referral for 504 program, if needed.
- Make referral for special education, if needed.
- Reconvene special education team for additional services, if needed.
- Review IEP for appropriateness, yearly and as needed.
- Provide cognitive and academic testing yearly and after any severe medical trauma to determine changes in cognitive function.

Monitor changes in physical mobility. (N.D. 13)
- Compare to student's baseline strength and limitations of mobility.
- Note physical therapy involvement, progress toward and attainment of goals.
- Note occupational therapy involvement, progress toward or attainment of goals.
- Assist with range of motion on days with no therapy.
- Teach student and caregivers proper exercises and frequency.
- Educate the student and parent for the purpose of the exercises.
- Develop a weekly scheduled and give to teacher, parent, and student.
- Help child choose strengthening and endurance activities.
- If the child is able, encourage participation in team, including academic team activities, and contact sports.

Help student maintain positive body image. (N.D. 15, 16, 17)
- Provide privacy and assistance with toileting, if needed.
- Provide oral care during feeding.
- Provide oral care for drooling, avoid use of bibs.
- Elaborate on student's strengths.

Offer counseling for student. (N.D. 15, 16)

Expected Student Outcomes

The student will:
- participate in regular education classes, when able. (N.D. 12, 15, 16)
- participate in regular physical education classes with modifications made, as needed. (N.D. 3, 4, 5,6, 7, 13, 14)
- increase knowledge and choose alternate activities, if unable to participate in regular gym class or recess. (N.D. 7, 13, 14)
- maintain a good school attendance record. (N.D. 12, 13, 14, 15)
- demonstrate a good understanding and describe the disease process and list reasons for medications and treatments. (N.D. 2, 3, 15, 17)
- eat a balanced diet. (N.D. 1, 8, 14)
- participate in prioritizing school-day activities. (N.D. 12, 15)
- list signs and symptoms of a respiratory or viral illness. (N.D. 2, 4)
- report signs and symptoms of having a respiratory infection to parents and school nurse. (N.D. 4)

- dress appropriately for the weather. (N.D. 4)
- describe the need for regular physical therapy. (N.D. 13, 14)
- do exercises as prescribed and instructed. (N.D. 13, 14)
- report any changes in vision. (N.D. 10)
- wear glasses as prescribed. (N.D. 10)
- report any changes in hearing. (N.D. 10)
- wear hearing devices, if prescribed. (N.D. 10)
- assist in monitoring his or her weight. (N.D. 1, 8)
- will rest for regular intervals, as needed. (N.D. 7, 13, 14, 15)
- demonstrate avoidance of exposure to respiratory and other infections. (N.D. 4)
- report migraine or pain when it occurs. (N.D. 6)
- follow prescribed pain management plan, if migraine or pain occurs. (N.D. 6)
- wear helmet and/or orthotics, if needed. (N.D. 7, 13)
- demonstrate alternate ways to carry out activities. (N.D. 7, 13)
- assist in caring for his or her skin. (N.D. 9)
- demonstrate proper hand washing. (N.D. 2, 4, 9, 17)
- make regular position changes. (N.D. 9, 13, 17)
- communicate needs to teacher, aide, nurse, and parents. (N.D. 11, 15, 16, 17)
- demonstrate speaking slowly and clearly. (N.D. 11)
- participate in speech therapy if needed. (N.D. 11)
- finish all assigned class work with modifications made, as needed. (N.D. 12)
- ask for extra class help, when needed. (N.D. 12)
- complete assigned homework. (N.D. 12)
- have a consistent bedtime. (N.D. 14)
- participate in counseling, if needed. (N.D. 15)
- describe physical limitations due to disease. (N.D. 13, 14, 15)
- voice feelings, questions, or concerns regarding disease and/or treatments to parents, school nurse, and/or physician. (N.D. 15)
- interact with peers in school. (N.D. 16)
- assist in choosing appropriate work or travel buddies. (N.D. 16)
- demonstrate ability to self-care. (N.D. 17)
- follow prescribed rest and exercise plan. (N.D. 1, 3, 4, 6, 7, 13, 14, 17)
- demonstrate ability to modify rest and exercise plan based on activity tolerance. (N.D. 1, 3, 4, 6, 7, 13, 14, 17)

CASE STUDY

Sarah is a 10-year-old white female diagnosed with Leigh disease at the age of 4 years. She has one older sibling who was also diagnosed with the same disease. She lives at home with her mother and sees a specialist at Boston Children's Hospital.

Sarah's sitting, crawling, and walking developed slowly. She crawled at 9 months and walked at 16 months. She was toilet trained at 3 1/2 years of age. She became unsteady and began to fall regularly at age 3 1/2. After multiple tests and a muscle biopsy, she was diagnosed with Leigh disease. Since that time she has been gradually weakening. She was placed on Carnitine, co enzyme Q and vitamin C and carbamazepine (Tegretol).

She appears happy and answers questions appropriately. Her speech is difficult to understand. She drools continuously. She is small for her age with very thin arms and legs. She has constant fine tremors in her arms. She is able to follow commands. Breath sounds are clear. Apical pulse is 94 and regular. Blood pressure is 102/58mm Hg. Abdomen is soft and nontender with good bowel sounds. She is diapered. Her urine is clear amber. Bowel movements are once every two to three days. She is wheelchair bound, nonambulatory, but can stand to pivot, with assist. She wears ankle foot orthatics (AFO) on both lower extremities. Her last tonic clonic seizure was one year ago. She enjoys school. She attends some special education and some regular education classes.

EMERGENCY CARE PLAN

Date: January 18, 1999

Name: Sarah Jones   Birthdate: Grade: School:

Address: Phone:

Mother's name: Home phone   Day phone

Father's name: Home phone   Day phone

Emergency contact: Phone:

Healthcare provider: Phone:

Hospital preferred: Phone:

Child-Specific Emergencies

If You See This:	Action to take:
Seizure Activity:	Remove from danger
New Onset	Maintain airway
Prolonged	Activate 911 system
Cyanosis present	Nursing care as needed
	Notify parent
	Transport to hospital with nurse
	Send a copy of the student's medical history, medications, and emergency contacts to the hospital

Emergency Care Plan written by: School Nurse

Parent(s) Signature   Date:

Student Signature (if appropriate)

Individualized Healthcare Plan*
Mitochondrial Disorders

Assessment Data	Nursing Diagnosis	Goals	Nursing Interventions	Expected Outcomes
ND1 Small for age - weight 55 lb. Extremities thin.	Alteration in nutritional status. (NANDA 1.1.2.2) related to chewing and fatigue.	Sarah will maintain good nutritional intake of fluids and food.	1) Monitor student with meals at school 2) Provide supplements as ordered 3) Monitor for dyshagia—notify doctor 4) Provide proper consistency of food and drinks	Student will have a slow, steady weight gain.
ND4 Breath sounds clear, short of breath after activity. Occasional dry cough. No cyanosis.	Ineffective breathing pattern (NANDA 1.5.1.3) related to lung involvement and low energy.	Sarah will increase knowledge of activities that cause shortness of breath and avoid or choose alternate activities.	1) Position for good respiratory effort 2) Assess breath sounds, rate, rhythm of respiration weekly and prn and document 3) Notify parent/doctor of any change in respiratory status 4) Rest when needed.	Sarah will avoid activities that trigger shortness of breath.

ND5 Alert. Arms tremulous. Follows commands. Speech slightly garbled.	Risk for alteration in neurologic status (NANDA 1.6.1.3) related to seizure activity.	Sarah will maintain baseline neurologic status.	1) Do baseline neurologic assessment & document 2) Reassess neuro status 9 month & prn; compare to baseline assessment 3) Notify parent and physician of any change in neuro status.	Sarah will inform teacher/nurse of any aura headache.
ND 9 Diapered for stool and urine. Transported by wheelchair. AFO's on bilateral lower extremities. Frequent drooling.	Risk for impaired skin integrity (NANDA 1.6.2.1.2.2) related to immobility, incontinence, and orthotics.	Sarah will maintain proper skin integrity.	1) Shift weight once per class 2) Change diaper every three hours 3) Provide skin care with each diaper change 4) Check for redness/broken areas; document and notify parents 5) Remove AFO's for one hour each day and check skin.	Sarah's skin will remain intact with no redness.

*See Appendix for student profile information to include on an IHP form.

REFERENCES

1. Bailey I. "Living with Mitochondrial Disorders." Klehm M. "Medications for patients with Mitochondrial Disease." Portales A. "Neurodevelopmental and Educational Issues of Mitochondrial Disease." Presented at the Conference of Mitochondrial Disorders, Boston children's Hospital; May 18, 1995; Boston, Mass.
2. Downie J. *Mitochondrial diseases*. Available at: www.hmtnet.com/users/cobrown. Accessed 8/4/98.
3. *Mitochondrial Disorders*. Washington University School of Medicine. St. Louis, Mo. Available at: www.neuro.wusl.edu/neuromuscular/mitosyn.html. Accessed 8/4/98.

BIBLIOGRAPHY

Doenges ME, Moorhouse MF, Geissler A, Jeffries MF. *Nursing Care Plans: Guidelines for Planning Patient Care,* 2nd ed. Philadelphia, Pa: FA Davis Company, 1989.

Downie J, *Mitochondrial diseases,* Available at: www.hmtnet.com/users/cobrown. Accessed 8/4/98.

Mitochondrial Disorders, Harbor UCLA Medical Center. Available at: http://www.humc.edu Accessed 8/4/98.

North American Nursing Diagnosis Association. *NANDA Nursing Diagnoses: Definitions & Classification 1999-2000.* Philadelphia, Pa: North American Nursing Diagnosis Assn, 1999. (NANDA, 1211 Locust Street, Philadelphia, PA 19107. 800-647-9002; fax 215-545-8107; e-mail: NANDA@nursecominc.com)

Preston P, *Mitochondrial diseases: information for patients and parents.* Available at: www.netcentral.co.uk/last. Accessed 8/4/98.

21 | IHP: Neurofibromatosis

Sally Zentner Schoessler

INTRODUCTION

Neurofibromatosis is a genetically determined developmental disorder that is present at birth. Neurofibromatosis takes many forms in that many patients have very mild cases with little symptomatology, while other patients display dramatic and disfiguring effects. The disorder seems to be a result of a defect that alters peripheral nerve differentiation and growth[1] and affects equal numbers of males and females with no common racial, ethnic, or geographical denominators.[2]

The severity and complications involved in each form of neurofibromatosis create a unique challenge for the school nurse caring for that child. Each case must be evaluated on an individual basis with an individual plan of care.

Pathophysiology and Management

Neurofibromatosis has several distinct characteristics. Although these distinguishing findings are indicative of the disorder, it is important to stress that the symptoms will vary in severity in each child. The condition derives its name from neurofibromas, the most common type of tumor seen in the condition.

Neurofibromatosis is categorized into two distinct disorders. They are both autosomal dominant genetic disorders and while approximately half of the cases of neurofibromatosis are passed to the child from a parent, an equal number occur due to a spontaneous mutation in the sperm or egg cell. [3]

Neurofibromatosis Type 1 (NF1) —Peripheral NF

This is the more prevalent form of neurofibromatosis and has been associated with von Recklinghausen's disease. The following are signs of NF1:
>   Occurs in 1:4000 births
>   Multiple café au lait spots
>   Neurofibromas under the skin
>   Enlargement of bones and bone deformity
>   Scoliosis
>   Tumors of the brain and spinal cord
>   Learning disabilites[4]

Neurofibromatosis Type 2 (NF2) —Bilateral Acoustic NF

>   Occurs in 1:40,000 births
>   Multiple tumors of the cranial and spinal nerves
>   Other lesions of the brain and spinal cord
>   Tumors of both auditory nerves[4]

Café au lait spots become prominent in over 90% of patients with NF. These flat pigmented spots are usually present at birth or appear by the child's second birth-day and increase in number and darken in color throughout childhood. Axillary freckling is also present in most cases.[5]

Patients with NF also have Lisch nod-ules develop on the iris surface that appear as clear to yellow or brown elevations and increase in number as the child grows older.[1] They have no effect on vision, and appear at puberty. While they are an indi-cator of NF, they have no medical signifi-cance.

Many complications can be present with NF. These include:

- Disfigurement from tumors
- Visual abnormalities due to optic nerve tumors
- Auditory difficulties due to auditory nerve tumors
- Scoliosis
- Learning disabilities
- Bone defects including an absence of the orbital wall and congenital bowing of the tibia and fibula (often see pseu-darthrosis if bones are fractured)
- Hypertension caused by renal artery stenosis

Treatment tends to be symptom-specific, but the student must be treated in a holistic manner to provide care for all aspects of NF. Many children with NF can function well within the school setting with slight modifications in their activity. The school nurse needs to be attentive to the physical limitations of each child and be aware of the psychosocial issues involved when the child's condition is obviously disfiguring.

INDIVIDUALIZED HEALTHCARE PLAN

Assessment

History

- What symptoms led to the diagnosis of neurofibromatosis?
- At what age was the child diagnosed?
- Has the genetic link to neurofibromatosis been identified?
- What course has the condition taken to this time?
- What treatments have been used?
- What is the child's surgical history?
- What is the current medical management?
- How do the child and family feel about the child's condition?
- Does the child use any orthotic devices? Which ones?
- What is the child's prognosis at this time?

Current Status and Management

- Presence of neurofibromas
- Presence of café au lait spots and/or axillary freckling
- Presence of iris nevi and other complications
- Vision screening results
- Hearing screening results
- Scoliosis screening results
- Child's and family's knowledge of disease process
- What management program is in place for the child? Does the student demonstrate an understanding of the management plan?

- What treatments are currently being used?
- How often does the child see his/her specialist(s) and/or healthcare provider?

Self-care

- Can student demonstrate understanding of condition?
- Child's ability to demonstrate correct and appropriate use of any orthotic devices

Psychosocial Status

- Does child have any outwardly disfiguring symptoms? Does he/she verbalize feelings about symptoms?
- What fears does the child have about how others will react toward him/her?
- Child's verbalization of feelings about course of condition?
- Self-esteem status (based on positive versus negative comments about self)
- How does student relate to peers? Siblings? Parents?
- What activities is the child involved in with peers outside of school? Sports? Church? Community?

Academic Status

- Academic achievement
- Attendance pattern - reasons for absences
- Use of orthotic at school?
- How does student feel about wearing orthotic at school?
- Does student have a strong peer group? Does student have friends at school? In classes? At lunch?
- Does student participate in after-school activities?
- Modifications needed in physical education program
- Need for 504 plan or Special Education services?

Nursing Diagnoses (N.D.)

N.D. 1 (Risk for) injury (NANDA 1.6.1) related to bone abnormalities and pseudarthrosis

N.D. 2 (Risk for) sensory/perceptual alteration—visual, (NANDA 7.2) related to (potential) tumors of the optic nerve

N.D. 3 (Risk for) sensory/perceptual alteration—auditory (NANDA 7.2) related to (potential) tumors of the auditory nerve

N.D. 4 (Risk for) altered growth and development (NANDA 6.6) related to (potentially) progressive skeletal abnormalities and complications

N.D. 5 (Risk for) body image disturbance (NANDA 7.1.1) related to numerous neurofibroma tumors, café au lait spots, and skeletal abnormalities

N.D. 6 (Risk for) self-esteem disturbance (NANDA 7.1.2) related to altered body appearance, physical limitations, and/or learning difficulties

N.D. 7 (Risk for) knowledge deficit (NANDA 8.1.1) regarding effective treatment of symptoms and possible progression of disease

Goals

Student will not experience injury or reinjury at school. (N.D. 1)

Student will develop and use/demonstrate adaptations that are needed to attain and maintain academic and social success in the school setting. (N.D. 1)

Student will maintain maximum potential for vision and hearing. (N.D. 2,3)

Student will identify any visual or auditory problems in early stages to promote early intervention. (N.D. 2,3)

Symptoms of skeletal involvement of tumors and/or scoliosis will be identified early to promote early intervention in care. (N.D. 4)

Student will demonstrate (increased) acceptance of and psychological comfort with body image. (N.D. 5)

Student will demonstrate (increased) self-acceptance and positive self-esteem. (N.D. 6)

Student will increase knowledge of disease process and possible progression of disease (as is age appropriate). (N.D. 7)

Nursing Interventions

Assist teacher to modify physical education program as needed. (N.D. 1)

Encourage participation in activities that do not increase risk for injury. (N.D. 1)

Monitor use of brace or orthotic in physical education and all physical activities (as prescribed). (N.D. 1)

Review brace or orthotic care with student (as needed). (N.D. 1)

Observe for signs of pressure on skin underneath brace. (N.D. 1)

Review injury prevention measures with physical education teacher(s) to decrease risk of injury. (N.D. 1)

Review injury prevention measures with faculty and staff to decrease risk of injury. (N.D. 1)

Screen student's vision twice a year and as needed. (N.D. 2)

Screen student's hearing twice a year and as needed. (N.D. 2)

Encourage student to report any problems with his or her ability to see. (N.D. 2)

Encourage student to report any problems hearing in the classroom. (N.D. 3)

Notify parents and assist them in accessing their healthcare provider if any alteration in screening results are noted. (N.D. 2,3,4)

Request teachers to inform you if they suspect the student has visual or hearing difficulties in the classroom. (N.D. 2)

Screen student for scoliosis twice/per year and as needed. (N.D. 4)

Monitor student's height and weight. (N.D. 4)

Allow student to verbalize feelings about condition and body alterations. (N.D. 5,6)

Arrange for private dressing area when changing clothes for physical education. (N.D. 5)

Provide positive feedback to student as needed. (N.D. 6)

Assist family in accessing counseling and other community resources as needed. (N.D. 6)

Encourage student to become active in school activities and community groups (appropriate to activity limitations). (N.D. 6)

Provide student with age-appropriate information about neurofibromatosis. (N.D. 7)

Discuss prognosis with family and student, help student to understand the potential body changes of adolescence as indicated. (N.D. 7)

Discuss treatment options that are available with family and student, as indicated (N.D. 7)

Expected Student Outcomes

Student will not experience injury. (N.D. 1)

Student will participate in school activities with modifications as needed. (N.D. 2,6)

Student will demonstrate understanding of measures necessary to prevent injuries. (N.D. 1)

Student will wear brace or orthotic during physical education classes and other activities that have potential for injury. (N.D. 1)

Student will maintain the maximum visual acuity as his/her condition allows. (N.D. 2)

Student will maintain the maximum auditory acuity as his/her condition allows. (N.D. 3)

Student will assist in bringing vision, hearing and scoliosis information to parents and healthcare provider. (N.D. 2,3,4)

Student will participate in scoliosis screening. (N.D. 4)

Student will experience adequate growth and development. (N.D. 4)

Student will verbalize feelings about body and self-image. (N.D. 6,7)

Student will increase involvement in school activities and/or community groups. (N.D. 7)

Student will demonstrate an age-appropriate understanding of his/her condition and prognosis. (N.D. 7)

CASE STUDY

Elizabeth Clarke is a 12-year-old student, diagnosed with neurofibromatosis as an infant. She has numerous neurofibromas and café au lait spots, but they are not pronounced on the visible parts of her body.

The primary cause for concern for Elizabeth's medical and nursing management is a pseudarthrosis of the left tibia. She has had numerous fractures of the bone and has been surgically treated several times including bone grafting. The last procedure was performed when Elizabeth was 5 years old and involved an Ilizarov brace which corrected the nonunion of the bone and allowed for proper growth of the left leg. She wears a brace at all times to protect her left leg. Her physical education activities need to be limited to noncontact, nonstress sports. She is allowed to run and enjoys modified physical activities.

Elizabeth is followed yearly by a pediatric neurologist and this includes MRIs every other year. Her parents have provided the school health office with the phone numbers of her doctors and emergency instructions should her leg become injured or should she report symptoms such as dizziness.

Individualized Healthcare Plan*
Neurofibromatosis

Assessment Data	Nursing Diagnosis	Goals	Nursing Interventions	Expected Outcomes
ND1 Elizabeth's left leg is susceptible to fractures. Elizabeth has had several surgeries, including use of the Ilizarov technique, to left leg.	Risk for injury due to bone abnormalities and pseudoarthrosis. (NANDA 1.6.1)	Elizabeth will not experience injury or reinjury at school. Elizabeth will develop and use/demonstrate adaptations that are needed to attain and maintain academic and social success in the school setting.	Assist PE teacher to modify physical education program as needed. Monitor use of leg brace in PE and all physically active settings. Encourage participation in activities that do not increase risk for injury. Review brace care with Elizabeth PRN. Observe for signs of pressure on skin underneath brace. Review injury prevention measures with PE teacher to decrease risk of injury. Instruct student and PE teacher in correct procedures should an injury occur. Review injury prevention measures with faculty and staff to decrease risk of injury.	Elizabeth will not experience injury. Elizabeth will participate in school activities with modifications PRN. Elizabeth will wear her brace during PE and other potentially injurious situations. Elizabeth will demonstrate understanding of measures necessary to prevent injuries.

ND2 Elizabeth is at risk for decreases in visual and auditory function.	Risk for sensory/ perceptual alterations: visual-related to potential tumors of the optic nerve. (NANDA 7.2)	Elizabeth will maintain maximum potential for vision and hearing.	Screen Elizabeth's vision twice a year. Notify parents and assist them in accessing their healthcare provider if any alteration in screening results are noted.	Elizabeth will retain the maximum visual acuity as her condition allows.
	Risk for sensory/ perceptual alterations: auditory-related to potential tumors of the auditory nerve. (NANDA 7.2)	Elizabeth will identify any visual or auditory problems in early stages to promote early intervention.	Screen Elizabeth's hearing twice a year. Request teachers to inform you if they suspect the student has visual or hearing difficulties in the classroom.	Elizabeth will retain the maximum auditory acuity as her condition allows.
ND4 Elizabeth is at an increased risk to develop scoliosis.	Risk for altered growth and development due to potentially progressive skeletal anomalies and complications. (NANDA 6.6)	Elizabeth will have any skeletal involvement of tumors and/or scoliosis identified early to promote early intervention in care.	Screen for scoliosis twice a year. Alert parents and assist them in accessing their healthcare provider if any alteration in results are noted.	Elizabeth will have signs of scoliosis identified early and be referred for medical intervention.

*See Appendix for student profile information to include on an IHP form.

REFERENCES

1. Wong DL Hockenberg-Eaton M, Wilson D, Winkelstein ML, Ahmann E, Divito-Thomas PA, eds. *Whaley and Wong's Nursing Care of Infants and Children* 6th ed. St. Louis, Mo: Mosby, 1999: 865, 856.
2. *Neurofibromatosis*, What is neurofibermatosis? [Online]. Available at: http://www.nfinc.org/whatisnf.html Accessed 1/23/99.
3. Rubenstein A, Korf FB. *A Handbook for Patients, Families, and Health-Care Professionals*. New York, NY: Thieme Medical Publishers, 1990.
4. National Neurofibromatosis Foundation, What is neurofibromatosis? *[Online]. Available at:* http://www.neurofibromatosis.pat1.htm Accessed 1/23/99.
5. Behrmann RE, Klingman RM. *Nelson Essentials of Pediatrics*. 2nd ed: Philadelphia, Pa: WB Saunders Company, 1994: 706.

BIBLIOGRAPHY

Behrmann RE, Klingman RM. *Nelson Essentials of Pediatrics*. 2nd ed. Philadelphia, Pa: WB Saunders Company, 1994.

National Neurofibromatosis Foundation, (1998) *What is Neurofibromatosis?* [Online]. Available at: http://www.neurofibromatosis.pat1.htm Accessed 1/23/99.

Neurofibromatosis, What is Neurofibromatosis? [Online]. Available at: http://www.nfinc.org/whatisnf.html Accessed 1/23/99.

North American Nursing Diagnosis Association. *NANDA Nursing Diagnoses: Definitions & Classification 1999-2000*. Philadelphia, Pa: North American Nursing Diagnosis Assn, 1999. (NANDA, 1211 Locust Street, Philadelphia, PA 19107. 800-647-9002; fax 215-545-8107; e-mail: NANDA@nursecominc.com)

Rubenstein A, Korf FB. *A Handbook for Patients, Families, and Health-Care Professionals*. New York, NY: Thieme Medical Publishers, 1990.

Serving Students with Special Care Needs. Hartford, Conn: State of Connecticut Department of Education, 1992.

Wong DL. *Clinical Manual of Pediatric Nursing*. 4th ed. St. Louis, Mo: Mosby-Year Book, 1996.

Wong DL, Hockenbery-Gaton M, Wilson D, Winkelstein ML, Ahmann E, Divito-Thomas PA, eds. *Whaley and Wong's Nursing Care of Infants and Children*. 6th ed. St. Louis, Mo: Mosby, 1999.

22 | IHP: Ophthalmic Conditions

Tamara Gonzalez Oberbeck

INTRODUCTION

Eye problems in the school setting range from an eyelash in the conjunctival cul-de sac the to pink eye to a penetrating eye injury from industrial education class. With the increased popularity and relatively inexpensive cost of soft contact lenses, eye infections and corneal abrasions related to contact lens use are being seen with increasing frequency. Dealing with eye problems and the potential loss of vision is a challenge for most school nurses. Although ocular complaints represent less than one fourth of all visits to the school health office, eye complaints represent the vital sense of sight. It is therefore imperative that the school nurse have a basic understanding of the anatomy, physiology, significant signs and symptoms, treatment, and prevention of eye problems.

The importance of prevention cannot be overstressed. School nurses have an opportunity to educate and promote prevention of eye injuries in the school setting. Conducting periodic checks in the industrial education classes to make sure that individual students are wearing eye protection, teaching hygiene and care of soft contact lenses, and discussing the prevention and spread of conjunctivitis during a presentation on infectious diseases in health class are a few ways that school nurses may become more involved in promoting eye care and prevention of blindness.

Pathophysiology

When a person looks at an object, the light rays are directed in parallel lines to the cornea of the eye where they pass through the cornea, the lens, and the vitreous. These rays of light are then bent to project an upside-down image on the retina of the eye where they are transmitted to the brain to be interpreted by the occipital lobe.

The tissue and structure surrounding the eye are referred to as the adnexa. The bony orbit provides protection for the eyes. Also in the bony orbit are the six extrinsic eye muscles, which move the eyeball. The lacrimal glands located in the upper eyelid secrete tears, which not only keep the cornea moist but also contain lysozomes. Lysozymes are a bactericidal enzyme. Without this tear film the cornea, which consists of five distinct layers of living cells, would dry out and become cornified.

The eyelid and, particularly, the strong tarsal plates protect the cornea from many possible foreign bodies. The eyelid works much like the protective cap of a delicate camera, protecting the more delicate interior structures of the eye.

The outer layer, which protects the fluid-filled center, is referred to as the sclera and the cornea. The cornea, which is located anteriorly, is transparent and must be kept moist by the tear film at all times. The cornea consists of five layers. The epithelium, which acts as the first line of defense against infection or injury; Bowman's membrane, an anchor for the epithelial layer; the stroma, which is the thickest body; Descemet's membrane, which gives rigidity and form to the cornea; and the endothelium, which works like a pump to maintain the proper fluid balance. The cornea is very sensitive, having many exposed nerve endings. Damage to the corneal epithelium results in pain, which generally prompts the patient to seek medical attention. The epithelium will heal and regenerate in 24 hours. Damage to the innermost corneal layers can cause serious infection and result in permanent scarring.

The middle layer of the eye is referred to as the uvea tract and consists of the iris, ciliary body, and the choroid. The iris and ciliary body consist of a muscular structure that aids in focusing the light. The choroid is the vascular system that provides nutrition to the outer half of the retina.

The innermost layer of the eye is the retina. The retina is often compared to the film of a camera. It is the structure that perceives both black and white (rods) and color (cones) light. The numerous layers of the retina are held tightly together to the choroid by a clear jellylike substance called the vitreous humor.

Common Eye Problems

Foreign Body—A complete detailed history is important when assessing a foreign body in the eye. Was the student in shop class working with high-powered drills or sanders? Was he or she outside on a windy day? Or did the student suddenly feel something in his or her eye?

The most common foreign body is an eyelash, most often found in the lower cul-de sac of the conjunctiva. These are easy to remove by irrigation using a sterile eye solution or by gently touching the tip of a wet applicator stick or wet gauze to the eyelash. To irrigate the eye ask the student to look up with both eyes while the student looks up, pull the lower lid down and place the sterile solution into the lower cul-de-sac of the eye. Remember that the cornea is very sensitive, and it is important to direct the stream of eye solution on the conjunctiva. Applying eye drops or eye solutions directly on the cornea will elicit a natural response of pulling away or squeezing the eyelids closed.

The second most common foreign body is dirt, dust, or gravel that has blown into the eye on a windy day. These small pieces of dirt frequently lodge under the upper lid in the palpebral conjunctiva. These small lodged pieces of dirt or gravel can cause a corneal abrasion by scratching the cornea with each blink of the eye. These are fairly easy to remove by turning the upper lid and touching gently with a wet applicator stick or irrigating them off with a stream of sterile eye irrigant.

Turning the upper lid is easily done if you remember to use the tarsal plate in the upper lid to aid in turning the lid. Ask the student to keep **BOTH** eyes open and to look down with both eyes. Using both eyes is the key to this trick. Gently grasp the eyelashes of the affected eye at the base of the lash line. Place the applicator stick horizontally on the upper rim of the tarsal plate and gently pull the lashes out and up over the applicator stick to expose the under side of the upper lid. Remind the patient to keep both eyes open and to continue looking down at his or her knees at all times. Look for the foreign body and remove with a wet applicator stick.

If the foreign body is lodged on the cornea, do not attempt to remove it. Lightly patch the eye, place a protective shield over it, and refer the patient to an ophthalmologist for removal.

Conjunctivitis—Conjunctivitis is an inflammation of the conjunctiva. This inflammation can affect the palpebral or bulbar conjunctiva. Any inflammation of the conjunctiva causes the small conjunctival blood vessels to swell and appear pink, hence the name pinkeye. The most common causes of conjunctivitis are bacteria, virus, or allergies.

Bacterial conjunctivitis is characterized by a mucopurulent discharge, a diffuse hyperemia of the conjunctiva, and sometimes swelling or discomfort of the preauricular node. The student will often state that his or her eyelids are sealed shut with a discharge upon waking in the morning. A broad-spectrum antibiotic eye drop is usually recommended and recovery is generally complete in fewer than two weeks. Keeping the hands away from the eyes and frequent hand washing will aid in preventing the spread of the bacteria from one eye to the other and from one person to another.

Viral conjunctivitis is caused by the adenovirus. Epidemic keratoconjunctivitis is a common form and is very contagious. It is characterized by a watery discharge, presence of preauricular nodes, and complaints of eyelids sticking together in the morning. Examine the conjunctiva by asking the student to look up while gently pulling the lower lid down. Note any changes in the palpebral conjunctiva. The palpebral conjunctiva may look as if it is covered with numerous small clear follicles.

Allergic conjunctivitis is usually seasonal and accompanied by other allergic symptoms. A history of allergies usually exists. Allergic conjunctivitis causes conjunctival edema, tearing, and itching. Redness and swelling of the lids may also be present. If this is a chronic problem, the palpebral conjunctiva may have a cobblestone appearance. Topical steroids may be needed, but an over-the-counter eye drop for red itchy eyes or cold compresses may be used for temporary relief. Referral to an allergist may be recommended if the problem is interfering with the student's school/classroom activities and performance or if it has become a chronic problem.

Blepharitis—Blepharitis is the most common inflammation of the eyelids. It usually involves a purulent discharge along the lid margin. It is frequently associated with conjunctivitis. Treatment usually consists of thorough cleansing of the eyelids, warm compresses to relieve discomfort and increase blood supply, and topical antibiotics.

Chalazions—A chalazion is an inflammation of the meibomian gland. It forms a nontender solid lump under the eyelid. They are easily visible on the outside of the eyelid. When the lid is lowered, a distinct red inflamed nodule can be noted. The chalazion can be surgically removed, but sometimes a warm compress several times a day to the area will aid in breaking up the congested gland.

Styes—A stye, also know as an external hordeolum, is caused by an infection of the eyelash follicle. It will appear as a small, red, tender nodule along the lash line. Hot moist packs and antibiotic drops are the most common treatment plans.

Corneal Abrasions—When the integrity of the corneal epithelium is disrupted, either by a foreign body or a scratch to the eye, the result is a corneal abrasion. Even a small scratch to the epithelium results in a very painful, uncomfortable eye, due to the numerous nerve endings beneath the corneal epithelium. The most common symptom is the feeling of something in the eye. This sensation is more noticeable when the student blinks his/her eye, as the upper eyelid rubs over the surface of the abrasion. A superficial corneal abrasion is very common and heals rapidly in 24 hours if there is no infection. A pressure patch prevents the upper eyelid from rubbing over the abrasion and aids the healing process.

Contact Lenses—Soft contact lenses are becoming increasingly more common at a younger age. More than 80% of contact lens users wear soft contact lenses. These soft contact lenses are more comfortable and easier to adjust to than the rigid contact lenses. They require meticulous care, cleaning, and disinfecting. Frequent hand washing is a must with contact lens wearers. In addition to hand washing, removing the soft contact lens each evening for careful disinfecting is required. The new cosmetic lenses are sometimes shared among students, a practice that should be discouraged at all times.

Any student seen by the school nurse with a pink, painful eye in which a contact lens is used must be suspected of a possible eye infection. The student should be advised to remove the contact lens and a parent should be notified of a potential eye infection. Wearing lenses too long, wearing lenses that have not been properly cleaned, or wearing lenses that are damaged can lead to serious corneal infections and permanent corneal damage.

Encourage students to keep an extra contact lens case and solution at school if they wear contact lenses at school.

Eye Emergencies

More than one million people suffer from eye injuries each year in the United States. More than 90% of these accidents could have been prevented. School nurses should encourage eye safety throughout the school. School nurses have the opportunity to teach about safety by promoting use of safety glasses in the industrial education classes, protecting the eyes from chemicals in the kitchen, and safely handling chemicals used in cleaning. The following situations constitute an eye emergency and should be referred for evaluation and treatment immediately.

Chemical Injuries—Chemical injuries to the eye are divided into two different

categories: *alkali or acid burns*, which can cause serious damage to the eye, and *chemical irritants*, which cause discomfort and irritation but are less severe. All chemicals should be irrigated with the eye fully open for at least 15 minutes. Flood the eye with water immediately, continuously and gently. Remember that the cornea is very sensitive. The eye should be kept wide open during irrigation, avoiding direct contact with the sensitive cornea. The important action is to dilute the chemical as quickly as possible.

Alkalines are very dangerous and will cause the most destructive damage to the cornea. Even a very small amount of alkaline left in the eye can cause severe injury to the cornea. (Alkaline compounds are found in plaster, cement, whitewash, and liquid or powders used to open clogged drain pipes.) If a student is suspected of having an alkaline solution splashed in his or her eye, continue to irrigate the eye for a full 15 to 20 minutes and refer him or her *immediately* to an ophthalmologist or emergency room for evaluation and care.

Penetrating Objects—High-powered equipment in the industrial education class can cause a small or large object to penetrate the eyelid, cornea, or globe of the eye. Never try to remove a penetrating object from an eye or eyelid. Reassure the student, place a large paper cup over the eye being careful not to exert any pressure on the eye or globe, call emergency care personnel for transport to nearest emergency room, and call parents.

Blunt Injuries—Severe, blunt injuries, with a fist, or small, hard balls can be potentially dangerous because they can cause hyphema (bleeding into the anterior chamber), or retinal detachment. Apply a cold compress immediately, and phone the parent(s) to inform them of the injury and the potential effects of the injury. Advise them to call their healthcare provider or ophthalmologist for evaluation and care.

INDIVIDUALIZED HEALTHCARE PLAN

Assessment

History

The history is important to determine the potential seriousness of the eye problem. The ocular history should describe any eye problem the student is having—usually in a reverse chronological order, from the present to the past. The following questions should be asked.

- What is the chief complaint?
- What were you doing at the time of the eye problem?
- When did the problem start?
- Do you wear glasses?
- Have you ever had any eye surgery or eye problems in the past?
- Have you ever been treated for a serious eye problem?
- Are you using any eye medication now?

An example is a complaint of a foreign body. A student who states that he or she was working in the industrial education shop without his/her safety goggles, using high-speed equipment, could have a serious penetrating injury. In contrast, a student who reports that he or she was walking outside on a windy day and suddenly felt "something" in the eye is likely to have a superficial foreign body found in the upper or lower eyelid.

Visual acuity—A test of visual acuity should be taken on any student with an ocular complaint. This is important for legal purposes later. A 20-foot Snellen chart is preferred; for young children an illiterate "E" chart or an HOTV chart may be used. The charts are inexpensive and come in ten-and twenty-feet room length size. After positioning the student the recommended distance from the chart, cover the left eye first, instructing the student to keep both eyes open. Ask the student to begin with the largest letter and read down as far as he or she can read without squinting or straining. Test the right eye first, then the left. It is important to obtain the visual acuity from both eyes even if only one is injured. Note the visual acuity on the health record.

After obtaining the visual acuity, assess the eye systematically, in the following order:

External Eye Exam—The eyelids cover and protect the eyeball. They protect the eye from serious injury. The eyelids aid in the lubrication of the ocular surface and produce the tear film. Carefully examine both the upper and lower eyelids. Check for any lacerations, redness, inflammation, crusting along the lid margin, styes, cyst, or chalazions.

Conjunctiva—The conjunctiva is a thin translucent mucous membrane that lines the inner surface of the upper and lower eyelid and the front surface of the eyeball, excluding the cornea. It consists of many blood vessels and becomes very red and inflamed upon any irritation or inflammation. Evaluate both the palpebral and bulbar conjunctiva. The palpebral conjunctiva covers the upper and lower lid. The bulbar conjunctiva covers the globe of the eye. Ask the student to look up and pull the student's lower lid down checking the palpebral conjunctiva for any redness, inflammation, follicular change, cobblestone appearance, exudate, or foreign body, such as an eyelash. To examine the bulbar conjunctiva instruct the student to look up, down, then to the right and then to the left. Note any inflamed blood vessels, hemorrhage, or irritation.

Cornea—The cornea is a tough, crystal clear membrane. It receives its nourishment from the tear film. It consists of numerous sensory nerve endings, which cause great pain and sensitivity if affected by a foreign body, scratch, or abrasion. A foreign body sensation is often present with an abrasion or scratch. To examine the cornea, ask the student to look straight ahead and look at the cornea and iris, working around in a clock-like pattern. Start at 12:00, l: 00, 2:00, and so on, checking for clarity of the cornea, scars, or foreign bodies. Carefully examine and observe the iris at the same time for abnormalities.

Pupil—The iris, ciliary body, and choroid come together to form the uveal tract. It is the center of these systems that forms the open window known as the pupil. A traumatic blow to the eye, a penetrating injury, infection of the uveal tract, or various neurologic problems may cause an abnormal pupil. To examine the pupil, dim the lights and ask the student to look straight ahead. Swing a light in from the side and note its size, shape, and reaction to light. Pupils should be round, symmetrical, and react to light and accommodation equally (PERLA).

Nursing Diagnosis (N.D.)

N.D. 1 Impaired tissue integrity (corneal, eyelid, etc.) (NANDA 1.6.2.1) related to:
- mechanical injury
- chemical injury
- infection

N.D. 2 Alteration in sensory perception (visual) (NANDA 7.2) related to:
- eye injury
- eye infection

N.D. 3 Pain (NANDA 9.1.1) related to:
- corneal abrasion
- eye, lid laceration
- eye injury
- conjunctival inflammation

N.D. 4 Noncompliance with medication or treatment plan (NANDA 5.2.1.1) related to:
- individual issues (wearing eye patch, remembering to use medication, etc.)
- family issues (financial, transportation for access to care, etc.)

N.D. 5 Alterations in sensory perception (depth perception) (NANDA 7.2) related to:
- eye being covered with a patch
- loss of vision in one eye (temporary or permanent)

N.D. 6 Risk for injury (NANDA 1.6.1) related to alteration in depth perception due to need for eye patch

N.D. 7 Knowledge deficit (NANDA 8.1.1) regarding:
- need for and use of eye protection glasses or goggles
- healing process of the eye tissue

Goals

The student will:
- participate in measures to prevent eye infections. (ND 1,2)
- participate in measures to prevent reinfection of his/her eye(s). (ND 1)
- participate in measures that promote healing of the eye injury. (ND 3,4,7)
- attain/maintain preinjury visual acuity. (ND 2,5)

- be compliant with the prescribed treatment and medication plan. (ND 4)
- access and utilize healthcare providers for eye problems, treatment, and follow-up care. (ND 1,2,3,4)
- safely move about and participate in activities in the school environment. (ND 6)
- increase knowledge regarding eye injuries and the healing process of the eye. (ND 7)
- increase knowledge of eye injury prevention. (ND 7)
- maintain eye safety by participating in measures to prevent eye injuries at school, at home, and in sports activities. (ND 5,6,7)

Nursing Interventions

Promote and provide information to school staff and students regarding maintaining eye safety in the classroom, in sports activities, and in the school environment. (ND 1,7)

Provide health reminders in all restroom facilities and in the health office educating students about the importance of frequent hand washing to reduce the risk of all types of infections, including eye infections. (ND 1)

Assess all eye complaints for signs of infection or trauma. (ND 1-3)

Assist parents with referral to an ophthalmologist / healthcare provider / emergency room, as needed. (ND 1-5)

Inform teachers of student's possible visual needs: (ND 1,2,4,6)
- preferential seating in the front of the classroom
- possible problems with depth perception if one eye is patched
- sensitivity to light (indoor and sunlight)
- need for time to take medication during school hours
- need for assignment modifications (due to eye pain/discomfort, fatigue)

Administer (or assist the student to administer) eye medications as directed by the physician. (ND 1,3)

Replace eye patch as needed or prescribed, note any: (ND 1,2,3,4)
- discharge
- new or increased pain
- increased sensitivity to light

Explain the importance of administering medication according to the physician's instructions, and the importance of wearing the eye patch and completing the follow-up care that was prescribed. (ND 1,4)

Assist the parents to obtain follow-up care as prescribed or as indicated by the physician. (ND 4)

Explain the role of healthcare providers (primary care physician, ophthalmologist, and school nurse) in treating the symptoms of an eye infection or injury. (ND 1,2,3,4,7)

Consult with the physical education teachers concerning physical activity limitations: (ND 1,2,5,6)
- visual acuity issues
- depth perception issues (catching and hitting activities)
- risk for reinjury of the eye (contact sports)
- sensitivity to light issues (need to wear sunglasses for outdoor activities)
- safety glasses for sports activities

Discuss with the student the necessity to report if photophobia or headaches accompany an injury or infection. (ND 1,2,3,6)

Educate the student regarding proper care of contact lenses: (ND 1,2,3)
- importance of hand washing prior to touching a lens or his or her eye
- proper disinfection and storage of the contact lenses

Assist the student in removing contact lenses as needed. (ND 1,2,3)

Discuss the importance of wearing safety glasses or goggles to protect the eyes from injury: (ND 1,2,3,7)
- industrial technology class
- science laboratory class
- sports activities

Expected Student Outcomes

The student will:
- remain free of infection. (ND 1,2)
- participate in classroom activities, with modifications made as needed. (ND 2,5)
- participate in physical education activities, with modifications made as needed. (ND 2,5.7)
- access and utilize health / ophthalmologic services and consultation for initial and follow-up care of eye injuries / infections. (ND 1,2,3,4)
- complete the full treatment plan including a medication plan and follow-up care. (ND 1,2,3,4,5)
- report incidence of increased or continuing pain / discomfort to the school nurse / parents / healthcare provider. (ND 3)
- describe his/her eye injury and the healing process that is or has been occurring. (ND 7)
- participate in the treatment plan for his or her eye injury / infection. (ND 1,4)
- successfully and safely move from class to class and up and down stairs in the school setting. (ND 6)
- wear safety glasses / goggles in classes / activities, as directed and as appropriate. (ND 1,7)
- describe the importance of wearing safety glasses or goggles in a particular class or activity. (ND 1,7)

CASE STUDY

Two days ago Charles Boulton, a 15-year-old sophomore, was escorted to the health office by his industrial art teacher. While working on a high-powered wood sander, Charles felt a sudden sharp pain in the left eye. Charles stated that he was not wearing glasses or safety goggles during class. Charles had no history of previous serious eye injuries or ophthalmic medication at this time.

Initial examination of the injury revealed a laceration of the left upper lid, disrupted corneal surface, profuse tearing, and photophobia. A small paper cup was taped over the eye and Charles was escorted to the emergency room by his parents.

Charles received a diagnosis of upper lid and corneal laceration of the left eye. Physician's orders include: use of gentle pressure patch for 1 week and antibiotic eye drops, one drop at 12:00 noon at school. After two days at home, Charles has returned to school.

Due to the eye patch, Charles is not able to see anything out of his left eye. Charles is concerned about how this will affect his ability to get around school and his ability to play basketball in physical education class. He is also very concerned about whether or not he will be able to see in his left eye even when it is healed and the patch is off.

Charles and his mom state that the physician really emphasized the importance of using the medication and the eye patch to prevent an infection. However, Charles feels embarrassed about wearing the eye patch in school. Charles also says he feels bad about not following the teacher's instructions about wearing safety goggles at all times when working with the equipment and is afraid the teacher is going to be really mad at him.

Individualized Healthcare Plan*
Ophthalmic Conditions

Assessment Data	Nursing Diagnosis	Goals	Nursing Interventions	Expected Outcomes
ND1 Left upper lid and corneal laceration	Impaired tissue integrity related to lid and corneal injury (NANDA 1.6.2.1)	Charles will participate in measures to prevent eye infection.	Assist Charles to administer eye drops as prescribed. Remind Charles to wash his hands prior to self-administering eye drops to prevent infection.	Charles properly self-administers his eye medication. Charles remains free of infection in his injured eye.
Use of pressure patch for one week		Charles will participate in measures to promote healing of the eye injury.	Assist Charles to change his eye patch: provide new eye patch and tape, provide waste container for proper disposal of used eye patch.	Charles demonstrates proper technique in changing his eye patch.
ND2 Due to the need to wear eye patch, Charles is unable to see with his left eye	Alteration in sensory perception (depth perception) related to left eye being covered (NANDA 7.2)	Charles will safely move about and participate in activities in the school environment.	Allow Charles extra time to get from class to class. Encourage Charles to use the hand rail at all times on the stairways during the time his eye is patched.	Charles successfully and safely moves from class to class and up and down stairs in the school building.
ND6 Charles is concerned about getting around school and playing basketball in phy. ed. class	Risk for injury, related to alteration in depth perception due to need for eye patch (NANDA 1.6.1)		Consult with phy. ed. teacher concerning physical activity limitations, esp. catching, running, and hitting activities.	Charles participates in physical education class with modifications made in activities and activity requirements.

ND7 Charles is concerned that he did not follow the teacher's instructions to wear safety goggles	Knowledge deficit related to eye injury, regarding need for and use of protective eye glasses or goggles in industrial technology and other activities (NANDA 8.1.1)	Charles will increase his knowledge regarding eye safety and use of protective eye wear.	Provide educational opportunities for Charles regarding eye safety measures, including when and how to use protective safety glasses and goggles.	Charles will describe the importance of wearing protective eyewear when working with machines. Charles will demonstrate the proper use of eye glasses/goggles in IT class.	
Charles is concerned his industrial technology (IT) teacher is mad at him for not following his instructions.	Ineffective individual coping related to choosing not to wear safety glasses that resulted in an eye injury (NANDA 5.1.1.1)	Charles will resolve his concerns and issues regarding his eye injury with his IT teacher.	Assist Charles to arrange a time to meet with his IT teacher. If needed, allow Charles the opportunity to practice what he would like to say and discuss with his teacher.		

*See Appendix for student profile information to include on an IHP form.

BIBLIOGRAPHY

Bates B. *Guide to Physical Examination and History Taking,* 5th ed. Philadelphia, Pa: JB Lippincott Company, 1991:176-180.

Friedberg M, Rapuano C. *Wills Eye Hospital Office and Emergency Room Diagnosis and Treatment of Eye Diseases.* Philadelphia, Pa: JB Lippincott Company, 1990.

Hass MB, ed. *The School Nurse's Source Book of Individualized Healthcare Plans*, Vol. I. North Branch, Minn: Sunrise River Press, 1993. (Sunrise River Press, 11605 Kost Dam Road, North Branch, MN 55056. 800-895-4585; fax 651-583-2023)

Kanski J. *Clinical Ophthalmology*. Boston, Mass: Butterworth/Heinemann, 1994.

Koller H. How does vision affect learning? *J Ophthalmic Nursing Technol.* 1999;18(1):12-18.

Kozier B, Herb G. *Fundamentals of Nursing*. White Plains, NY: Addison-Wesley, 1987: 817-828.

Newell F. *Ophthalmology: Principals and Concepts*. St. Louis, Mo: CV Mosby, 1992.

North American Nursing Diagnosis Association. *NANDA Nursing Diagnoses: Definitions and Classification 1999-2000*. Philadelphia, Pa: North American Nursing Diagnosis Assn, 1999. (NANDA, 1211 Locust Street, Philadelphia, PA 19107. 800-647-9002; fax 215-545-8107; e-mail: NANDA@nursecominc.com)

Pavan-Langston D. *Manual of Ocular Diagnosis and Therapy*. Boston, Mass: Little, Brown, 1991.

Saunders WH, Havener WH, Havener G. *Nursing Care in Eye, Ear, Nose and Throat Disorders.* St. Louis, Mo: CV Mosby, 1979.

Samper R, Wasson P. *Ophthalmic Medical Assisting.* San Francisco, Ca: American Academy of Ophthalmology, 1994.

23 | IHP: Organ Transplant

Mary Jo Martin

INTRODUCTION

Solid organ transplant has become an increasingly acceptable treatment for children with end-stage organ failure. The three most prevalent solid organ transplants for children are liver, kidney, and heart replacement. With the introduction of the immunosuppressive drug cyclosporine in 1983 and better surgical techniques, the number of organ transplant procedures has increased dramatically. However, this number has reached a plateau in the last five years.[1] This plateau is related to the shortage of organ donors and is an unfortunate situation for those candidates awaiting a lifesaving transplantation.

Successful kidney transplantation was first performed in the 1960s. Kidney transplantation is now more successful than ever using both living donor and cadaver organs. Estimates indicate that the 1-year and 2-year survival rates of living donor transplants are 90% and 86%, respectively. For cadaver donors, 1-year and 2-year survival rates are 78% and 72%. [2]

Renal transplantation clearly provides the optimum therapy for children with end-stage renal failure. Causes of kidney failure include congenital diseases such as renal hypoplasia or dysphasia; acquired diseases such as glomerulonephritis; and hereditary diseases such as Alport's syndrome and juvenile nephrophthisis. Clinical manifestations include: electrolyte abnormalities, hyperglycemia, anemia, congestive heart failure, and peripheral neuropathy.

In 1963, the first pediatric liver transplantation was performed on a child with biliary atresia. The 1-year survival rate in the 1960s was 34%. Pediatric liver transplantation and survival rates have increased in recent years with the development of reduced-size liver (cadaver donors) and living-related donor transplants. It is now estimated that the 2-year survival rate for children receiving partial livers from living-related donors is 92%. The survival rate for those who receive livers from cadavers is approximately 75%.[3]

Liver transplantation may result from the complications of acute or chronic liver failure. Common clinical manifestations include jaundice, ascites, hepatomegaly, hypoglycemia, hormone imbalance, and encephalopathy. Rapid progression of symptoms over days to a few months is characteristic of acute-onset liver disease. Fulminant liver failure or acute hepatitis may be the cause. Chronic liver disease may progress more slowly, with symptoms appearing gradually over a few months. Causes of chronic liver failure include biliary atresia, cystic fibrosis, Wilson's disease, and Alagille syndrome.

Heart transplantation also began in the 1960s. In recent years, it has become a treatment option for infants and children with worsening heart failure and a limited life expectancy despite maximum medical and surgical management. The International Society for Heart Transplantation (ISHT) registry data on survival of cardiac transplant recipients since 1982 indicate a 1-year survival rate of approximately 73% and a 3-year survival rate of 66%. Indications for heart transplantation in children include cardiomyopathy and end-stage congenital heart defects. Clinical manifestations include respiratory distress, congestive heart failure, cardiomegaly, arrhythmias, and growth retardation.[4]

Pathophysiology

Transplantation for children with end-stage organ failure is a hope for survival and a better quality of life. Evaluation for the procedure involves multiple diagnostic tests, blood work, and radiologic examination. Each child is evaluated individually and the child's compatibility for the particular organ is weighed against the presence of other ongoing health conditions.[4] Once approved to be a candidate, the child is matched for donor tissue. Kidney and partial liver organ donations come from either a living donor or a cadaver donor soon after death. The closer the genetic relationship between the donor and recipient the better the chances for long- term survival.[5] Donor matching for heart transplants is primarily by ABO blood type and body size.[4]

Once a child is typed and matched, his or her medical criteria for transplantation are entered into a computerized database. The United Network for Organ Sharing (UNOS) maintains a centralized computer network linking all organ procurement organizations and transplant centers. When an organ becomes available the information about the donor's organ is entered and a list of possible recipients is generated.[6] The pediatric transplant team reviews the list, considers several factors, and decides what would be best for their individual patient.

Posttransplant care involves not only the physical recovery from the surgery but the possibility of problems associated with immunosuppression and organ rejection. Immunosuppression is the artificial suppression of the immune response, usually through drugs, so that the body will not reject a transplanted organ or tissue. Immunosuppression is vital for long-term survival of the donated organ. Prednisone and cyclosporine are used along with other drugs specific to the type of transplant. However, the administration of these drugs is not without risk. Children are at risk for infection since the therapy not only suppresses the immune response to the grafted tissue but also suppresses the body's ability to fight off other infectious agents. Studies have shown that over 80% of these patients do not get serious infections and have the same risk as the general population. Ten percent become infected with viruses such as cytomegalovirus, Epstein-Barr virus, or the hepatitis B or C virus.[7]

Initially, immunosupresion drugs are administered intravenously for 14 days after the transplant. However, for long-term survival the transplanted child must take the drugs for the rest of his or her life. Careful monitoring of the possible side effects of cyclosporine and prednisone is required. Some of the more common side effects of cyclosporine are hypertension, renal dysfunction, gum hyperplasia, hirsutism, diarrhea, seizures, and tremors. Prednisone can interfere with calcium absorption and retard linear growth. Other corticosteroid-induced side effects include the characteristic cushingoid face, cataracts, fluid and sodium retention, gastric ulcer, and obesity.[5]

Despite successful transplantation, rejection of the new organ is a leading cause of graft failure.[4] It occurs when the body makes antibodies that work to eliminate the transplanted organ. Rejection can be one of three types, hyperacute, acute, and chronic. Hyperacute happens immediately or within a few hours of the surgery and is irreversible. This type of rejection is usually seen in second transplant cases where the individual body has already built up a supply of antibodies against the new tissue.

Acute rejection usually occurs between the first few days to 6 months after transplantation but can occur as long as 1 or 2 years later. These symptoms of rejection are very similar to the symptoms of organ failure. Early detection is essential to successful reversal of acute rejection. The child must be closely monitored in all settings and the transplantation team should be notified of any concerns.

Chronic rejection is characterized by a gradual deterioration of organ function and typically begins 6 months or more after transplantation. Typically this type of rejection is not reversible and is also a response to the child's immune system. Some organs lose complete function over time, some only partial and are able to provide adequate function. The best way to prevent chronic rejection is by taking antirejection medications exactly as prescribed.[8]

Symptoms of rejection are particular to the type of organs involved. Rejection of a transplanted kidney is characterized by fever, decreased urine output, weight gain over 2 pounds per day, hypertension, and pain over the site. Rejection can be determined by decreased blood flow on a renal flow scan. Signs and symptoms of liver rejection include: fever, fatigue, jaundice, darkening of urine, clay-colored stools, and pain. A liver biopsy is used to confirm the rejection process. Cardiac rejection is complicated by the fact that rejection has progressed to moderate or severe levels before signs and symptoms appear. Manifestations include: congestive heart failure, cardiomegaly, fever, arrhythmias, ventricular dysfunction, and pericardial effusion. Myocardial biopsy and lab and radiologic tests help confirm rejection.[4,8]

The school nurse is the recipient's advocate and health manager in the school setting. Posttransplantation care is demanding and complex. The physical and emotional needs of the child and family need to be continually monitored. A multidisciplinary approach to care is needed so that all needs can be assessed and met. Good communication skills are the key to establishing trust with the child, family and transplantation team. Compliance with posttransplant medications and treatments will give the child the second chance at life, which he or she deserves.

INDIVIDUALIZED HEALTHCARE PLAN

Assessment

History

- Symptoms experienced during end-stage organ failure
- Review of medical records and testing
- Review of previous illness
- Hospital experiences
- Age of child at the time of diagnosis
- Medical management routine

- Immunization history
- Growth and development history
- Individual response of child to treatment
- History from family
  - family knowledge base of posttransplantation care
  - family's concerns and needs
  - family's coping abilities

Current Status

- Current symptoms
  - related to transplant
  - related to other health conditions
- Management plan
  - medications
- Diet plan
- Healthcare procedures that need to be done in the school setting
  - medications
- Physical limitations in school environment
- Vision and hearing assessment
- Healthcare providers
  - transplant team contact
  - pediatrician/primary care physician

Self-Care

- Self-care abilities (independent, assisted, supervised, done by parent)
- Posttransplantation care compliance
- Motivators to self-care and compliance
- Barriers to self-care

Psychosocial Status

- Life stressors: terminal illness, hospitalization, medication requirements, physical activity limitations
- Coping abilities: successful coping strategies
- Level of knowledge
- Body image: changes related to
  - scars
  - drug side effects (obesity, cushingoid face)
- Interaction with peers
- Peer acceptance
- Level of self-esteem
- Family coping

Academic Issues

- Developmental and academic level and progress

- Consult with teacher, counselor, physical therapist, occupational therapist, or any other member of multidisciplinary team
  – assess current, or need for, 504 plan and/or Individual Education Program (IEP)
- Physical activity tolerance during the school day, including transportation to and from school
- Attendance pattern — past and current
- School health services needed

Nursing Diagnoses (N.D.)

N.D. 1 Altered nutrition: less than body requirements (NANDA 1.1.2.2) related to:
- poor or loss of appetite
- pain (abdominal)
- infection
- depressed body defenses

N.D. 2 Risk for infection (NANDA 1.2.1.1) related to:
- alteration in immune response
- immunosuppression
- medication (side effects)
- exposure to pathogens
- organ rejection
- infections in the school environment

N.D. 3 Risk for injury (NANDA 1.6.1) related to:
- lack of safety precautions
- lack of safety education
- photosensitive skin

N.D. 4 Risk for alteration in activity tolerance (NANDA 6.1.1.3) related to:
- fatigue
- chronic health condition

N.D. 5 Risk for altered growth and development (NANDA 6.6) related to:
- effects of chronic condition
- long-term effects of corticosteroids after transplantation

N.D. 6 Risk for body image disturbance (NANDA 7.1.1) related to:
- actual change in body part
- side effects of medication
- verbalization of:
  – fear of reaction by others
  – negative feelings about body
  – feelings of helplessness and hopelessness
  – lack of privacy
  – depression

N.D. 7 Risk for altered family processes (NANDA 3.2.2) due to:
- child's chronic health condition
- fear of organ rejection
- psychosocial stressors
  – feelings of isolation
  – financial burdens
  – role strain
  – family disruption

Goals

The student will:
- maintain adequate nutritional intake. (N.D. 1)
- remain free of infections. (N.D. 2)
- demonstrate good personal hygiene skills. (N.D. 2)
- remain free of injury. (N.D. 3)
- decrease energy expenditure as needed based on activity tolerance level. (N.D. 4)
- maintain adequate growth pattern. (N.D. 5)
- demonstrate positive behaviors that indicate a good body image. (N.D. 6)
- participate in school/classroom activities with modifications as needed
  – maintain academic progress. (N.D. 1-6)
- develop and/or maintain effective individual and family coping behaviors. (N.D. 7)
- seek, obtain, and maintain community support for self and his/her family. (N.D. 7)

Nursing Interventions

Teacher/School Interventions

Implement prescribed diet at school. (N.D. 1)

Monitor eating habits. (N.D. 1,5)

Monitor for and teach staff to recognize signs and symptoms of bacterial, fungal, viral, and protozoan infections. Signs and symptoms include: fever, fatigue, pain. (N.D. 2)

Monitor school environment for infectious diseases, especially chickenpox, influenza, pneumonia, pertussis. (N.D. 2)

Teach students, classmates, and staff good hand-washing and illness prevention techniques. (N.D. 2)

Encourage student to bring own water bottle and instruct him/her not to drink from drinking fountains. (N.D. 2)

Maintain current emergency information with current emergency contacts (eg., phone or pager number of parents, medical care providers). (N.D.3)

Coordinate communication between medical care provider, organ transplant team, parents, and school staff. (N.D. 3)

Develop emergency care plan (ECP) regarding what to do if signs of possible rejection or infection occur. (N.D. 3)

Notify parent of any signs or symptoms of infection that occur. Decide with parent whether student goes home or stays in school. (N.D. 3)

Assist staff in modifying activities appropriate to activity tolerance. (N.D. 3)

Encourage sun safety measures such as: use of a sunscreen with sun protection factor of at least 15, avoid exposure to direct sunshine, wear a hat. (N.D. 3)

Encourage exercise within child's limitations. (N.D. 4)

Inform staff about student's limitations. (N.D. 4)

Inform staff of signs and symptoms to report such as: respiratory difficulties, cyanosis, fatigue. (N.D. 4)

Discuss with student signs and symptoms that need to be reported to the teacher or health office as soon as they occur. (N.D. 4)

Assist student to set own physical limitations based on tolerance. (N.D. 4)

Assist student to rest as needed. (N.D. 4)

Certain activities are not recommended for students having had solid organ transplant; these include: contact sports, downhill sledding, and hanging from the waist on a bar. (N.D. 4)

Monitor height and weight as requested by parent and/or healthcare provider. (N.D. 1,5)

Assess vision and hearing annually. (N.D. 5)

Encourage routine dental visits with prophylactic antibiotics administered before dental work to prevent infection. (N.D. 2, 5)

Monitor gums for signs and symptoms of gum hyperplasia in children taking cyclosporine. (N.D. 5)

Assess change in:
- social involvement with family, peers, and school staff
- verbalization of negative body image
- signs of depression and noncompliance with health plan (N.D. 6)

Assess student for successful coping mechanisms, reinforce as needed. (N.D. 6)

Establish caring atmosphere to keep communication open. (N.D. 6)

Demonstrate sense of acceptance regardless of health condition. (N.D. 6)

Encourage interactions with peers and other students with same diagnosis (i.e., support group). (N.D. 6)

Encourage verbalization of feelings. (N.D. 6)

Assist the student to share his/her feelings about self with family and staff. (N.D. 6)

Student/Family Interventions

Notify parents if student is exposed to measles, mumps, varicella, shingles, herpes, or influenza. (N.D. 2)

Discuss diet guidelines with student and family. (N.D. 1,5)

Encourage student to verbalize feelings of self and body image to family. (N.D. 6)

Assess family dynamics: communication and coping patterns. (N.D. 7)

Assess need for student and family to seek counseling to help deal with stressors. (N.D. 7)

Refer to community resources and local organ transplant support group as needed. (N.D. 7)

Supply information and emotional support to cope with fears, future milestones, and financial aspects of organ transplant. (N.D. 7)

Expected Student Outcomes

The student will:
- maintain a well-balanced diet as prescribed. (N.D. 1,5)
- remain free of infection in the school setting. (N.D. 2)
- demonstrate good (independent, assisted) personal hygiene skills. (N.D.2)
- demonstrate compliance with activity limitations as prescribed. (N.D. 2,4,6)
- not experience physical injury in the school setting. (N.D. 3)
- demonstrate good activity tolerance with modification made as needed. (N.D. 4)
- rest as needed. (N.D. 4)
- participate in school/classroom activities with modifications made as needed. (N.D. 4)
- maintain academic progress. (N.D. 1-5)
- be able to verbalize feelings of body image. (N.D. 6)

- develop and demonstrate positive coping strategies. (N.D. 6)
- assist in notifying parents if signs and symptoms of infection/organ rejection develop. (N.D. 2,6)
- receive support from family. (N.D. 7)
- monitor eating habits. (ND 1,5)
- monitor for and teach staff to recognize signs and symptoms of bacterial, fungal, viral and potozoan infections. Signs and symptoms include: fever, fatigue pain. (N.D.2)
- monitor school environment for infectious diseases, especially chickenpox, influenza, pneumonia, pertussis. (N.D.2)
- teach students, classmates, and staff good hand-washing and illness prevention techniques. (N.D. 2)
- encourage student to bring own water battle and instruct him/her not to drink from drinking fountains. (N.D. 2)
- maintain current emergency information with current emergency contacts (eg., phone or pager number of parents, medical care providers). (N.D.3)
- coordinate communication between medical care provider, organ transplant team, parents, and school staff. (N.D. 3)
- develop ECP regarding what to do if signs of possible rejection or infection occur. (N.D. 3)
- notify parent of any signs or symptoms of infection that occur. Decide with parent whether student goes home or stays in school. (N.D. 3)
- assist staff in modifying activities appropriate to activity tolerance. (N.D. 3)
- encourage sun safety measures such as: use of a sunscreen with sun protection factor of at least 15, avoid exposure to direct sunshine, wear a hat. (N.D. 3)
- encourage exercise within child's limitations. (N.D. 4)
- inform staff about student's limitations. (N.D. 4)
- inform staff of signs and symptoms to report such as: respiratory difficulties, cyanosis, fatigue. (N.D. 4)
- discuss with student signs and symptoms that need to be reported to the teacher or health office as soon as they occur. (N.D. 4)
- assist student to set own physical limitations based on tolerance. (N.D. 4)
- assist student to rest as needed. (N.D. 4)
- certain activities are not recommended for students having had solid organ transplants; these include: contact sports, downhill sledding, and hanging from the waist on a bar. (N.D. 4)
- monitor height and weight as requested by parent and/or healthcare provider. (N.D. 1,5)
- assess vision and hearing annually. (N.D. 5)
- encourage routine dental visit with prophylactic antibiotics administered before dental work to prevent infection. (N.D. 2,5)
- monitor gums for signs and symptoms of gum hyperplasia in children taking cyclosporine. (N.D. 5)
- assess change in:
  – social involvement with family, peers, and school staff
  – verbalization of negative body image
  – signs of depression and noncompliance health plan (N.D. 6)
- assess student for successful coping mechanisms, reinforce as needed. (N.D. 6)
- establish caring atmosphere to keep communication open. (N.D. 6)

CASE STUDY

Name: Emily
DOB: 5-15-93
Age: 5 years 4 months

Health History:

History was obtained from Emily's parents at an informational meeting on September 2, 1998, and from a review of health records.

Emily was delivered at 40 weeks via cesarean section after a prolonged labor. Apgar scores were 7 at one minute and 9 at five minutes. Records show a slightly elevated serum bilirubin and the doctor told her parents to put her in the sunlight for a couple of hours a day. Mother and baby were discharged 48 hours after birth.

Mom describes Emily as a "fussy" baby. Feeding was difficult and she only slept for short periods of time. Her stomach seemed bloated and her parents thought she had colic. The yellow color of her skin was a concern to her doctor and tests were conducted at age 4 weeks. Blood and urine studies, ultrasound, and a liver biopsy confirmed that Emily had biliary atresia (inflammation and obstruction of the ducts which carry the bile from the liver to the intestine). On June 20, 1993, a Kasai procedure was performed.

Emily seemed to "feel better" after the surgery. Her parents describe this time as stressful and they were concerned about her growth. She was initially put on a low-fat diet with vitamin supplements but progressed to a regular diet in 6 months. She took a variety of medications including oral antibiotics, diuretics, and phenobarbital. Developmental milestones included sitting up at 9 months, crawling at 11 months, and walking at 18 months. Dad states that Emily began cooing at 3 months and said her first word at 10 months.

Her parents' concerns grew greater when at the age of 3 1/2 Emily's weight had dropped to 28 pounds. She had increasing episodes of stomachaches, loss of appetite, and fatigue. Medical tests found Emily's liver to be damaged further. Records show that complications from cirrhosis would require a liver transplant

Emily received one-fourth of her mother's liver on November 28, 1996. Recovery was described as slow, but Emily has now regained her strength and has gained 10 pounds in the past 18 months.

Current Health

Emily has no known allergies. Her immunizations are up to date. Early childhood screening records indicate that Emily passed her vision and hearing screen 6 months ago. Emily currently attends a morning kindergarten program and has never been in a daycare setting.

Emily eats a low-fat diet. She is described as a "picky" eater and often has to be encouraged to eat. She takes medication daily which includes cyclosporine and prednisone. Her parents describe her as an active child and that she sometimes becomes tired after a lot of physical activity. After a short rest period Emily is then able to resume activity. Emily is described as a good "sleeper." She falls asleep easily and sleeps 8 to 10 hours per night.

Individualized Healthcare Plan*
Organ Transplant

Assessment Data	Nursing Diagnosis	Goals	Nursing Interventions	Expected Outcomes
ND1 Student has had a liver transplant.	Risk of infection related to: 1) immunosupression; 2) medication (side effect); 3) exposure to pathogens in the school environment; 4) organ rejection. (NANDA 1.2.1.1)	Student will remain free of infection.	Monitor for and teach staff to recognize signs and symptoms of bacterial, fungal, viral and protozoan infections including: fever, fatigue, pain. Monitor school environment for infectious diseases, especially chickenpox, influenza, pneumonia, pertussis. Notify parents if student is exposed to measles, mumps, varicella, shingles, herpes, or influenza.	The student will remain free of infection in the school setting.
			Teach student, classmates and staff good hand-washing and illness prevention techniques. Encourage student to bring own water bottle and instruct him/her not to drink from drinking fountains.	The student will demonstrate good (independent, assisted) personal hygiene skills.

| ND3 Student attends school. She takes immunosuppression medication daily and continually needs to be monitored for signs and symptoms of infection and/or organ rejection. | Risk for injury related to: 1) lack of safety precautions; 2) lack of safety education; 3) photosensitive skin. (NANDA 1.6.1.) | The student will remain free of injury. | Maintain current emergency information with current emergency contacts.

Coordinate communication between medical care provider, organ transplant team, parents, and staff.

Develop an emergency care plan regarding what to do if signs/ symptoms of possible rejection or infection occur.

Notify parents of any signs/ symptoms of infection that occur. Decide with parent whether student should remain in school or not.

Assist staff in modifying activities appropriate to activity tolerance.

Encourage sun safety measures, such as: use suncreen with sun protection factor of at least 15, avoid exposure to direct sunshine, wear a hat. | The student will not experience physical injury in the school setting. |

*See Appendix for student profile information to include on an IHP form.

REFERENCES

1. Hanton LB. Caring for children awaiting heart transplantation: pychosocial implications. *Pediat Nurs*. 1998;24(3): 214-215.
2. Salvatierra O, Alfrey E, Tanney DC, et al. *Superior Outcomes in Pediatric Renal Transplantation* [online]. Available at: http://www.med.stanford.edu. 1997. Accessed 1/29/99.
3. Rochell A. Mother-son transplant makes Georgia history: liver donor takes organ tissue from living donor. *The Atlanta Constitution*. 1997;3(12): 5.
4. Jackson PL, Vessey JA. *Primary Care of the Child with a Chronic Condition*. St. Louis, Mo: Mosby-Year Book, 1992.
5. Wong DL. *Whaley & Wong's Nursing Care of Infants and Children*. 5th ed. St. Louis, Mo: Mosby, 1995.
6. *The Transplant Process* [online]. (1998). Available at: http://www.unos.org. Accessed 1/18/99.
7. Fishman JA, Rubin RH. Infection in organ transplant recipients. *N Engl J Med*. 1998;338(24): 174.
8. The University of Iowa Hospitals and Clinics, Department of Surgery. *Rejection.* [online]. Available at: http://www.vh.org.1998.Accessed 1/18/99.

BIBLIOGRAPHY

Johnson AB. *Pediatric Transplantation*. Philadelphia, Pa: WB Saunders Company, 1992.

Nolan MT, Augustine SA. *Transplantation Nursing: Acute and Long Term Management.* Norwalk, Conn: Appleton & Lange, 1995.

Norris MK, House MA. *Organ Transplantation: Nursing Care for Procurement Through Rehabilitation*. Philadelphia, Pa: FA Davis Company, 1991.

North American Nursing Diagnosis Association. *NANDA Nursing Diagnoses: Definitions & Classification 1999-2000.* Philadelphia, Pa: North American Nursing Diagnosis Assn, 1999. (NANDA, 1211 Locust Street, Philadelphia, PA 19107. 800-647-9002; fax 215-545-8107; e-mail: NANDA@nursecominc.com)

Williams BH, Grady KL, Sandiford-Guttenbeil DM. *Organ Transplant: A Manual for Nurses*. New York; NY: Springer Publishing Company, 1991.

Williams BH, Sandiford-Guttenbeil DM. *Trends in Organ Transplantation*. New York; NY: Springer Publishing Company, 1996.

ORGANIZATIONS/AGENCIES

American Heart Association
National Center
7272 Greenville Avenue
Dallas, TX 75231
1-800-AHA-USA1
http://www.americanheart.org

American Liver Foundation
75 Maiden Lane
New York, NY 10038
1-800-GO-LIVER
http://www.liverfoundation.org

American Lung Association
http://www.lungusa.org

American Red Cross Tissue Donation
http://www.redcross.org/tissue/index.html

American Share Foundation
http://www.asf.org

CenterSpan
http://www.centerspan.org

Children's Liver Alliance
3835 Richmond Avenue, Box 190
Staten Island, NY 10312
718-987-5200
http://www.livertx.org

Children's Organ Transplantation Association
1-800-366-2682
http://www.cota.org

National Kidney Foundation
30 East 33rd Street
New York, NY 10016
1-800-622-9010
http://www.kidney.org

Trans Web
1327 Jones Drive, Suite 105
Ann Arbor, MI 48105
734-998-7314
http://www.transweb.org

United Network for Organ Sharing (UNOS)
1100 Boulders Parkway, Suite 500
PO Box 13770
Richmond, VA 23225-8770
1-888-TXINFO1

24 IHP: Pervasive Developmental Disorders and Autism

Jeanette H. Williams

INTRODUCTION

Pervasive Developmental Disorders (PDD) consist of a group of disorders that have some similar characteristics. Included in this category in the *DSMR-IV*[1] are autism, Asperger's syndrome, Rett syndrome, and PDD NOS (not otherwise specified). Common symptoms include poor social skills, impaired communication, and lack of imaginative skill.[1] Some of these children have limited cognitive ability. Autism is the best known of this group of disorders. Treatment for these disorders is primarily educational.[2]

Autism

Kanner added the diagnosis of autism to the psychiatric literature in 1944, 55 years ago. He described it as a syndrome defined by behaviors and a characteristic history,[3] as a peculiar and emotional detachment from people and the world.[4] Autism is now generally accepted as a syndrome related to a neuropathology of the central nervous system, the etiology of which is unknown[5] although a strong genetic basis is suggested by the fact that siblings of autistic persons have autism or milder symptoms at a rate of 50 to 100 percent higher than normal.[4] Autism is a lifelong, nonprogressive neurologic developmental disorder.[2,5] It is a spectrum disorder with varying degrees of severity. Its expression ranges from the very severely involved to those who are only mildly affected and may appear very close to normal. It can be a severe and incapacitating lifelong developmental disability. Seventy-five percent of children with autism are boys.[4] However, females are likely to exhibit more severe retardation .[1]

Signs may appear in the early months. Infants with autism do not like to cuddle and may shrink from touch.[4] Symptoms may be subtle during infancy and go unnoticed, but it is apparent before age 30 months that something is wrong. They have little interest in other people, do not maintain eye contact, and may not distinguish their parents from strangers.[4] They have a narrow and restrictive range of interests.[1]

Impaired development in social interaction, communication, speech, and language, a narrow interest in activities, and extreme reactions to changes in the immediate environment are major characteristics of the syndrome. Most autistic children are mentally retarded with IQ scores lower than 70 to 75 (80%),[2] and IQs of 35 to 50 are common.[6]

Children with autism are attracted to objects rather than people. They may experience violent and extreme reaction to a slight change, hyperactivity, short attention spans, impulsivity, aggressiveness, and a range of behavioral symptoms.

Sleeping and eating disorders may also be present. Their play is ritualistic and repetitive. Imaginative play may be absent or impaired. They have a narrow and restricted range of interests. Language may be absent or development of language is delayed. [1,4] Children with autism have a high threshold for pain, oversensitivity to sounds or being touched, exaggerated reactions to light or odors, lack of fear in response to real dangers, and variety of self-injurious behaviors (head banging or finger, hand, or wrist biting). [1,7]

A wide variety of neurologic disorders have been reported in children with autism, including cerebral palsy, maternal rubella, toxoplasmosis, tuberous sclerosis, cytomegalovirus infection, demyelinating disease, lead encephalopathy, meningitis, encephalitis, severe brain hemorrhage, phenylketonuria, and many types of epilepsy. Many studies also show that children with autism have an excess of congenital minor physical anomalies. [6] Although data does not suggest a unifying pathologic process in autism, it indicates that some type of physical damage may produce autism. Twenty-five percent of children with autism develop seizures as adults. [4]

Pervasive Developmental Disorder NOS (Not Otherwise Specified)

Pervasive Developmental Disorder NOS is described as severe and pervasive impairment in the development of reciprocal social interaction or verbal and nonverbal communication, or when stereotyped behavior, interests, and activities are present. The criteria are not met for a specific PDD, [8] however, are not met.

Autism and PDD NOS share many of the same characteristics. Both are neurologic disorders that affect a child's ability to communicate, understand language, play, and relate to others. [8] Children with PDD have abnormal responses to sensations. Any one or a combination of senses or responses may be affected: sight, hearing, touch, balance, smell, taste, reaction to pain. Speech and language are absent or delayed and these children relate to people abnormally. Children with PDD have stamina and well-developed gross and fine motor skills. They enjoy routines, have good long-term memory, and can accurately perform tasks well once they have learned them. [9] The condition may occur by itself or in association with other disorders that affect the function of the brain, such as viral infections, metabolic disturbances, and epilepsy. [10]

Rett Syndrome

Rett syndrome is described as profound withdrawal from contact with people and obsessive desire for preservation of sameness. Victims are extremely regressed in severe cases. It is a genetic neurologic disorder of unknown cause affecting only females. [10, 11] Development appears normal until about the age of 5 months. [4] Rett syndrome is characterized by dementia with autistic behavior, apraxia of gait, loss of facial expression, stereotyped movements, shakiness of the torso and possibly limbs, breathing difficulties, seizures, teeth grinding and difficulty chewing, and loss of purposeful hand movements. The child's functioning level is between severely and profoundly mentally retarded. [12,13]

An essential feature of the condition is loss of normal development and regression after a relative period of normal functioning. Normal development takes place until ages 6 to 18 months. Deceleration of head growth occurs between 6 months and 4 years and early behavioral, social, and psychomotor regression occurs. Regression in cognition, motor skills, and social development occurs throughout life. [12]

Music, rocking, and car riding may have a calming effect. A ketogenic diet has been reported to improve clinical seizures. [14] Autopsies on the brains of victims indicate pathology different than autism. Prevalence of Rett syndrome is l in 12,000 to 15,000 girls.[11,12]

Asperger's Syndrome

Asperger's syndrome is one of a group of diagnoses included under the general term "Pervasive Developmental Disorders." It is sometimes compared to high-functioning autistic disorder. Asperger's syndrome is used to describe persons with severe deficits in social interaction who display a restricted pattern of activities and repetitive stereotyped behaviors without significant delays in the acquisition of language or cognitive functioning.[1]

Motor delays or motor clumsiness may be seen in the preschool period. Asperger's disorder is characterized by an impairment in social interaction, a restricted pattern of interests and activities and stereotyped behaviors.[1] A variety of medications are used to treat the symptoms. [15]

Management

Management of PDD is primarily educational, with medications used as needed for associated problems (seizures, behaviors, etc.) Services for children vary greatly depending on the community and the quality of programs available in the school district.[2] The treatment may vary but should always be highly structured and geared to the child's developmental level of functioning.[6] The following paragraphs describe some of the therapies being used for children with autism.

Facilitated communication. This educational intervention is based on the theory that children with autism cannot control their movements to communicate what they think and feel. The child works with a facilitator who isolates the index finger of the child and teaches him or her how to type responses. In this way, the child learns to communicate. The program has met with both praise and criticism.[4]

Applied behavior analysis (ABA) is an intensive behavior modification program being used. It requires dedication and makes heavy demands on the parents. Most therapy is home based. The children are enrolled as early as age 3 in an intense program for most of their waking hours. The program is aimed at changing the child's environment and patterns of reinforcement. According to a 1987 article written by Dr. Ivar Lovaas and published in the *Journal of Counseling and Clinical Psychology,* 47% of a group of nineteen children with autism were functioning normally in intellectual and academic areas following ABA training. Nine of the children had completed first grade in a regular classroom.[4] Much controversy exists as to the effectiveness of this treatment and research has been extremely limited. More studies are being done, and children are being followed over a period of time to determine the long-term success of the program.[4, 14,15]

Medical management of the child with autism has centered around controlling the associated problems that develop because of the condition. If seizures develop, seizure medication is indicated. Neuroleptic drugs are used to reduce behavioral symptoms. Anticholinergic drugs may be used to treat the extrapyramidal symptoms that are sometimes a side effect of some neuroleptic drugs (e.g., haloperidol). Megavitamin therapy has also been tried. [5]

Education, counseling, and extended family support are necessary to help parents raising a child with a PDD. Having a child with PDD significantly affects all family members. Families need support groups and access to new findings and research to help them cope with the concerns, questions, and problems they incur daily living with a child with one of these conditions.[16] Respite care should be available to families to assure that they may continue to care for the child in the home, especially in severe cases.

INDIVIDUALIZED HEALTHCARE PLAN

History

- Age and developmental level
- At what age was the diagnosis made?
- Diagnosis, severity of condition and prognosis
- Growth and weight gain pattern
- Medications
- Illnesses
- Injuries
- Seizures (may or may not be present)

Current Status

- Current developmental level of student including:
  - physical
  - cognitive, evidence of mental retardation
  - social
  - communication skills
- Student's temperament
- Student's ability to interact with peers and adults
- Student's current height and weight
- Student's current vision status
- Student's current hearing status
- Healthcare providers involved in management of child's condition (neurologist, psychiatrist, psychologist, pediatrician)
- Seizures (may or may not be present)
- Medications and side effects
- Eating habits
- Sleeping habits

Self-Care

- Student's perception of health
- Self-care skills
- Decision-making skills
- Parents' perception of student's condition

Psychosocial Issues

- Student's temperament
- Student's perception of stressors
- Student's fears, anxieties
- Student's coping skills
- Level of family functioning
- Parents' coping skills
- Family education, and counseling; modifications in family environment
- Family resources, socioeconomic, extended family, friends
- Availability and involvement of support system

Academic Issues

- Educational providers involved in management of child's education (teacher, occupational therapist, physical therapist, speech and language therapist, school nurse)
- Review of special education assessments/interventions
- Behavior management plan
- Classroom modifications necessary for child's participation in class
- Parents' and teachers' knowledge of specific PDD condition affecting student

Nursing Diagnoses (N.D.)

N.D. 1   Impaired and altered thought processes (NANDA 8.3) related to:
- Abnormal processing of input
- Possible mental retardation
- Decreased ability to focus
- Sensory perceptual alterations

N.D. 2   Sensory/perceptual alterations (NANDA 7.2) related to
- Decreased ability to sort for relevant data
- Decreased ability to control sensory input
- Decreased ability to choose which sensory data to consider relevant
- Incomplete processing of sensory inputs (auditory, kinesthetic, tactile, olfactory)

N.D. 3   Knowledge deficit (NANDA 8.1.1) related to mental retardation and/or impaired thought processes (N.D. 1) and sensory perceptual alterations (N.D.2)

N.D. 4   Ineffective individual coping skills (NANDA 5.1.1.1) related to:
- Decreased ability to plan
- Decreased ability to self-limit behaviors (self-control)
- Decreased ability to anticipate consequences of actions
- Limited cognitive skills and social functioning

N.D. 5   Impaired verbal communication (NANDA 2.1.1.1) related to syndrome limitations

N.D. 6   Anxiety (NANDA 9.3.1) and fear (NANDA 9.3.2) related to minimal understanding and abnormal sensory input

N.D. 7   Diversional activity deficit (NANDA 6.3.1.1) related to narrow range of interests

N.D. 8   Risk for injury (NANDA 1.6.l) related to inability to recognize dangers and understand consequences, and potential self-injurious behaviors

N.D. 9   Risk for violence: self-directed (NANDA 9.2.2.2) or directed at others (NANDA 9.2.2) related to high tolerance for pain and altered thought processes (N.D. 1)

N.D. 10   Impaired social interaction (NANDA 3.1.1) and isolation (NANDA 3.1.2) related to abnormal sensory input, processing, limited language and communication skills and lack of understanding of social interaction

N.D. 11   Risk for sleep pattern disturbance (NANDA 6.2.1) related to chronic health condition

N.D. 12   Risk for altered nutrition: less than body requirements (NANDA 1.1.2.2) related to narrow selection of foods child will eat and high activity level

N.D. 13   Risk for self-care deficits (NANDA 6.5.2, .3, & .4) related to limited ability in self-care skills required and attentions in sensory perceptual

N.D. 14   Risk for alterations in family processes (NANDA 3.2.2) and risk for altered parenting (NANDA 3.2.1.1.2) related to difficulty adjusting to family member with chronic condition

N.D. 15   Risk for ineffective family coping: disabling (NANDA 5.1.2.1.1) and/or family coping compromised (NANDA 5.1.2.1.2) related to stressors and anxiety

N.D. 16   Family coping: potential for growth (NANDA 5.1.2.2) related to acquiring knowledge and support and becoming aware of resources available

Goals

Student will utilize mental and emotional strengths. (N.D. 1-5)

Student will decrease anxieties and fears. (N.D 6)

Student will try new activities. (N.D. 7)

Student will remain safe and uninjured. (N.D. 8)

Student will decrease outbreaks of violent behavior. (N.D. 9)

Student will participate in social/recreational activity, as tolerated. (N.D. 10)

Student will maintain normal sleep pattern. (N.D. 11)

Student will maintain normal growth. (N.D. 12)

Student will participate in personal care. (N.D. 13)

Family will increase/maintain family functions/processes; for example, parenting, family interaction. (N.D. 14)

Family will utilize positive coping strategies in dealing with student's disability. (N.D. 15 & 16)

Nursing Interventions

Refer for special education testing if student is not receiving services. (N.D. 1-5)

Consult with education staff regarding need for safe, consistent, routine environment. (N.D. 1-5)

Find out what causes anxiety and fears in student and collaborate with staff to eliminat or minimize these situations. (N.D. 6)

Collaborate with educational staff/parents to encourage student to explore various activities. (N.D. 7)

Provide for safe environment with adequate personnel and enclosed areas as deemed appropriate. (N.D. 8 and 9)

Develop calming techniques. (N.D. 4, 6, 8 and 9)

Identify factors leading to outbursts of violent behavior. (N.D. 4, 8 and 9)

Use appropriate restraints as necessary. (N.D. 8 and 9)

Suggest medical consultation for possible use of medication if self-injurious behavior or violence toward others is exhibited. (N.D. 8 and 9)

Identify social/recreational interests of child and encourage participation. (N.D. 10)

Consult with parents/physician regarding sleep patterns. Assist parents in exploring strategies for dealing with the problem (medication, calming techniques). (N.D. 11)

Offer variety of foods and encourage child to try new foods. Weigh monthly if indicated. (N.D. 12)

Assist the student in developing self-care skills, especially grooming and hand washing. Instruct and supervise in self-care, especially hand washing. (N.D. 13)

Provide educational opportunities for staff regarding PDD and specific syndrome of student in collaboration with parents and special education staff. (N.D. 1-13)

Consult with staff, physician, and parents as needed. (N.D. 14, 15 and 16).

Provide resources for parents for education, counseling, support groups, and respite care. Be available to parents as resource. (N.D. 14, 15 and 16)

Encourage parents to attend behavior management classes and support groups for parents of children with PDD. (N.D. 14, 15 and 16)

Expected Student Outcomes

Student will increase cognitive, social, processing, language, and self-control skills. (N.D. 1–5)

Student will feel comfortable in school setting. (N.D. 6)

Student will develop interest in several activities. (N.D. 7)

Student and peers will remain safe in the school environment. (N.D. 8 and 9)

Student will have decrease in inappropriate behavioral episodes. (N.D. 8 and 9)

Student will participate in social/recreational activities. (N.D. 10)

Student will maintain/improve sleep pattern. (N.D. 11)

Student will maintain normal growth. (N.D. 12)

Student will take care of personal hygiene needs independently or with minimal assistance while at school. (N.D. 13)

Education staff will be knowledgeable about PDD and student's specific syndrome. (N.D. 1-13)

Normal parenting will be maintained in family. Parents will increase understanding of student's condition. (N.D. 14, 15 and 16)

Family will remain stable. (N.D. 14, 15 and 16)

Parents will utilize positive coping strategies. (N.D. 14, 15 and 16)

CASE STUDY

Jamie is a 7-year-old girl who attends Windsor Elementary School. She has a diagnosis of Pervasive Developmental Disorder – Not Otherwise Specified (NOS) from her neurologist. She is in the second grade and is doing fairly well academically She has an educational diagnosis of language impairment and receives therapy from the therapist five hours a week.

She has few friends and usually plays alone at recess. This does not seem to bother her and she seems very content at amusing herself. She does not like to try new foods and is a poor eater. She is below the fifth percentile in weight for her age. She is easily upset by the unexpected or a change in any routine. She sometimes refuses to participate in new activities introduced in physical education and prefers to do the same thing over and over.

Her parents are very concerned about her lack of friends and her reluctance to try new activities. They also worry about her outbursts when her routine is changed.

IEP Recommendations For Student with
Pervasive Developmental Disorder
Based on the above IHP

Jamie should be weighed monthly until her weight falls within the fifth percentile for height and age.

Nurse will consult with parents regarding Jamie's nutritional requirements.

Nurse will consult with parents regarding available resources, support groups, and so on.

Nurse will collaborate with educational staff regarding efforts to help Jamie interact with peers and form friendships.

Weekly School Nursing Time Required

Total weekly nursing - indirect services needs = 30 minutes per week

Individualized Healthcare Plan*
Pervasive Developmental Disorders and Autism

Assessment Data	Nursing Diagnosis	Goals	Nursing Interventions	Expected Outcomes
ND10 Student's lack of friends and interaction with peers.	Impaired social interaction (NANDA 3.1.1) and isolation (NANDA 3.1.2) related to abnormal sensory input processing, limited language and communication skills, and lack of understanding of social interaction.	Develop student's ability to interact with peers and have friends.	Collaborate with educational staff to determine student interests, how to involve her in group activity, promote friendships. Consult with parents about having student join after-school activities (Brownies, sports, etc.).	Student will interact with peers. Student will develop friendly relationships with peers.
ND12 Weight is abnormally low for age and height.	Altered nutrition: less than body requirements (NANDA 1.1.2.2) related to narrow selection of foods.	Student will eat a wider variety of foods and will gain weight to meet criterion for 5th and 10th percentiles for weight within one year.	Weigh student monthly. Consult with parents regarding nutritious high-calorie foods, student's likes and dislikes. Educate parents about nutrition requirements of student to maintain growth and development. Allow student to eat in quiet calm area at lunch. Introduce peers slowly if indicated.	Student will attain normal weight for age and height.

ND6 Upset by change in routine.	Anxiety (NANDA 9.3.1) and fear (NANDA 9.3.2) related to minimal understanding and abnormal sensory input.	Student will be able to comfortably make changes as necessary.	Collaborate with staff to tell student before changes will occur and be available to reassure her. Ex. Substitute teacher, student teachers, fire drills, assemblies, field trips.	Student will adjust to change in routine as needed.
ND15 Parental concerns about student's problems.	Family coping: Potential for growth (NANDA 5.1.2.2) related to acquiring knowledge and support and becoming aware of resources available.	Parents will increase knowledge of child's condition. Parents will learn and utilize positive coping strategies in dealing with Jamie's behavior.	Consult with parents. Provide list of resources and support groups. Be available to help with concerns and questions. Inform parents of behavior management classes available. Encourage parents to utilize special education teachers for strategies for dealing with PDD-related behavior.	Parents will increase knowledge of condition. Parents will successfully utilize positive coping strategies for dealing with Jamie's behavior.

*See Appendix for student profile information to include on an IHP form.

REFERENCES

1. American Psychiatric Association. *Diagnostic and Statistical Manual of Mental Disorders* 4th ed. Washington, DC: American Psychiatric Association, 1994: 66-71.
2. Thoene JG, ed. *Physicians Guide to Rare Diseases*. Montvale, NJ: Dowden Publishing Company, 1992:315-317.
3. Kanner L. Autistic disturbances of affective contact. Nervous Child.1943; 2: 217-280 In: Freeman BJ. *Diagnosis of the Syndrome of Autism: Questions Parents Ask*. Available at: http://www/autism – society.org/packages/getstart_diagnosis.html Accessed 2/20/98.
4. *Autism*. Harvard Mental Health Letter. Available at: http://www.mentalhealth.com/mag/1/1997/h97-aut.6.html Accessed March/April 1997.
5. Schopler E, Mesibov GB. *Neurobiological Issues in Autism*. New York: Plenum Press, 1987: 83-86, 373-385.
6. Campbell M, Geller B, Small AM, Petti TA, Ferris SH. Minor physical anomalies in young psychotic children. *Am J Psychiatry*, 1987;135:573-575.
7. Freeman BJ. *Diagnosis of the Syndrome of Autism: Questions Parents Ask*. Available at: http://www/autism-society.org/packages/getstart_diagnosis.html. Accessed 6/96.
8. National Information Center for Children and Youth with Disabilities.(NICHY). *Autism/PDD*. Washington, DC: NICHY, 1995.
9. Gotera MA, Johnson C, Plew GT. *Introduction to Autism*. Bloomington, Ind. Indiana Resource Center for Autism, Institute for the Study of Developmental Disabilities, 1987.
10. Autism Action Committee, Special School District of St. Louis County. *An Introduction to Autism*. St. Louis, Mo: Special School District of St. Louis County, 1991.
11. Edelson SM. *Rett Syndrome*. Salem, Ore: Center for the Study of Autism, 1995.Available at: http://www.awtismorg.rett.html
12. *Rett Syndrome*. from Pediatric Database. Available at: http://www.icondata.com/health/pedbase/files/RETTSYND.HTM (PEDBASE) Accessed 10/21/94.
13. Holm VA. *Notes from Rett Syndrome Conference*, October 1986; Vienna, Austria.
14. Bowers B. Cracking the shell – an intensive therapy for autistic children yields gains and hope. *Wall Street Journal* May 20, 1992: Al and A5.
15. Bell P. Autism: even the experts debate treatment. *Pacesetter*. Winter 1996:9-11.
16. Sigman M Capps L. *Children with Autism: A Developmental Perspective*. Cambridge, Mass: Harvard University Press, 1997:186.

BIBLIOGRAPHY

Autism Society of America. *General Information on Autism*. Silver Spring, Md: Autism Society of America (no date).

Carpenito LJ. *Handbook of Nursing Diagnoses*. 4th ed. Philadelphia, Pa: JB Lippincott Company 1991.

Grandin T. *Teaching Tips for Children and Adults with Autism*. Fort Collins, Colo: Colorado State University, 1996.

Haas MB, ed. *The School Nurse's Source Book of Individualized Healthcare Plans*. North Branch, Minn: Sunrise River Press, 1993. (Sunrise River Press, 11605 Kost Dam Road, North Branch, MN 55056. 800-895-4585; fax 651-583-2023)

Hootman J. *Nursing Diagnosis: Application in the School Setting*. Scarborough, Me: National Association of School Nurses, 1996.

Indiana Resource Center for Autism. *Characteristics of the Person with Autism*. Bloomington, Ind. Indiana University (no date).

North American Nursing Diagnosis Association. *NANDA Nursing Diagnoses: Definitions & Classification 1999-2000*. Philadelphia, Pa: North American Nursing Diagnosis Assn, 1999.

(NANDA, 1211 Locust Street, Philadelphia, PA 19107. 800-647-9002; fax 215-545-8107; e-mail: NANDA@nursecominc.com)

Schopler E, Mesibov GB, eds. *High Functioning Individuals with Autism.* New York, NY: Plenum Press, 1992.

RESOURCES

Asperger Syndrome Support Newsletter
Mark Bebbengton, Editor
National Autistic Society
276 Willesden Lane
London England NW2 5RB

Autism Research Institute
Bernard Rimland, PhD, Director
4182 Adams Avenue
San Diego, CA 92116

Autism Society of America
8601 Georgia Avenue
Suite 503
Silver Spring, MD 20910

Center for the Study of Autism
3904 SE Clinton Street
Portland, OR 97202
    (Auditory training research)

Division TEACCH
    (Treatment and Education of Autistic and
    related Communication Handicapped Children)
Eric Schopler, PhD, Director
Gary Mesibov, PhD, Co-Director
CB 7180, 310 Medical School Wing E
The University of North Carolina at Chapel Hill
Chapel Hill, NC 27599-7180

Temple Grandin, PhD
2915 Silver Plume Drive, #C3
Fort Collins, CO 80526
    (Autistic adult)

Illinois Society for Autistic Citizens
2200 South Main Street
Suite 317
Lombard, IL 60148

Indiana Resource Center for Autism
Institute for the Study of Developmental Disabilities
Indiana University

Bloomington, IN 47405

International Rett Syndrome Association
9121 Piscataway Road, Suite 2B
Clinton, MD 20735
1-800-818-7388
301-856-3334
irsa@paltech.

National Organization for Rare Disorders
The National Society for Children and
Adults with Autism
Autism Society of America
7910 Woodmont Avenue, Suite 650
Bethesda,MD 20814-3015
Phone: 800-3-AUTISM

National Information Center for Children
and Youth with Disabilities (NICHCY)
P.O. Box 1492
Washington, DC 20013-1492
1-800-695-0285
    202-884-8200
nichcy@aed.org

Progress ACCESS
Southwest Missouri State University
901 South National Avenue
Springfield, MO 65804
    (Has large lending library)
417-836-6755

PDD/Asperger Syndrome Support Group
49 Ascolese Road
Trumbull, CT 06611-2330
kkr74a@prodigy.com

25 | IHP: Prader-Willi Syndrome

Linda L. Solum

INTRODUCTION

Prader-Willi syndrome (PWS) is a neurobehavioral genetic disorder affecting 1 in 10,000 live births. The most dominant characteristics of PWS are an insatiable appetite (resulting in obesity) and aberrant behaviors. Individuals with PWS are suspected to have a functional defect in the hypothalamus, which is the part of the brain that determines hunger and satiety. [1]

Historical Background

In 1956, Prader, Labhart, and Willi described a new syndrome characterized by obesity (due to hyperphagia), short stature, lack of muscle tone in infancy, undescended testicles, and mental retardation. Since then, other researchers have noted additional characteristics of a tendency toward diabetes, strabismus, orthopedic problems (scoliosis and hip dislocation among others), gross motor developmental delay, and severe personality problems. [2]

It is interesting to note that in 1680 a six-year-old female who weighed 120 pounds was the subject of a painting by Juan Carreno de Miranda, a painter to the Spanish Court. The painting entitled Eugenia Martinez Vallejo, "La Monstura" was ordered by King Charles II and depicts some of the common features of PWS, that of obesity, small triangular mouth, and small hands and feet. The painting is located in the Prado Museum in Madrid, Spain. [2]

Clinical Features

Prader-Willi syndrome has two distinct clinical stages.

Stage I – Failure to Thrive

Infants with PWS have a low birth weight and may be referred to as "floppy babies." Along with weak muscles (hypotonia), these babies often are unable to suck and demonstrate delayed developmental progress in lifting their head, sitting up, crawling, walking and speaking.

Stage II – Thriving Too Well

An insatiable appetite and excessive weight gain usually become apparent during toddlerhood. Children with PWS do not feel full and can eat great amounts of food without becoming nauseated. They also gain weight on relatively few calories. Between the ages of 3 and 5 years, behavior problems may develop that include stubbornness, temper tantrums, acts of violence, and perseveration, or the uncontrollable repetition of a particular word, phrase, or gesture. These behaviors may be spontaneous or initiated by withholding food. [1]

People with PWS also share some common physical features. They may have almond-shaped eyes, narrow forehead, downturned mouth, thin upper lip, small chin, and small hands and feet. Other common features that may be present include a tendency to pick at their skin, thick saliva, scoliosis, daytime sleepiness, sleep abnormalities due to obesity, small penis in boys, and small clitoris in girls.

Management

The one thing that all people with PWS need is 24-hour-a-day supervision of their access to food and consumption of food. They have been known to gorge, hoard, and forage for food. Families have reported that whole batches of cookies have disappeared and raw hamburger that was defrosting was eaten. Cupboards, refrigerators, freezers, and garbage cans need to be locked up. People with PWS may also steal money to have access to more food. Even though people with PWS may have a lower IQ, they can still demonstrate cleverness in seeking food.

Everyone in the child's food environment needs to be aware of monitoring food intake. Children with PWS may ask others for food or trade food at lunchtime. They cannot use school snack bars and they need to be monitored during school lunch. Special occasions like parties at school should be planned in advance so children with PWS can eliminate 50 to 100 calories a day for a week ahead of the social.

Other considerations in the school setting may include adaptations to physical education because of orthopedic concerns, weight loss or maintenance, and special education involvement because of the tendency to have a lower IQ and negative behavior issues.

INDIVIDUALIZED HEALTHCARE PLAN

Assessment

History

- Healthcare providers involved
- When was PWS diagnosed, age of child at time of diagnosis
- Involvement of support systems/groups for child and family
- Past experiences concerning obsession with food
- Past experiences concerning behavior problems/issues
- Management methods concerning food intake which are successful
- Medications: types, reason, efficacy
- Behavioral issues management, behavior modification, social skills training

Current Status and Management

- Current symptoms
- Last assessment with healthcare providers
- Knowledge of student's general health
- Level of intellectual functioning
- Current management of sleep disturbances
- Current behavioral issues and current management plan
- Current height and weight
- Current daily caloric intake

- PWS management plan, including problems and successes in:
  - Medication
  - Behavior management
  - Counseling/therapy
  - Child/family education
- Current scoliosis screen
- Presence of orthopedic problems and any physical limitations
- Skin integrity

Self-care

- Student's decision-making skills
- Student's perception about PWS
- Student's level of cooperation and participation in food management plan
- Student's level of personal self-care-oral hygiene, bathroom cues, skin picking
- Child's motivation to be involved in self-care, self-management

Psychosocial Status

- Student's locus of control—health, school, activities of daily living
- Student's concerns about health condition, behaviors, sleep problems

Academic Issues

- Barriers to food management control in school
- Individual Education Program (IEP) or Section 504 plan
- Monitoring food intake in school classroom/education/hallway-locker, etc.
- Staff awareness and knowledge of PWS
- Behavior management issues/plan (inclusion of teachers, psychologist, social worker, paraprofessionals, etc.)

Nursing Diagnoses (N.D.)

N.D. 1 Alteration in nutrition: more than body requirements (NANDA 1.1.2.1) related to excessive appetite (PWS)

N.D. 2 Risk for noncompliance (NANDA 5.2.1.1) with food management plan related to:
  - behavior patterns
  - lack of ability to feel satiety

N.D. 3 Altered thought processes (NANDA 8.3) related to:
  - appropriate eating behaviors
  - mental retardation (mild to severe)

N.D. 4 Knowledge deficit (NANDA 8.1.1 and 8.3) related to:
  - mental retardation (mild to severe).

N.D. 5   Risk for violence: self-directed (NANDA 9.2.2.2) or directed at others (NANDA 9.2.2.) related to aberrant behaviors associated with PWS.

N.D. 6 Altered growth and development (NANDA 6.6) related to lack of adolescent growth spurt in PWS.

N.D. 7   Fatigue (NANDA 6.1.1.2.1) related to:
- sleep disturbances
- decreased metabolic rate

N.D. 8   Risk for impaired physical mobility (NANDA 6.1.1.1) related to skeletal impairments associated with PWS.

N.D. 9   Alteration in activity tolerance (NANDA 6.1.1.2) related to:
- obesity
- decreased physical stamina/endurance
- gross motor delay
- hypotonicity

N.D. 10   Risk for impaired skin integrity (NANDA 1.6.2.1.2.2) related to skin-picking behaviors

N.D. 11   Disturbance in self-esteem (NANDA 7.1.2) related to:
- looking different from peers

Goals

Participate and cooperate in food management plan in the school setting. (N.D. 1, 2)

Increase compliance with food management plan. (N.D. 1, 2)

Increase appropriate eating behaviors. (N.D. 1, 2)
- Choice of food
- Amount of food

Make appropriate decisions regarding food choices. (N.D. 1, 2)

Maintain stable and appropriate weight. (N.D. 1, 6)

Participate in physical education activities, with modifications made as needed. (N.D. 1, 8)

Participate in classroom activities, with modifications made as needed. (N.D. 3, 4, 5, 8)

Increase knowledge of PWS and increase knowledge in alteration in growth and development. (N.D. 3, 4, 6)

Decrease in violent/injurious behavior to others. (N.D. 5)

Decrease in self-injurious behavior (skin picking). (N.D. 5, 10)

Prevent fatigue during the school day. (N.D. 7)

Decrease sleeping in the classroom. (N.D. 7)

Increase activity tolerance. (N.D. 9)

Maintain skin integrity and prevent infection. (N.D. 10)

Participate in social club activities with peers. (N.D. 11)

Nursing Interventions

Encourage parents to send appropriate school lunches from home to control portions. (Standard school lunches are usually too high in calories.) (N.D. 1)

Monitor weight on a basis agreed upon with parents and healthcare provider and alert family of weight gain. (N.D. 1)

Inform staff that educational plan should include thirty minutes of daily physical activity to prevent fatigue, raise metabolism, and help maintain or promote weight loss, and discuss possible ways of scheduling physical activity into the student's schedule. (N.D. 1, 2, 3)

Inform staff and administration that one-to-one supervision during the school day may be necessary to monitor food intake, especially in the cafeteria, and discuss possible ways of providing supervision. (N.D. 1, 2, 3)

Assist the student to learn which behaviors are associated with PWS. (N.D. 1, 2, 3, 4, 5)

- gorging, hoarding, and foraging for food
- stubbornness
- temper tantrums
- acts of violence
- perseveration
- skin picking

Assist student to learn and understand the limits or boundaries that are needed to: (N.D. 1, 2, 3, 4, 7, 9)

- control food intake
- control behavior
- promote adequate sleep
- exercise

Educate everyone working with the student about PWS and the PWS management plan, including food restriction, food-related activities, behavior modification, and physical activity. (N.D. 1, 2, 3, 5, 9)

Update healthcare plan annually to provide current student concerns. (N.D. 1-11)

Assist the student in realistic goal setting and positive, effective problem solving regarding the condition. (N.D. 2, 3, 4)

Communicate with family regarding behavior modification techniques that are successful and inform staff of these interventions in the school setting. (N.D. 2, 3, 4, 5)

Initiate collaboration between families and educators regarding educational plan, which should be based on intellectual functioning and behavioral needs. (N.D. 2, 3, 4, 5)

Develop and implement measures for behavior modification plan that are consistent and oriented toward intervention and prevention. (ND 3,4,5)

Refer to special education team for assessment if behaviors significantly impact ability to learn or if the student is having difficulty academically. (N.D. 4, 5)

Assist the student to learn what PWS is

- a genetic disorder resulting in a desire to eat food without control (N.D. 4, 11)

Assist the student to learn alterations in growth and development associated with PWS. (N.D. 6)

- delayed growth spurt

Screen for scoliosis annually or as necessary. (N.D. 8)

Review student's daily schedule. (N.D. 9)

- academic classes
- movement around the school environment
- pattern of activities: sitting, moving around, physical education

Assist student to identify and participate in activities with peers outside of class time, for example: school newspaper, student bulletin board, after-school sports (adaptive sports). (N.D. 9,11)

Observe, clean, and bandage skin lesions as necessary. (N.D. 10)

Expected Student Outcomes

The student will maintain a stable weight or appropriate weight as defined by his or her healthcare provider. (N.D. 1)

The student will list three or more behaviors associated with PWS. (N.D. 1, 2, 3, 4, 5)

The student will cooperate with the food and behavior management plan in the school setting. (N.D. 2, 3)

- Does not take food from other students
- Does not get food from the snack bar
- Does not trade his or food for other people's food

The student will describe alterations in his/her growth and development related to PWS (at the level of the student's understanding). (N.D. 4, 6)

The student will describe what PWS is. (N.D. 4, 11)

The student will not demonstrate self-injurious or inappropriate behaviors in the school setting. (N.D. 5)

The student will not sleep in school. (N.D. 7)

The student will follow the physical activity plan to prevent fatigue. (N.D. 7)

The student will describe his/her physical limitations. (N.D. 8)

The student will participate in physical education activities (with modifications as needed). (N.D. 8, 9)

The student will be involved in activities with other students outside of the school day. (N.D. 8, 9, 11)

The student will self-manage activities and mobility in the school setting. (N.D. 9)

The student will decrease skin-picking episodes. (N.D. 10)

CASE STUDY

Peter is 12 years old and in the fifth grade. Currently his height is 59 inches and his weight is 150 pounds. When Peter was born, he was a "floppy baby" with poor muscle tone. When he was around 2 years old, he gained 20 pounds in four months. He was then diagnosed with Prader-Willi syndrome. Since then he has needed to be on a strictly monitored diet.

Because of the neurologic disabilities associated with Prader-Willi syndrome, Peter demonstrates poor judgment and difficulty understanding abstract concepts. He has been known to crawl out of his bedroom window in the middle of the night to walk to a grocery store to get extra food. He also struggles with obsessive-compulsive behaviors, skin picking, temper tantrums, and a tendency to be argumentative. His mental abilities are at the level of a 7-year-old. At times he is frustrated because of the inability to live a normal lifestyle.

Individualized Healthcare Plan*
Prader-Willi Syndrome

Assessment Data	Nursing Diagnosis	Goals	Nursing Interventions	Expected Outcomes
ND1 Excessive continual overeating leading to obesity.	Alteration in nutrition: more than body requirements (NANDA 1.1.2.1) related to excessive appetite.	Participates and cooperates in the food management plan in the school setting.	Inform staff and discuss with administration that one-to-one supervision during the school day may be necessary to monitor food intake. (Meals monitored by a school staff member.)	Student will cooperate with the food and behavioral management plan in the school setting.
		Makes appropriate decisions regarding food choices.	Record weights weekly and alert family of weight gain.	The student will maintain a stable weight or appropriate weight as defined by his healthcare provider.
			Food intake must be monitored in the school setting, especially during school lunch. The student cannot use the school snack bar.	The student does not use the snack bar during lunch.

ND3 The student has been known to ask other students for food, trade food and badger other students for food.	Altered thought processes (NANDA 8.3) related to: inappropriate eating behaviors and mental retardation (mild).	Increase compliance with the food management plan.	Educate everyone working with the student about PWS, the management plan including food restrictions, food-related activities, behavior modification, and physical activity.	The student will cooperate with the food and behavioral management plan in the school setting: will not take food from other students; will not trade food with other students.
ND4 It is difficult for the student to understand PWS and the boundaries that need to be followed during the school day.	Knowledge deficit (NANDA 6.1.1.2.1) related to: mental retardation (mild).	Increases knowledge of PWS.	Assist the student to learn and understand what PWS is and the limits or boundaries that are needed to control food intake boundaries.	The student will describe what PWS is) at appropriate development level).

*See Appendix for student profile information to include on an IHP form.

REFERENCES

1. Angulo MA. Prader-Willi syndrome: a guide families and others. For information, contact the Prader-Willi Foundation USA, 5700 Midnight Pass Road, Sarasota, FL 34242. 800-926-4797.
2. Prader-Willi Perspectives (eds). Prader-Willi syndrome FAQ. For information, contact the Prader-Willi Foundation USA, 5700 Midnight Pass Road, Sarasota, FL 34242. 800-926-4797.

BIBLIOGRAPHY

Angulo MA. Prader-Willi syndrome: A Guide for Families and Others. For information, contact the Prader-Willi Foundation USA, 5700 Midnight Pass Road, Sarasota, FL 34242. 800-926-4797.

Hanchett J, Greenswag L. Health care guidelines for individuals with Prader-Willi syndrome. [online] Available at: http://www.pwsausa.org/postion/HCG_ doc.htm Accessed November 11, 1998.

North American Nursing Diagnosis Association. *NANDA Nursing Diagnoses: Definitions and Classification 1999-2000.* Philadelphia, Pa: North American Nursing Diagnosis Assn, 1999. (NANDA, 1211 Locust Street, Philadelphia, PA 19107. 800-647-9002; fax 215-545-8107; e-mail: NANDA@nursecominc.com)

Prader-Willi Perspectives (eds). Prader-Willi syndrome FAQ. For information, contact the Prader-Willi Foundation USA, 5700 Midnight Pass Road, Sarasota, FL 34242. 800-926-4797.

Pipes, PL. Nutrition and weight management for individuals with Prader-Willi syndrome. [online] Available at: http://www.pwsyndrome.com/pub/pipes./html Accessed July, 1993.

Prader-Willi syndrome. [online] Available at: http://www.icondata.com/com/pedbase/files/ PRADER-W.HTM Accessed January 21, 1994.

Prader-Willi syndrome: basic facts and medical alert. [online] Available at: http:// www.pwsausa.org/medalert.htm November 5, 1998.

Prader-Willi California Foundation – Prader-Willi syndrome (PWCF-PWS) diagnostic criteria, Clinical Features Treatment. [online] Available at: http://www.pwcf.org/diagnostic.html http://

al.html; http://www.pwcf.org/treatment.html. Accessed September 30,

...ursing Care of Infants and Children. St. Louis, Mo: CV Mosby, 1999.

...linical Manual of Pediatric Nursing. St. Louis, Mo: CV Mosby, 1990.

...tion, USA

Sarasota, FL 34242
800-926-4797
941-312-0400
941-312-0142, fax
e-mail pwsausa@aol.com

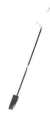

26 | IHP: Prenatal Alcohol and Drug Exposure

Mariann Smith

INTRODUCTION

Historically, society has always used herbs, plants, and other substances to relieve pain and/or alter mental perceptions. Prior to the passage of the Harrison Narcotic Act in 1914 (which made narcotics illegal), opium was a common ingredient in patent medications easily obtained without prescriptions and given to women to prevent miscarriages.[1]

This increased the incidence of addiction in women because of the standard of practice at the time. Still, these women faced more public censor, more punitive responses, and less access to treatment.

Today, women are still abusing drugs—before, during, and after pregnancy. The National Institute on Drug Abuse (NIDA) estimated that in 1988, 15% of the women of childbearing age (15 to 44 years of age) were substance abusers.[2] Thirty-four million of the above women drank alcohol, 18 million smoked, and 6 million used illegal drugs. The current drug of choice is alcohol (which many in society do not consider a drug); however, prenatal exposure to alcohol can result in fetal alcohol syndrome (FAS) or fetal alcohol effects (FAE). fetal alcohol syndrome is the leading *preventable* cause of birth defects.[1]

Substance abuse covers all socioeconomic groups and has become a very costly burden on our social, health, and educational services. Treatment for these women continues to be a problem because many of the treatment facilities do not accept pregnant women or their children. These children are often shifted from foster family to foster family while the mother is in treatment. Grandparents also may be asked to take over the care of these children.

One study concluded that 25% of drug-affected children have developmental delays, and 40% have neurologic abnormalities that might affect their ability to socialize and function appropriately in a school setting.[3] It is also estimated that 42% to 52% will need special education services.[4] Even with special education services, the prognosis is not good. Intelligence scores of children with FAS do not improve over time.[5] Using the Vineland Adaptive Behavior Scales, a study of adolescents and adults (chronological age 17 years) also found that overall adaptive functioning was only at the level of a 7-year-old.[6]

Pathophysiology

Alcohol directly affects brain growth and differentiation of embryonic and fetal tissue.[7] The brain is smaller in size with enlarged ventricles, decreased white matter, and cell groups located in the wrong places. A particular pattern of abnormal features of the eyes, face, and head is possible. It is not the degree of alcohol intake of the mother that is related to the presence of abnormalities in the fetus. Rather, it is the amount consumed in excess of the fetal liver's ability to detoxify it.[8] When the fetal liver receives more alcohol than it is able to handle, the excess is continually recirculated until it can be converted to carbon dioxide and water. Circulating alcohol has a special affinity for brain tissue.

Exposure to cocaine can result in decreased uterine blood flow, especially in the placenta.[9] This can lead to uterine irritability, abruptio placenta, and premature birth. Cerebral infarcts after birth can occur. Hypotonia and tremors can also occur. Often these women have a general lack of interest in self-care. Because of the fear of being discovered using illegal drugs, they often avoid the medical system and receive little or no prenatal care. The effects on the fetus are secondary to maternal problems for example, maternal hypertension can result in decreased uterine blood flow.

Maternal smoking is related to significant deficits in birth weight. Twenty-one to thirty-nine percent of the incidence of low-birth-weight infants is attributable to maternal smoking.[8] Smoking also results in more miscarriages, premature births, increased perinatal mortality, and respiratory concerns. Exposure to marijuana is similar to the effects of tobacco smoking. There is also some increase in precipitate labor and meconium staining.

Heroin exposure often results in first trimester spontaneous abortions, premature delivery, intrauterine growth retardation, and meconium aspiration. Maternal and/or neonatal infections are also prevalent (sexually transmitted diseases, hepatitis, human immune deficiency virus, cytomegalovirus, herpes, chlamydia, etc.).

Prenatal exposure to alcohol, tobacco, and illegal drugs is harmful to babies. These babies may be born prematurely and may, have a low birth weight, a small head circumference, cardiac concerns, and neurologic concerns. They may be retarded. They are often hyperactive, irritable, and highly sensitive to sensory stimuli. They may have to remain in the hospital longer following their birth. Bonding and feeding problems are common. These problems, along with the mother's continued substance abuse, place these babies at an increased risk for physical abuse and/or neglect.

During the preschool years, drug-affected children are affectionate but also distractible. Many display poor fine motor skills. As these children enter elementary school, they often have inadequate communication skills, are impulsive, and have difficulty with social interactions. When these same students enter adolescence, they may exhibit poor judgment, trouble with abstract reasoning, and limited problem-solving skills (see figure 1).

FIGURE 1

Characteristics Often Observed in Students Exposed to Prenatal Substance Abuse

- mental retardation or learning disabilities
- hyperactivity/impulsiveness
- distractible
- microcephaly
- developmental delays
- fine and gross motor difficulties
- expressive language difficulties
- poor peer interactions
- visual/motor difficulties
- low tolerance for frustration
- facial abnormalities, especially with fetal alcohol syndrome
- hearing loss
- heart murmur
- heightened response to sensory/motor stimuli

Compiled from material obtained from "Workshop on Drug-Affected Children," Wichita, Kansas, Summer, 1992.

Management

Managing students exposed to prenatal substance abuse is challenging. Substance abuse does not occur in a vacuum. The child may have been exposed to a combination of drugs — often in a chaotic and violent environment. Restructuring the child's environment at home and at school is the primary intervention technique used.[5] It is best to have the same home caregiver for the child rather than frequent changes in foster care placements or being moved from relative to relative. A consistent, highly structured routine as well as consistent limits on behavior is very important at home and school. Classroom stimuli and noise need to be kept to a minimum. Pictures and other clues need to be posted throughout the classroom to provide information on how to use materials, etc.

Many of these students have cardiac, neurologic, visual, hearing, and speech and perceptual concerns. Medical management involves monitoring and treating the various symptoms in order to maximize the child's potential. Medical management for any of these problems may be lifelong.

Because of numerous health and/or developmental concerns, these students usually require special education services, including health-related services such as medication administration. The student's teachers will need to know each student's health status, activity restrictions, medication effects, and possible side effects.

The school nurse is a critical liaison between the educational and the medical community. Close communication with the teacher and healthcare provider is necessary so that the most appropriate medications, dosage schedule, and so on can be obtained. The school nurse is also an important member of the Individual Education Program team if special education services are needed or as part of a 504 team if a 504 plan is needed.

INDIVIDUALIZED HEALTHCARE PLAN

Assessment

History

- Prenatal care
- Type of prenatal substance abuse of mother
- Birth weight
- Birth trauma
- Length of baby's hospital stay
- Physical abnormalities
- Neurologic abnormalities
- Cardiac abnormalities
- Attainment of developmental milestones
- Social and Rehabilitation Services involvement (e.g. foster care)
- Concurrent diagnoses (e.g., Attention Deficit Hyperactivity Disorder, Oppositional Defiant Disorder, Obsessive Compulsive Disorder)
- Any early medical/educational interventions

Current Status and Management

- Current medications
- Healthcare provider(s)
- Current health status

Self-care

- Current developmental level
- Ability level in independent activities of daily living
- Level of responsibility in complying with medication plan
- Willingness and interest in participating in self-care activities

Psychosocial Status

- Peer relations
- Family support systems
- Social interactions in school, in small groups, etc.
- Parent(s) realistic expectations regarding health concerns
- Parent(s) realistic expectations about educational concerns
- Feelings of being different, needing to take medications, etc.

Academic Issues

- Early educational interventions
- School attendance
- Academic performance patterns
- Regular education and special education issues
- Need for 504 plan
- School staff perceptions
- Healthcare needs during the school day: medications, special procedures, etc.

Nursing Diagnoses (N.D.)

N.D. 1   Body image disturbance (NANDA 7.1.1) related to:
  - physical anomalies
  - increased activity level
  - hyper reactions to sensory stimuli

N.D. 2   Risk for altered parenting (NANDA 3.2.1.1.2) related to:
  - bonding difficulty; hard to console
  - increased activity level; impulsiveness

N.D. 3   Impaired verbal communication (NANDA 2.1.1.1)

N.D. 4   Altered growth and development (NANDA 6.6)

N.D. 5   Risk for injury (NANDA 1.6.1)

N.D. 6   Self-esteem disturbance (NANDA 7.1.2)

N.D. 7   Sensory/perceptual alterations (N.D.7.2)

N.D. 8   Impaired social interaction (NANDA 3.1.1)

N.D. 9   Thought processes, altered (N.D.8.3)

N.D.10   Knowledge deficit (NANDA 8.1.1) related to effects of prenatal drug exposure

Goals

The student will:
- increase knowledge about current medical status, including any disabilities and need for medications. (N.D.1,4,10)

- increase ability to participate in school activities with accommodations as needed in order to maximize intellectual potential by:
  - increasing appropriate participation in social interactions with adults and peers. (N.D.5,8)
  - increasing appropriate participation in educational activities. (N.D.3,7,9)
- maintain good school attendance pattern. (N.D.4,8)
- participate in medication plan at school. (N.D.1,9)
- participate in IHP development. (N.D.1-10)
- increase self-awareness and acceptance of self. (N.D.6)

The school staff will:
- provide appropriate school curriculum and activities in order for student to maximize intellectual potential. (N.D.1,3-9)

Caregiver(s) will:
- demonstrate realistic understanding of student's potential regarding growth and development (physical and psychosocial) and his or her education. (N.D.2)

Nursing Interventions

In-service school staff about effects of exposure to prenatal substance abuse. (N.D.10)
- outline characteristics of students prenatally exposed to drugs
- discuss methods of restructuring classroom environment to minimize distractions
- stress need for routine and calmness
- cite specific health needs, including medications and specific healthcare needs
- outline specific educational needs – including special education services if needed
- discuss psychosocial needs

Develop and implement IHP. (N.D.1-10)
- include student, parents/guardians, appropriate school personnel, and healthcare provider in process

Obtain written authorization from healthcare provider(s) for medications and specialized healthcare procedures, if indicated. (N.D.1-10)

Assist parents to maintain supply of medication at school. (N.D.2)

Assist in providing a safe environment at school. (N.D.5,7,8,9)

Maintain open communication with parents/caregivers. (N.D.1-9)
- educate regarding student's physical and psychosocial needs
- educate regarding realistic goals and expectations
- educate regarding respite care and utilization of support systems

Expected Student Outcomes

The student will:
- participate in all school activities with modifications as necessary. (N.D.3,5,7,8,9)
- comply with medication regimen if indicated. (N.D.1,4)
- demonstrate self-acceptance by working toward maximizing his/her potential (educational and psychosocial). (N.D.6)
- maintain regular school attendance. (N.D.1,2,6)
- maintain academic progress, with modification made as needed (per IEP or 504 plan).

The school staff will:
- describe characteristics of students prenatally exposed to drugs. (N.D.10)
- modify classroom as needed to minimize distractions, etc. (N.D. 1,3,4,5,7,8,9)
- teach appropriate educational and social skills. (N.D. 1,3,4,5,7,8,9)
- assist student to comply with medication needs (e.g., remind student when time for medication, etc.). (N.D. 10)

The caregivers will:
- encourage student to work toward his/her potential. (N.D. 1-10)
- describe and realistically accept student's strengths and weaknesses. (N.D.2)
- comply with medical management. (N.D.1-10)
- effectively manage student's health needs according to the medical management plan. (N.D. 2,10)

CASE STUDY

Janson is a 6-year-old kindergarten student at Place Elementary School. Jason was exposed prenatally to cocaine. Diagnoses of attention deficit hyperactivity disorder (ADHD) and oppositional defiant disorder (ODD) were made after being evaluated by a developmental pediatrician. Adderall and Tegretol were prescribed.

Janson currently lives with his third set of foster parents. His biological mother is incarcerated due to cocaine dealing. The whereabouts of the biological father is unknown.

Janson is having difficulty in school because of his impulsive behavior and very short attention span. In addition, he often hits and/or kicks other children, but denies that he did it. He also frequently uses inappropriate language and does not respond well when corrected. He hates school and everyone at school.

His foster parents have started Janson in private counseling. They have also attended several parent work sessions where math and reading games, etc. can be made to be used at home. They have been consistent in maintaining the medication plan; however, they do admit that it is a challenge trying to get Janson to take his medications. He often hides them in his mouth and then spits them out when his foster parent is not looking.

Lately, he has complained of frequent headaches and/or stomachaches in the morning and tries to convince his foster mother that he needs to stay home from school. When at school, Janson frequently visits the health room with minor complaints. Janson and his school nurse are beginning to trust each other and have decided to decrease health room visits through a reward system and contract.

Individualized Healthcare Plan*
Prenatal Alcohol and Drug Exposure

Assessment Data	Nursing Diagnosis	Goals	Nursing Interventions	Expected Outcomes
ND2 Student in hew foster home. Diagnoses: ADHD, ODD. Medications: Ritalin, Tegretol	Potential for altered parenting related to new foster placement, hyperactivity, impulsiveness, and defiance (NANDA 3.2.1.1.2)	New foster parents will provide stability and a nurturing environment for student.	Establish trusting, open communication with foster parents. Liaison between foster parents, school and physician to monitor medications, dosages, and schedules.	Foster parents will provide nurturing environment. Foster parents will effectively manage health needs at home.
Private family counseling. Complaints of physical symptoms - wants to stay home from school.			Encourage continuation of family counseling with student and foster parents. Encourage foster parents to send student to school every day.	Student will participate in counseling. Student will consistently attend school. Foster parents will maintain a supply of medication at school. Student will maintain a good school attendance pattern.
ND6 Student hates to take medication.	Self-esteem disturbance and altered body image related to hyperactivity, impaired communication skills, impaired social interactions, sensory/perceptual alterations, altered thought process, and potential for injury (NANDA 7.1.2)	Student will utilize support systems at school. Student will increase skills in effectively compensating and coping regarding learning and behavior problems.	Establish trusting relationship with student. Introduce student to school counselor and other support personnel.	Student will participate in classroom activities. Student will increase appropriate behavior in classroom/school. Student will participate in medication plan (comes on time for medications, comes independently, etc.).

Student hates school because he is "different" and "dumb, no one likes me, I have no friends"		Student will increase acceptance of self.	Implement reward system to help student participate and comply with medication plan. Initiate preassessment process with teacher to document possible academic/ behavior concerns.	Student will feel acceptance and reassurance from school staff. Student will increase acceptance of self.
ND10 Student unaware of reason for medications and why he is always "getting into trouble"	Knowledge deficit related to effects of prenatal drug exposure, ODD, ADHD, and need for taking medication to manage the effects of the prenatal drug exposure (NANDA 8.1.1)	Student will continue to increase knowledge about his health and need for mediation. Staff will learn about effects of prenatal substance abuse on students. Student will increase his participation in the medication plan.	In-service staff regarding effects of prenatal drug exposure. Discuss medications, potential side effects, etc. to enable staff to be part of his school support system. Health teaching with student regarding health status and the need for how medications can help improve behavior and school work.	Student will increase knowledge about his health conditions. Student will be able to identify methods to help cope and/or compensate for lifelong deficits. Student will describe need for his medications. Student will swallow his medication immediately upon taking it at school.

*See Appendix for student profile information to include on an IHP form.

REFERENCES

1. Lewis KD. *Infants and Children with Prenatal Alcohol and Drug Exposure: A Guide to Identification and Intervention* North Branch, Minn: Sunrise River Press, 1995. (Sunrise River Press, 11605 Kost Dam Road, North Branch, MN 55056. 800-895-4585; fax 651-583-2023)
2. Bureau of Child Research, University of Kansas. *Juniper Gardens Children's Project - Maternal Substance Abuse and Infant Drug Exposure* Kansas City, Kan: University of Kansas, February 1991.
3. US General Accounting Office. Publication HRD 90-138. *Drug Exposed Infants* Washington, D.C: US General Accounting Office; 1991.
4. Kansas Department of Social and Rehabilitation Services. *Alcohol and Other Drug Exposed Babies: A Preventable Tragedy.* Topeka, Kan: Kansas Dept of Social & Rehabilitation Services, June 1990.
5. Weiner L, Morse BA. Intervention and the child with FAS. *Alcohol Health Res World,* 1994;18(1): 67-72.
6. Streissguth AP. A long-term perspective of FAS. *Alcohol Health Res World,* 1994;18(1): 74-81.
7. Aase JM. Clinical recognition of FAS. *Alcohol Health Res World,* 1994;18(1): 5-9.
8. Wong DL, Hockenbery-Eaton M, Wilson D, Winkelstein ML, Ahmann E, Divito-Thomas PA, eds. *Whaley & Wong's Nursing Care of Infants and Children,* 6th ed. St. Louis, MO: Mosby, 1999.
9. Peterson P. *Pregnancy and Drug Facts,* Santa Cruz, Calif: ETR Associates, 1992.

BIBLIOGRAPHY

Aase JM. Clinical recognition of FAS. *Alcohol Health Res World,* 1994;18(1): 5-9.

Brunette EA. Management of ADHD in the school setting. *J School Nurs,* 1995;11(3): 33-38.

Bureau of Child Research, University of Kansas. *Juniper Gardens Children's Project— Maternal Substance Abuse and Infant Drug Exposure* Kansas City, Kan: University of Kansas, 1991.

Coleman WS. *Attention Deficit Disorders, Hyperactivity and Associated Disorders,* Madison, Wis: Callipoe Books, 1993.

Heagarty MC. Crack cocaine: a new danger in children. *Am J Dis Child.* 1990;144: 756-757.

Kansas Department of Social and Rehabilitation Services. *Alcohol and Other Drug Exposed Babies: A Preventable Tragedy* Topeka, Kan:Kansas Dept of Social & Rehabilitation Services, June 1990.

Lewis KD. *Infants and Children with Prenatal Alcohol and Drug Exposure: A Guide to Identification and Intervention* North Branch, Minn: Sunrise River Press, 1995.(Sunrise River Press, 11605 Kost Dam Road, North Branch, MN 55056. 800-895-4585; fax 651-583-2023)

North American Nursing Diagnosis Association. *NANDA Nursing Diagnoses: Definitions & Classification 1999-2000.* Philadelphia, Pa: North American Nursing Diagnosis Assn, 1999. (NANDA, 1211 Locust Street, Philadelphia, PA 19107. 800-647-9002; fax 215-545-8107; e-mail: NANDA@nursecominc.com)

Odom SE, Herrick C, Holman C, Crowe E, Clements C. Case management for children with attention deficit hyperactivity disorder. *J School Nurs,* 1994;10(3): 17-21.

Peterson P. *Pregnancy and Drug Facts* Santa Cruz, Calif: ETR Associates, 1992.

Streissguth AP. A long-term perspective of FAS. *Alcohol Health Res World.* 1994;18(1):74-81.

United States General Accounting Office. *Drug Exposed Infants* Washington, DC:US General Accounting Office; 1991 Publication HRD 90-138.

Weiner L, Morse BA. Intervention and the child with FAS. *Alcohol Health Res World.* 1994;18(1): 67-72.

Wong DL, Hockenbery-Eaton M, Wilson D, Winkelstein ML, Ahmann E, Divito-Thomas PA, eds. *Whaley & Wong's Nursing Care of Infants and Children,* 6th ed. St. Louis, Mo: Mosby, 1999.

Yates SR. The school nurse's role: early intervention with preschool children. *J School Nurs,* 1992;8(4): 30-36.

27

IHP: Rett Syndrome

Charlotte R. Gorun

INTRODUCTION

Rett syndrome is a neurologic, developmental disorder that usually affects females regardless of race or ethnic background. It was first recognized by a German physician, Dr Andreas Rett, in a presentation of a paper in 1966.[1] Since Dr Rett's presentation, more research is available and more attention has been focused on this disorder.

Diagnosis of Rett syndrome is made by the child's physician following the established criteria. Parents are very aware of their child's development and may begin to notice changes in the child's skills and growth. After the diagnosis has been established, a multidisciplinary approach must be established to maintain optimal health. As the stages progress, the child's medical needs will be reassessed and changes made when needed.

Pathophysiology

There are several theories as to the cause of Rett syndrome. Dr Rett suspected elevated ammonia levels. Another theory suggested an abnormal neurotransmitter function.[2] At present there are no biological tests that establish the diagnosis of Rett syndrome.

Diagnosis is made through a comprehensive history, documentation of developmental milestones, and elimination of other developmental and metabolic disorders. A definitive diagnosis is usually not made until 2 to 5 years of age to avoid a misdiagnosis.

Diagnosis of Rett syndrome is dependent upon meeting the diagnostic criteria established by Hagburg.[1] The infant develops normally for approximately 6 to 18 months. The infant has a normal head circumference at birth, but the head's growth rate slows between 3 months to 4 years of age. The child loses the ability for expressive, communicative, and receptive language. There is a decline in acquired skills between 6 and 30 months. The classic appearance of handwringing, squeezing, clapping together, mouthing, and rubbing take the place of purposeful hand movements. The child's gait becomes stiff legged, and unsteady and the habit of toe walking develops.[2]

Other symptoms also support the initial diagnosis. Breathing dysfunction such as periodic apnea while awake, intermittent hyperventilation, and forced expulsion of air or saliva occur. Abnormalities in EEG testing, with the possible development of seizures, contractures of limbs related to muscle rigidity and spasticity, scoliosis, growth retardation, and decreased body fat and muscle mass also occur. A child may also experience abnormal sleep patterns and irritability and agitation. Eating becomes difficult due to difficulty with chewing and swallowing. Due to poor circulation, the extremities may feel cold and develop a bluish discoloration. Constipation becomes an issue as well as decreased mobility.[1]

The progression of Rett syndrome is identified through clinic stages that were established by Hagberg.[1] Stage I, known as Early Onset, occurs from ages 6 to 18 months. Symptoms of Rett syndrome may begin but are often difficult to detect. Parents may describe a child as easygoing. The baby may lose interest in toys and exhibit decreased eye contact. Developmental milestones may be delayed. The characteristic hang wringing may begin and head growth slows.

Stage II, or Rapid Destructive Stage, may occur from ages 1 to 4 years and last for weeks to months. Symptoms during this stage may progress rapidly or gradually. Purposeful hand skills are lost with the increase of hand wringing or mouthing of hands. These movements do not occur in sleep. Acquired verbal communication skills are lost. Breathing characteristics of apnea, irritability, and hyperventilation occur. Ambulating skills decline and become unsteady. The child with Rett syndrome becomes irritable at times, has frequent crying spells, and has difficulty sleeping.[1]

Stage III, or Plateau Stage, occurs from 2 to 10 years of age and may last for years. This stage is characterized by increased difficulty performing automatic movements; motor coordination is poor and seizures may occur. There appears to be less autistic-type behavior, and irritability and crying decrease.[1] There may be more awareness of the environment and a willingness to interact with others.

Stage IV, or Late Motor Deterioration, is divided in two subcategories: 1) where the child is presently walking; and 2) where the child has never walked.[1] Stage IV begins when Stage III ends, which could be up to 25 years. Some children may never exit Stage III, and Stage IV may last for decades. The child will stop walking. There is leveling off of cognitive, communication, and hand skills. The characteristic hand movements may decrease. Scoliosis may develop. Overall rigidity and spasticity are common, which will affect ambulating skills.

Management

- Modification of environment—eliminating barriers to prevent injury
- Medication: anticonvulsant for seizure control; laxative for bowel elimination management
- Physical therapy: negotiating school environment safely
- Occupational therapy: for motor planning, fine motor control, self-care skills, adaptive equipment
- Speech therapy: establish communication system to express wants and needs
- Nutritional modification: to accommodate risk of aspiration; increase fiber and fluid
- Assistance with activities of daily living
- Parent / guardian education for maintenance of health
- Counseling: assist student and family in coping with Rett syndrome
- Staff and peer education for understanding Rett syndrome

INDIVIDUALIZED HEALTHCARE PLAN

Assessment

History

- When was diagnosis made? Which stage is child in?
- Respiratory status: apnea, reaction to upper respiratory infection, hyperventilation
- Level of ambulating mobility, orthotic use
- Level of fine motor coordination
- Nutritional status; difficulty swallowing or chewing; reflux, need for gastrostomy tube feedings
- What type of seizure activity is present; duration of seizure; behavior observed prior to the seizure
- History of bowel and bladder training
- Sleep patterns
- Physical development

Current Status

- Current status of seizure activity: duration, frequency, behavior observed
- Current medication's therapeutic effects and adverse side effects
- Nutritional status: assess type of food toleration for texture, consistency, ability to chew, ability to swallow, oral feedings
- Bowel and urinary elimination pattern: toileting schedule; frequency of diaper changes
- Monitor urination: toileting schedule; frequency of diaper changes
- Monitor height and weight
- Assess respiratory status: periods of apnea; hyperventilation; coloration of skin
- Assess dental status
- Assess for scoliosis
- Ambulation status: walking or wheelchair mobility
- Classroom environment: safety for ambulation and seizure activity
- Emergency information with current contact names, phone numbers, medical needs
- Emergency care plan: seizures, apnea, hyperventilation

Self-care

- Toileting: assistance needed
- Dental hygiene: assistance needed
- Meals and snacks: assistance needed
- Ambulation or wheelchair mobility: assistance needed
- Ability to communicate needs
- Ability of child to participate in decisions about himself/herself

Psychosocial Status

- Orientation to time and place, especially after seizure
- Ability to participate in classroom activities, especially activities with other children, groups

- Interactions with peers: in and outside of school
- Assistance needed in activities with other students to prevent accidental injury
- Targeted socialization activities with staff and peers

Academic Issues

- Mobility around the school and classroom: assistance needed
- Transportation needs to and from school
- Communication needs: assistance needed, speech/language therapy, facilitated language
- Ability to process information and respond
- Nutritional needs during the school day: snacks, lunch
- Bathroom facilities: privacy assistance, storage of supplies
- Academic schedule: courses in morning; better able to attend
- Functional skills development
- Academic classes
- Physical education: modification needed, assistance needed
- Special education services
- Implement facilitated communication
- Adaptations needed for field trips

Nursing Diagnoses (N.D.)

N.D. 1 Altered nutrition: less than body requirements (NANDA 1.1.2.2) related to intake versus increased metabolism

N.D. 2 Constipation (NANDA 1.3.1.1) related to functional disorder

N.D. 3 Ineffective breathing pattern (NANDA 1.5.1.3) related to hyperventilation and apnea

N.D. 4 Risk for injury (NANDA 1.6.1) related to possible orthopedic fractures when interacting with other children; seizure activity

N.D. 5 Risk for aspiration (NANDA 1.6.1.4) related to difficulty swallowing, chewing, nasal regurgitation, and seizure activity

N.D. 6 Impaired verbal communication (NANDA 2.1.1.1) related to loss of expressive language

N.D. 7 Impaired social interaction (NANDA 3.1.1) related to communication barriers

N.D. 8 Social isolation (NANDA 3.1.2) related to decreased mobility; delay in accomplishing developmental tasks

N.D. 9 Impaired physical mobility (NANDA 6.1.1.1) related to increased muscle spasticity, ataxia, postural instability, and need for wheelchair

N.D. 10 Fatigue (NANDA 6.1.1.2.1) related to interruption of sleep cycle at night

N.D. 11 Feeding, self-care deficit (NANDA 6.5.1) related to loss of purposeful hand skills

N.D. 12 Impaired swallowing (NANDA 6.5.1.1) related to Rett syndrome

N.D. 13 Dressing/grooming, self-care deficit, (NANDA 6.5.3) related to loss of purposeful hand skills, muscle spasticity

N.D. 14 Toileting, self-care deficit (NANDA 6.5.4) related to loss of purposeful hand skills; need for total daily care

N.D. 15   Altered growth and development (NANDA 6.6) related to difficulty swallowing, reflux; difficulty maintaining caloric intake

Goals

- Participation in school/ classroom activities with modifications made as needed (N.D. 7, 8)
- Maintenance of communication through facilitated language (N.D. 6)
- Prevention of injury during seizure activity (N.D. 4, 9, 10)
- Prevention of injury during interactions with peers (N.D. 4, 9, 10)
- Prevention of injury from aspiration (N.D. 1, 3, 5, 12)
- Prevention of choking while eating (N.D. 1, 3, 5, 12)
- Promote good personal care (N.D. 2, 11, 13, 14)
- Maintenance of adequate nutrition (N.D. 1, 5,15)
- Utilization of a period of relaxation between activities (N.D. 3, 9, 10)
- Maintenance of ambulation/mobility in the school/classroom setting (N.D. 9)
- Maintenance of bowel elimination pattern (N.D. 1, 2, 9)
- Maintenance of urinary elimination pattern (N.D. 6, 9, 14)

Interventions

- Assist student with all areas of personal care (toileting, dental care, grooming, applying outerwear) (N.D. 2, 13, 14)
- Monitor eating behaviors, food tolerance (N.D. 3, 5, 9, 11,12)
- Instruct paraprofessionals working with student on assistance required with meals and snacks (N.D. 3, 5, 11, 12)
- Monitor height and weight (N.D. 1, 12, 15)
- Collaborate with therapists to instruct staff on proper feeding technique (N.D. 3, 5, 9, 11, 12)
- Instruct school staff working with the student on what to do if a seizure occurs as outlined in Haas[3] (N.D. 4, 5)
- Develop Emergency Care Plan (ECP): seizures, apnea, hyperventilation (N.D. 3, 4, 5, 9)
- Assess nutritional intake (N.D. 1, 2, 15)
- Promote relaxation periods between work sessions (N.D. 3, 9, 10)
- Monitor activity tolerance (N.D. 3, 4, 9, 10, 15)
- Monitor respiratory status during activities which require increased energy expenditure (N.D. 1, 3,)
- Assess classrooms for safe environment, barriers to mobility (N.D. 4, 9)
- Develop Emergency Evacuation Plan (EEP) to assure safe and expedient exit from the school building if needed (N.D. 4, 9)
- Participate in the school multidisciplinary team regarding special educational services required and development of Individual Education Program (IEP) (N.D. 4, 6, 8, 9)
- Assist in determining and providing appropriate bathroom facilities: storage of supplies, privacy room to assist with toileting needs (N.D. 2, 9, 11,13, 14)
- Assist in establishing appropriate activity restrictions in cooperation with parent/ guardian and physician to prevent injury (N.D. 3, 4, 9, 10, 15)

- Allow student adequate time to process and respond to information (N.D.6)
- Utilize facilitated communication when interacting with student (N.D. 6, 7, 8)
- Encourage parent/ guardian to maintain semiannual dental evaluation with dentist (N.D. 5)
- Annual scoliosis screenings (N.D. 9)
- Instruct staff working with student on how to perform Heimlich maneuver (N.D. 3, 4, 5, 6)
- Administer prescribed medication monitor therapeutic and adverse effects (N.D. 4, 5)
- Maintain communication with parent/guardians regarding child's adjustment to school activities and modify school programs as needed (N.D. 3-10)
- Provide only two choices in assisting the student to make decisions (N.D. 6, 7, 8)

Expected Student Outcomes

- The student will not aspirate during meal and snack periods. (N.D. 3, 5, 9, 12)
- The student will use facilitated communication to interact with staff and peers. (N.D. 6, 7, 8)
- The student will participate in school/ classroom activities with peers. (N.D.6, 7, 8, 9)
- The student will maintain good hygiene with assistance as needed. (N.D. 11, 13, 14)
- The student will participate in classroom activities without injury to self and with assistance from staff as needed. (N.D. 3, 4, 9, 10)
- The student will participate in health screenings. (N.D. 1, 5, 9, 15)
- The student will receive good nutrition orally or by gastrostomy feedings. (N.D. 1, 3, 5, 12, 15)
- The student is mobile in the school/ classroom environment. (N.D. 3, 4, 8, 9, 10)
- The student will exit the school building safely and quickly in an emergency (fire, etc.). (N.D. 6, 8, 9)

Collaborative Problem

Potential complication: Gastrostomy

CASE STUDY

The IHP was initiated for Anne, who is 10 years old. She was diagnosed at 18 months with Rett syndrome. Prior to this age she was achieving the normal developmental milestones. According to Anne's mother, she was speaking in two-to three-word phrases and feeding herself. One morning the child was participating in a routine interaction with her mother, asking for a pretzel, but she only stared at the cabinet and was unable to verbalize the request. Self-injurious behavior began, which consisted of banging her head on the cabinet. She lost the ability to create phrases. Eye contact diminished. She became incontinent after having been toilet trained prior to this episode.

The child was examined by several physicians. A complete physical examination was performed including an EEG. She was diagnosed with Rett syndrome at 22 months of age. Starting at age 25 months, she was enrolled in an Early Intervention Program. During the early stage, Anne had periods of irritability, crying, and screaming. She also lost purposeful hand skills. At age 3, she was enrolled in a private school for special needs students which she still attends. At the age of 9 years 6 months, she was diagnosed with partial complex seizures and is currently taking medication for the seizures, which appears to be effective. Eye contact has improved and periods of irritability have also diminished. The student is able to ambulate while in school, with assistance. She uses a wheelchair during family outings that require longer periods of ambulation. Complete care is required for all activities of daily living. The school district has arranged for a one-to-one classroom aide. Her educational program is multidisciplinary, involving a physical therapist, occupational therapist, speech therapist, and music therapist as well as a classroom teacher experienced with special needs students. Anne's placement is in an out-of-district school specific to students with special needs.

Individualized Healthcare Plan*
Rett Syndrome

Assessment Data	Nursing Diagnosis	Goals	Nursing Interventions	Expected Outcomes
ND4 Frequency 6-8 times per hour. Occurs daily. Stops activity and has staring spell and blinking eyes (similar to daydreaming) Unable to determine if child experiences aura No loss of consciousness	Risk for injury related to random staring spells (seizures) (NANDA 1.6.1)	Prevent injury during seizures.	Protect child during seizure and educate staff. Provide supervision during all school activities. Establish appropriate activity, restrictions in cooperation with parents/physician in order to prevent injury during seizure. Provide documentation of seizure activity in school. Communicate such activity to parents. Administer first aid as needed. Instruct staff in proper ambulation technique.	Student will not experience injury during seizure.

ND5 Frequent drooling. Needs to eat small amounts of food at a time, occasionally gags on food while eating. Is able to cough at present	Potential for aspiration related to seizure activities (NANDA 1.6.1.4)	Prevent aspiration during seizure.	Assist with eating activities - small mouthfuls of food. Consult with parents as to which foods are appropriate for student. Position child on side, if necessary, to prevent aspiration.	Student will not aspirate during seizure.
Responds well with consistent staff member	Fear related to loss of stability due to medical diagnosis (NANDA 9.3.2)	Identify source of fear and assist to reduce or eliminate.	Provide emotional support for staff so they are comfortable working with student. Provide for continuity of staff working with student so each staff member assists the student in the same manner.	Relates less anxiety, fear of loss of control. Appears secure participating in class activity.
Consistent staff member is able to understand student's communication	Alteration of daily living. Personal, recreational, hygiene, toileting, eating, walking, stair climbing, relating to physical disabilities. (NANDA 6.6)	Student will acquire adaptations necessary to experience activities commensurate with capabilities in school setting.	Arrange for assistance as necessary for daily school activities, i.e., opening doors, getting on and off bus, toileting, extra time for passing between classes.	Student will be able to manage mobility around school and perform as many activities in the educational setting as possible.

Individualized Healthcare Plan*
Rett Syndrome

Assessment Data	Nursng Diagnosis	Goals	Nursing Interventions	Expected Outcomes
Incontinence of urine 3-4 times a day. Student wears orthotic.	Alteration in urine elimination related to effects of physical disability and self-care deficit: toileting (NANDA 1.3.2 and NANDA 6.5.4) Potential for skin injury related to use of orthotic (NANDA 1.6.2.1.2.2)	Student will have successful bladder elimination program. Student will have skin maintained in good condition.	Provide access to bathroom in close proximity to classroom. Instruct physical education teacher in motor expectations appropriate with level of limitations. Classroom teacher establishes time schedule appropriate with classroom activity. Provide appropriate nursing supervision to all personnel assisting student with toileting. Arrange for space and time to perform urinary activity. Observe pressure points for early signs of tissue breakdown. Avoid prolonged pressure of orthotic/follow schedule established by mother. Hot and cold prevention when performing hygiene.	Student will receive assistance for those activites with which she requires assistance. Student will not experience tissue breakdown relating to orthotics and decreased sensory awareness.

*See Appendix for student profile information to include on an IHP form.

REFERENCES

1. Braddock SR, Braddock BA, Graham JM Jr, Rett syndrome: an update and review for the primary pediatrician. *Clin Pediatr*, 1993; 32. October: 613-626.
2. Iyama CM. Rett syndrome. *Adv Pediatr*. 1993; 40: 217-245.
3. Haas MB, ed. *The School Nurse's Source Book of Individualized Healthcare Plans*. North Branch, Minn: Sunrise River Press, 1993: 385. (Sunrise River Press, 11605 Kost Dam Road, North Branch, MN 55056. 800-895-4585; fax 651-583-2023)

BIBLIOGRAPHY

Gerber MJ. IHP: Gastrostomy. In: Haas, MB, ed, *The School Nurse's Source Book of Individualized Healthcare Plans*, North Branch, Minn: Sunrise River Press, 1993:269-273. (Sunrise River Press, 11605 Kost Dam Road, North Branch, MN 55056. 800-895-4585; fax 651-583-2023)

Goodship S. Games and play in the Rett syndrome *Brain Development.*1990;12(1): 164-168.

Hootman J. *Quality Nursing Interventions in the School Setting: Procedures, Models, and Guidelines*. Scarborough, Me: Natl Assn of School Nurses, 1996.

Lieb-Lindell C. The therapist's role in the management of girls with Rett syndrome. *Child Neurol.* 1988; 3: S31-S34.

Lindberg B. *Understanding Your Child With Rett Syndrome: An Approach to Education* . Presented at the Sixth Annual Conference of the International Rett Syndrome Association; May 26, 1990.Washington, DC.

North American Nursing Diagnosis Accociation. *NANDA Nursing Diagnoses: Definitions & Classification 1999-2000*. Philadelphia, Pa: North American Nursing Diagnosis Assn, 1999. (NANDA, 1211 Locust Street, Philadelphia, PA 19107. 800-647-9002; fax 215-545-8107; e-mail: NANDA@nursecominc.com)

Swaiman KF. *Pediatric Neurology: Principles and Practice. Vol II*. St. Louis, Mo: C.V. Mosby Company, 1989:783-786.

Tams-Little S, Holdgrafer G. Early communication development in children with Rett syndrome. *Brain & Development* 1996; 18:376-378.

von Tetzchner S, Jacobson KH, Smith L, Skjeldal OH, Heiberg A, Fagan JF. Vision, cognition and developmental characteristics of girls and women with Rett syndrome. *Developmental Med Child Neurol.* 1993; 38: 221-225.

RESOURCES

International Rett Syndrome Association
9121 Piscataway Road, Suite 2-B
Clinton, MD 20735
(301) 856-3334   1-800-818- RETT
(301) 856-3336 FAX
online: irsa@paltech.com
http://www.2.paltech.com/irsa.htm

28

IHP: Scoliosis

Sally Zentner Schoessler

INTRODUCTION

Scoliosis is a condition that results from alterations in a child's spinal alignment. It is the most common spinal deformity.[1] The child is typically an otherwise healthy child and the spinal curvature is usually an isolated health concern. The cause of scoliosis is unknown, although it can be congenital, secondary to an underlying neuromuscular disorder, or a compensatory disorder resulting from a discrepancy in the lengths of the child's legs.[2]

Pathophysiology

Scoliosis is defined as a curvature of the spine.[3] Although the exact cause of the condition is unknown, there is an increased incidence in young females, who are also more prone to having the problem progress to the point that treatment will be required. Some cause for concern also exists if there is a family history of spinal abnormalities. Heredity plays a part in the diagnostic process because approximately 20% of children with scoliosis have a family member that has scoliosis.[3]

Scoliosis can be classified into two different types, structural and functional, each with unique characteristics. It is very important that the child is carefully examined to determine the origin and severity of the child's spinal curvature as well as how the condition impacts the child's gen-

eral health and mobility. Diagnosis is made by direct observation of the child's exposed back and by radiographic evaluation.

Structural Scoliosis

1. Idiopathic

This is the most common form of scoliosis and is a painless disorder that is most commonly characterized by a right thoracic curve.[2] It occurs more often in children over the age of 10[4] and is the form of scoliosis most often diagnosed following a positive finding from school screenings. Many idiopathic spinal deformities are nonprogressive and never advance to the stage of requiring medical intervention.

2. Congenital

In congenital scoliosis, spinal abnormalities have their origin in the first trimester of fetal formation. The symptoms of spinal problems are evident early in the child's life. There can be a partial or complete curvature of the spine, and the scoliosis may be a single deformity or in combination with other bone or soft tissue anomalies. The risk for progression is dependent on many factors specific to the child's overall condition. A tethered spinal cord or menigomyelocele may also be associated with scoliosis and should be considered in symptoms that appear to develop dramatically over a short period of time.[5]

3. Neuromuscular

Neuromuscular scoliosis is caused by a muscle imbalance and is often only one factor involved with the child's disabilities. This category usually presents along with Duchenne's muscular dystrophy, cerebral palsy, or another significant health problem that is involved in the child's overall condition.[2] Students who are ambulatory tend to have a milder spinal deformity than those who are wheelchair dependent. Students who are nonambulatory can suffer changes in their pulmonary function as a result of the drastic changes that their spinal curvature can cause. The treatment plan for this category of student should involve maintaining the student's current condition and preventing increased spinal abnormality.

4. Neurofibromatosis

Scoliosis is also seen as a complication of neurofibromatosis. Skeletal abnormalities are seen in other parts of the body, but spinal curvature is also seen with this disorder.[6]

5. Traumatic

Trauma to the spine, including fracture, irradiation for treatment of a tumor, or surgical displacement can also cause the condition.[4]

6. Mesenchymal Disease

Congential disorders, such as mesenchymal disease, with dwarfism, connective tissue and bone diseases can be responsible for spinal curvatures. Rheumatoid arthritis is an example of an acquired disorder responsible for a diagnosis of scoliosis.[4]

7. Miscellaneous

Finally, a child may present with idiopathic spinal symptoms, for several other reasons, and these are as follows:
    Tumor
    Inflammation
    Nutritional deficit - rickets
    Metabolic - renal osteodystrophy
    Intraspinal[4]

Functional Scoliosis

Functional scoliosis is caused by a nonspinal condition, such as unequal leg length. The curve is flexible and correction is seen on bending or in compensating for the unequal leg length.

Some states require scoliosis screening for students annually (between 8 and 16 years of age) whereas other states do not make this the responsibility of the school's health services. There is some controversy as to whether or not the school nurse (or physical education department) should be using his or her time to screen for scoliosis. On the other hand, the school nurse is a valuable individual to be assessing questionable spinal curvatures because he/she has a high level of contact with the student and is able to identify and confirm students at risk for developing problems related to scoliosis.

Therapeutic Management

Nonoperative

Treatment for cases of scoliosis that are progressive may include the use of braces, or orthotics, which can be an effectual nonsurgical method of correcting a worsening spinal curve or serve to stabilize the spine. Orthotics, including use of the "Milwaukee brace" (which is to be worn 23 hours a day) can be effective, but the adolescent student often exhibits a low compliance level with this form of therapy. In cases where the scoliosis is caused by a specific condition, treatment of that underlying condition is necessary to correct the scoliosis.

Operative

Several surgical methods can be employed to straighten and secure the spine. These often include the implantation of metal rods or a form of spinal fusion to correct the misalignment. Recovery time for these procedures varies, and can impact the student's mobility and physical education and/or sports program for up to a full school year.

INDIVIDUALIZED HEALTHCARE PLAN

Assessment

History

- Is there a family history of scoliosis?
  If yes, what member of the family has been diagnosed with scoliosis?
- At what age was the alteration in the student's spine first noticed?
- At what age was the student diagnosed with scoliosis?
- Is the curve thoracic? Lumbar? Sacral?
- Is kyphosis (an accentuated backward rounding of the upper spine) seen?
- Is lordosis (an accentuated forward curvature of the lower spine) present?
- Have orthotics been prescribed?
- Take detailed family and student history in regard to general health, but especially for symptoms related to scoliosis.

Current Status and Management

- Has surgery been planned? Has the student had surgery to correct scoliosis?
- Check student physicals and/or scoliosis screening results to validate history and current findings.
- Assess and chart in detailed notations location of curve, kyphosis, and/or lordosis.

Self-Care

- Can student verbalize his/her scoliosis management plan?
- Is student aware of status of his/her scoliosis?
- Does student use orthotic appropriately (if prescribed)?

Psychosocial Status

- Discuss student's perceptions of body and body image.
- Discuss student's feelings in regard to diagnosis of scoliosis.

Academic Issues

- Does student require a modified physical education program?
- Does student require homework assistance during postsurgical period?

Nursing Diagnoses (N.D.)

N.D. 1 (Risk for) impaired physical mobility (NANDA 6.1.1.1) related to spinal alignment abnormalities and /or use of orthotic brace, spinal surgery, and instrumentation.

N.D. 2 (Risk for) body image disturbance (NANDA 7.1.1.1) related to defect in body structure, pronounced spinal curves or as related to scarring from surgical procedures.

N.D. 3 (Risk for) self-esteem disturbance (NANDA 7.1.2) related to visible spinal abnormalities and potential long-term treatment of condition.

N.D. 4 (Risk for) knowledge deficit (NANDA 8.1.1) related to pathophysiology scoliosis and treatment plan.

N.D. 5 (Risk for) impaired skin integrity (NANDA 1.6.2.1.2.1) related to orthotic brace.

Goals

Student will retain or attain maximum level of physical mobility with classroom/school modifications in activities as needed. (N.D. 1)

Student will participate in physical education classes and sports with modifications in physical education program as needed. (N.D. 1)

Student will demonstrate use of orthotic and describe its therapeutic value. (N.D. 1)

Student will express feelings about his/her body. (N.D. 2,3)

Student will express feelings about how his/her scoliosis affects his/her feelings about self. (N.D. 3)

Student will demonstrate understanding of scoliosis and treatment modalities. (N.D. 4)

Student will demonstrate understanding of his/her scoliosis treatment plan. (N.D. 4)

Student will demonstrate understanding of use of orthotics and/or appropriate surgical procedures. (N.D. 4)

Student will demonstrate methods to prevent skin irritation and breakdown with use of orthotic brace. (N.D. 5)

Nursing Interventions

Screen student as needed, at least twice a year, to assess condition of spine and/or curvature. (N.D. 1)

Assist parent and student to access their healthcare provider as needed for assessment of positive screening findings. (N.D. 1)

Communicate with healthcare provider, with parental permission, to document treatment plan and prognosis for student's condition. (N.D. 1)

Encourage student to identify and discuss activities that are difficult and/or strenuous for him/her due to spinal abnormalities. (N.D. 1)

Encourage student to identify and discuss activities that are difficult and/or strenuous for him/her due to limitations from use of orthotics. (N.D. 1)

Encourage student to identify and discuss activities that are difficult and/or strenuous for him/her due to limitations due to spinal surgery instrumentation. (N.D. 1)

Encourage student to identify and discuss activities that are pleasurable and manageable for him/her. (N.D. 1)

Encourage student to identify and discuss activities that are pleasurable and manageable for him/her even with the use of orthotics. (N.D. 1)

Collaborate with physical education teachers to modify physical education program as needed with approval of healthcare provider. (N.D. 1)

Arrange for extra books as needed so the student does not have to carry books to class or home. (N.D. 1)

Arrange for early release between classes and at the end of the day (for two to four weeks) following surgery to avoid getting bumped or pushed in the hallway. (N.D. 1)

Arrange for use of elevator, as needed. (N.D. 1)

Assist in arranging for homebound services, as needed, following surgery. (N.D. 1)

Encourage student to verbalize feelings about body image and self as related to scoliosis. (N.D. 2,3)

Encourage student to verbalize feelings about body image and self as related to use of orthotic brace. (N.D. 2,3)

Encourage student to write a journal to record his/her feelings about his/her condition, treatment, and how it relates to his/her life. (N.D. 2,3)

Encourage student to share his/her understanding of his/her condition and treatment with his/her parents and the school nurse. (N.D. 4)

Assist student and parents to understand the scoliosis management plan appropriate to age and level of understanding. (N.D. 4)

- Screening procedure
- Screening results
- Pathophysiology of scoliosis
- Treatment options
- Personal treatment plan
- Use of orthotics prescribed and self-care as related to their use (if appropriate)
- Surgical procedures and recovery process (if appropriate)

Discuss school scoliosis management plan with parents, as needed. (N.D. 4)

Review and revise school scoliosis management plan as needed with parents and student to provide a unified approach to management. (N.D.4)

Discuss with student and parent the need to monitor skin integrity and proper care of areas of skin irritation. (N.D. 5)

Assist student to notify parents of any alteration in skin integrity related to orthotic use. (N.D. 5)

Expected Student Outcomes

Student will attend classes regularly without absences related to scoliosis symptoms. (N.D. 1)

Student will participate in classroom and school activities with modifications made as needed. (N.D. 1)

Student will participate in regular physical education classes with modifications in activities as needed. (N.D. 1)

Student will use orthotic with 100% reliability. (N.D. 1)

Student will verbalize feelings about body image, whether positive or negative, in a safe and comforting environment. (N.D. 2)

Student will write feelings about body image, whether positive or negative. (N.D. 2)

Student will verbalize positive feelings about himself/herself and what he/she is capable of doing well. (N.D. 3)

Student will write positive feelings about himself/herself and what he/she is capable of doing well. (N.D. 3)

Student will accurately describe what scoliosis is. (N.D. 4)

Student will demonstrate self-limitation of activities based on scoliosis management plan in physical education classes/sports activities. (N.D. 4)

Student will accurately describe his/her treatment plan. (N.D. 4)

Student will describe to the school nurse any changes made in the treatment plan. (N.D. 4)

Student will demonstrate use of his/her orthotic. (N.D. 4)

Student will describe methods utilized to prevent skin breakdown (when using the orthotic). (N.D. 4)

Student will explain any surgical procedure(s) that he/she has undergone or will undergo. (N.D. 4)

Student will describe the postoperative course he/she can expect to experience. (N.D. 4)

Student will express his/her concerns about upcoming scoliosis treatments. (N.D. 4)

Student will experience minimal skin breakdown due to proper use of orthotic brace. (N.D. 5)

Student will experience minimal skin breakdown due to early identification and intervention. (N.D. 5)

Student will report skin irritation problems to his/her parents or school nurse, upon occurrence. (N.D. 5)

CASE STUDY

Stephanie Blake is a 16-year-old girl who has undergone several surgeries at ages 5 months and 18 months to repair a cleft lip and palate, as well as surgery at 14 months to remove and repair her toes. She continues to have minimal facial scarring from these surgeries but is a student who is bright and quick to smile despite her ongoing health concerns.

Stephanie was screened annually for scoliosis from age 8 until the current time. Until age 12, her screening results were negative, at which time the school nurse found her to have a 8 to 9° thoracic spinal curvature using a scoliometer. A referral was sent home and returned with the report that she had already been seen by an orthopedic scoliosis specialist after the curvature was noticed by her healthcare provider at her seventh grade physical. She has undergone a series of x-rays as well as a computed tomographic scan. At the time the specialist indicated that no restrictions on her activity were indicated, but she would be followed and evaluated for possible surgical intervention. Her parents indicated that they would be seeking a second and third opinion in the coming months.

In the summer preceding this school year, Stephanie underwent surgery to have a full metal rod inserted along her spine. She has been recuperating in a brace and can expect to wear the brace for two to three months. Her surgeon has requested no physical education classes or sports for the full school year. Stephanie should also avoid lifting heavy objects. It has been arranged to issue her three sets of books so that she will not need to carry any textbooks. She may use the stairs, but an elevator pass has been issued for use as she feels the need.

Individualized Healthcare Plan*
Scoliosis

Assessment Data	Nursing Diagnosis	Goals	Nursing Interventions	Expected Outcomes
ND1 Stephanie has difficulty ambulating and maneuvering with brace in place at school.	Impaired physical mobility due to spinal alignment abnormalities and use of orthotic brace (NANDA 6.1.1.1)	Stephanie will retain maximum level of physical mobility with modifications in classroom/school activities as needed. Stephanie will demonstrate use of orthotic and describe its therapeutic value.	Communicate with healthcare provider, with parental permission, to document treatment plan and prognosis for Stephanie's condition. Encourage Stephanie to identify and discuss activities that are strenuous for her due to limitations form use of orthotics. Encourage Stephanie to identify and discuss activities that are pleasurable and manageable for her even with the use of orthotics.	Stephanie will attend classes regularly without absences related to scoliosis symptoms. Stephanie will participate in classroom and school activities, with modifications made as needed. Stephanie will participate in modified physical education program as needed. Stephanie will use orthotic with 100% reliability.

Assessment	Nursing Diagnosis	Goal	Interventions	Expected Outcomes
ND2 Stephanie has had numerous surgeries with resulting scarring.	Body image disturbance due to scarring from surgical procedures (NANDA 7.1.1.1)	Stephanie will express feelings about her body.	Collaborate with PE teachers to modify PE program as needed with approval of healthcare provider. Arrange for extra books as needed so Stephanie does not have to carry books to class or home. Arrange for use of elevator, as needed. Encourage Stephanie to verbalize feelings about body image and self as related to scoliosis. Encourage Stephanie to verbalize feelings about body image and self as related to use of orthotic brace. Encourage Stephanie to write a journal to record feelings about her condition, treatment and how it relates to her life.	Stephanie will verbalize feelings about body image, whether positive or negative, in a safe and comforting environment. Stephanie will write feelings about body image, whether positive or negative.

Individualized Healthcare Plan*
Scoliosis (continued)

Assessment Data	Nursing Diagnosis	Goals	Nursing Interventions	Expected Outcomes
ND4 Stephanie occasionally asks questions about treatment plan.	Knowledge deficit related to pathophysiology of scoliosis and treatment plan (NANDA 8.1.1)	Stephanie will demonstrate understanding of her treatment plan. Stephanie will demonstrate understanding of use of orthotic and her recent surgical procedure.	Encourage Stephanie to share her understanding of her condition and treatment with her parents and the school nurse. Assist Stephanie and parents to understand her scoliosis management plan as appropriate to age and level of understanding. Discuss, review and revise the school scoliosis management plan as needed with parents and student to provide a unified approach to management.	Stephanie will accurately describe her treatment plan. Stephanie will describe any changes that are made in the plan to the school nurse. Stephanie will demonstrate use of her orthotic. Stephanie will describe methods utilized to prevent skin breakdown (when using the orthotic). Stephanie will explain the surgical procedure that she has undergone. Stephanie will describe the postoperative course she can expect to experience.

*See Appendix for student profile information to include on an IHP form.

REFERENCES

1. Wong DL. *Clinical Manual of Pediatric Nursing.* 4th ed. St. Louis; Mo: Mosby-Year Book, 1996:522.
2. Behrmann RE, Klingman RM. *Nelson Essentials of Pediatrics.* 2nd ed. Pennsylvania, Pa: WB Saunders Company, 1994:731,733-734.
3. Children's Hospital, Oakland, Calif. *Scoliosis treatment.* [online]. Available at: http://www.scoliosisrx.com Accessed 1/27/99.
4. Wong DL, Hockenbery-Eaton M, Wilson D, Winkelstein ML, Ahmann E, Divito-Thomas PA, eds. *Whaley and Wong's Nursing Care of Infants and Children.* 6th ed. St. Louis, Mo: Mosby, 1999:1941, 1943.
5. Epstein F. *Complications of spina bifida.* [online]. Available at: http://www.bethisraelny.org/inn/myelo/mye_com.html Accessed 1/27/99.
6. Rubenstein A, Korf FB. *A Handbook for Patients, Families, and Healthcare Professionals.* New York, NY: Thieme Medical Publishers, 1990.

BIBLIOGRAPHY

Behrmann RE, Klingman RM. *Nelson Essentials of Pediatrics.* 2nd ed. Philadelphia, Pa: WB Saunders Company, 1994.

Children's Hospital, Oakland, Calif. *Scoliosis treatment* [online]. Available at: http://www.scoliosisrx.com Accessed 1/27/99.

Epstein F. *Complications of spina bifida* [online]. Available at: http://www.bethisraelny.org/inn/myelo/mye_com.html Accessed 1/27/99.

MedHelp International. *What is scoliosis? And how is it treated?* [online]. Available at: http://www.medhelp.org/lib/scolio.htm Accessed 1/27/99.

North American Nursing Diagnosis Association. *NANDA Nursing Diagnoses: Definitions & Classification 1999-2000.* Philadelphia, Pa: North American Nursing Diagnosis Assn, 1999. (NANDA, 1211 Locust Street, Philadelphia, PA 19107. 800-647-9002; fax 215-545-8107; e-mail: NANDA@nursecominc.com)

Rubenstein A, and Korf FB. *A Handbook for Patients, Families, and Healthcare Professionals.* New York, NY: Thieme Medical Publishers, 1990.

Wong DL. *Clinical Manual of Pediatric Nursing.* 4th ed. St. Louis, Mo: Mosby-Year Book, 1996.

Wong DL, Hockenbery-Eaton M, Wilson D, Winkelstein ML, Ahmann E, Divito-Thomas PA, eds. *Whaley and Wong's Nursing Care of Infants and Children.* 6th ed. St. Louis, Mo: Mosby, 1999.

29

IHP: Sickle Cell Disease

Carolyn F. Holman

INTRODUCTION

Sickle cell disease is an inherited chronic illness that affects approximately 50,000 Americans. In the African-American population: 1 in 357 live births have sickle cell anemia (HbSS), 1 in 835 live births have hemoglobin SC disease (HbSC), and 1 in 1,667 live births have sickle beta thalassemia disorders. Other ethnic groups that are affected include Hispanic, Mediterranean, Caribbean, Arabian, and East Indian. [1,2]

Children with sickle cell anemia require careful monitoring and coordination of their care. The signs and symptoms of sickle cell disease can range from mild to life threatening. Knowledge and appropriate management of this disease can have a significant impact on the life of the child with sickle cell disease.

Recent advances include a decrease in infant morbidity and mortality caused by overwhelming pneumococcal infections. The administration of prophylactic penicillin until the age of 5 years is responsible for this decrease. Bone marrow transplants have been reported to cure some patients of their disease. Improved testing of blood products has decreased the number of complications resulting from blood transfusions.[1,2] Administration of hydroxyuria has been shown to decrease the incidence of painful events by 50%.[2] The use of regular blood transfusions (every three weeks) for children at high risk of stroke has been proven to reduce the incidence of stroke in children with sickle cell disease. [2,3] Comprehensive sickle cell programs that are easily accessible and administered by qualified people have also had a positive impact. [1,2]

Pathophysiology

Sickle cell disease is the term used to describe a group of genetic disorders characterized by the presence of abnormal sickle hemoglobin S (HbS), hemolytic anemia, and acute and chronic tissue injury secondary to blockage of blood flow by abnormally shaped erythrocytes. Sickle cell anemia (HbSS) is the most prevalent type of sickle cell disease. [1,2,4]

Normal hemoglobin (HbA) is composed of two alpha globin chains. In HbS, the alpha chain is the same as in HbA. The beta chain is different due to the substitution of valine for glutamic acid on the sixth position. [1,2,4]

Chronic hemolytic anemia is caused by the amino acid substitution on the beta globin of HbS. This results in the polymerization of the HbS molecules within the erythrocyte upon deoxygenation. This produces a change in the erythrocyte's shape from a biconcave disc to a crescent or sickle shape. When the erythrocyte is reoxygenated, it initially resumes a normal shape, but with repeated cycles of "sickling and unsickling," the erythrocyte is damaged permanently and hemolyzes. The anemia is the result of this hemolysis, which reduces the normal life span of the erythrocyte from 120 days to 10 to 20 days. [1-3]

The lowered hematocrit actually helps reduce the blood viscosity and deoxygenation, which decreases the incidence of polymerization of HbS to its abnormal form. Hypoxemia, acidosis, erythrocyte dehydration, hyperosmolality of the renal medulla (which dehydrates the erythrocyte), and viral infections can result in increased sickling. Other risk factors that affect the above are: hemoglobin (Hgb) higher than 8.5 gm/ml, elevated reticulocyte count, cold weather, fever, menstruation, sleep apnea, obstructive snoring, infection, pregnancy, and deoxygenation (i.e., high altitude). [2]

The acute and chronic tissue injury is a result of hypoxia, secondary to vaso-occlusion caused by the abnormally shaped erythrocytes. All tissues within the body are susceptible to damage. At greatest risk are the spleen, bone marrow, eye, head of the femur and humerus. The lung may be at special risk for vaso-occlusion and infarction since receives any deoxygenated erythrocytes that leave the spleen or bone marrow. Acute hypoxic injury may present as painful events or acute chest syndrome. Aseptic necrosis of the hip and sickle cell retinopathy are examples of insidious hypoxic injury. Acute and/or chronic tissue injury usually results in organ damage, especially as the person ages. [2]

Management

A definitive diagnosis should be made based on clinical history, blood counts, peripheral blood smear, and hemoglobin electrophoresis, including measurement of the minor hemoglobins A2 and F1. Family studies that include electrophoresis and measurement of Hb A2 and Hb F1 are helpful if available. [2]

Immunizations should follow guidelines of the American Academy of Pediatrics and/or the American Academy of Family Practice. In addition, the pneumococcal vaccine should be given at 2 years of age, with a booster at 4 years. Begining of the age of 14 years, yearly influenza vaccine is recommended.

Birth (or first visit)	Hepatitis B vaccine #1 or hepatitis B immunoglobulin if the mother is HBsAg
1 month old (or 4 weeks after first visit)	Hepatitis B vaccine #2
2 months old	DTaP #1, HbcV #1 or Tetrammune, IPV #1
4 months old	DTaP #2, HbcV #2 or Tetrammune, IPV #2
6 months old	DTaP #3, HbcV #3 or Tetrammune, OPV #3 Hepatitis B vaccine #3 (or six months after Hepatitis #2 vaccine)
12 to 15 months old	MMR (measles, mumps, rubella) #1
15 months old	HbcV booster
15 to 18 months old	DTaP booster #1, IPV #3
24 months old	Pneumococcal vaccine
4 to 6 years old	DTaP booster #2, pneumococcal vaccine booster, OPV #4, MMR booster
14 to 16 years old	TD booster, annual influenza vaccine [2]

Oral prophylactic penicillin is recommended twice a day for children until the age of 5 years. This is given to reduce the risk of pneumococcal infections. Tablets often are used due to their increased shelf life over liquid penicillin. Injectable bicillin can be used intramuscularly if indicated. Erythromycin ethyl succinate is used for children allergic to penicillin.[2]

Maintaining adequate hydration is very important to reduce sickle cell episodes (painful events) and vaso-occlusive complications. Due to the inability to concentrate urine, the child will need access to fluids throughout the day and restroom privileges as well. Fluid requirements are calculated on the basis of 150cc/kg/day. Water and juices containing electrolytes are recommended. An illness with vomiting and/or diarrhea could have serious consequences if appropriate care is not provided.[2] It is essential that the child and teacher understand their responsibilities related to this and work together.

Many times the child will know he or she is beginning to have trouble. The child should feel comfortable discussing this with parent, teacher, or school nurse so appropriate interventions can be taken. Utilizing a self-rating scale for pain management is helpful. It is important for the child with sickle cell to access medical care if his/her temperature exceeds 101 degrees F (38.5 degrees C). Early treatment of infections is imperative.[1,2,5]

A decline in academic performance could indicate the pressence of cardiovascular disease and the need for further medical evaluation. If the child is hospitalized, absent frequently, or taking narcotic pain medications, changes in performance may be noted. An Individualized Education Program (IEP) may recommend tutoring, homebound, or hospital-based instruction.[2]

A "Sickle Cell Crises Action Plan" appears as Table 1 and is a resource for the school setting. Priapism is a painful, prolonged penile erection that was not included in this action plan. The initial interventions for this are to empty the bladder and increase fluid intake. Taking a warm bath and/or using exercise to divert blood flow may also be helpful. If the painful erection persists for several hours, this is considered a medical emergency. This condition can adversely affect the reproductive function in the male.[2]

Dietary counseling should recommend a well-balanced diet. No supplemental iron is recommended. Folic acid is not necessary unless the diet seems to be low in folate. Extensive nutritional counseling may be necessary if the child comes from a high-risk environment such as limited education or low income.[2]

Regular dental care is indicated, including topical fluoride. Prophylactic antibiotics are indicated prior to procedures to reduce the risk of rheumatic fever, septicemia, or sepsis. Blood transfusions may be necessary if general anesthesia or extensive surgery is needed.[2,5]

Blood pressure screening is recommended every six months after 2 years of age.[5] Routine hearing and vision screening are indicated for young children. Older children and adolescents should have yearly eye examinations by an ophthalmologist due to the increased risk of retinopathy. Periodic tuberculosis skin tests are also recommended.[2,5]

Counseling should include the dangers of illicit drugs, tobacco, and alcohol use. Abstinence, safe sex, and contraception should also be discussed.[2] Contraception for the female with sickle cell disease may include low-dose estrogen, oral birth control pills, since there is a theoretical risk of thrombosis. Depo-Provera, given every twelve weeks intramuscularly, may have inhibitory effects on sickling with improved hematologic function during treatment. The decrease in menstrual flow may decrease the anemia. Other benefits include reduced risk of pelvic inflammatory disease (PID), endometriosis, uterine fibroids, ectopic pregnancies, and ovarian cysts. The diaphragm and gel are less effective for contraception than the oral or intramuscular medications. Intrauterine devices (IUDs) are not recommended for women with sickle cell due to the risk of bleeding and infections. Condoms are unreliable for contraception but do offer barrier protection against sexually transmitted diseases. Abstinence should be strongly advocated with preteens and adolescents. [2,6]

Genetic counseling is recommended at the appropriate developmental level. Academic and vocational counseling are needed to assist the individual in making life choices. Patients with sickle cell disease will also need information on recreational activities, which can help them develop a positive self-esteem and self-image and promote self-reliance. They will need guidance on travel arrangements that are appropriate for their situation. Parents, family, and the school community should be counseled on the advantages of treating children with sickle cell disease as normally as possible. [2]

Please refer to Table 2, a Summary of Primary Care Needs of the Child with Sickle Cell Disease. It provides a concise overview of primary care needs.

INDIVIDUALIZED HEALTHCARE PLAN

Assessment

History

- When did you find out your child had sickle cell disease?
- Do you know the specific type of sickle cell disease your child has?
- Who is your child's primary healthcare provider?
- Does your child see a specialist or attend any special clinics?
- What immunizations has your child received?
- What problems, hospitalizations, or emergency department visits has your child experienced?
- How has your child been doing in school up to this point? (grades, attendance, physical education class participation, special interests/achievements)
- Is there a previous individualized healthcare plan (IHP)?
- Is there an individualized educational program (IEP)?
- What modifications have been made in his/her school program?

Current Status and Management

- Is he/she currently experiencing any problems?
- What is your current management routine at home, including medications and fluid requirements?
- Does your child use a pain management rating scale? (If yes, which one)-Does he/she require any immunizations during this school term, and if so when are they due?
- Which of these interventions do we need to provide while your child is at school?
- If there was an emergency, who would you want us to call if we could not reach you?
- What are the medical phone numbers in case of an emergency?
- Perform physical assessment appropriate for setting, including but not limited to height, weight, blood pressure, hearing, and vision.

Self-care

- What areas of care does your child manage alone?
- What does he/she do with your supervision?
- What things do you manage or do for the child?
- Assess student's age-appropriate knowledge about sickle cell disease.
- Assess student's perception about sickle cell disease and his or her locus of control.
- Assess student's knowledge about risk factors.
- Assess student's knowledge of preventive measures to decrease risk factors for complications (diet, fluid requirements, rest, exercise, hygiene, reporting symptoms promptly).
- Assess student's self-care skills, barriers to self-care, self-medication and treatment.
- Assess student's medical records and treatment plans obtained from the healthcare provider.

Psychosocial Status

- What are your child's strengths?
- Does your child seem well adjusted to the problems he/she experiences with sickle cell (medical visits, medications, other related problems)?
- Who makes up the family support system for this child?
- Does your child have friends and what social activities does he/she enjoy?

Academic Issues

- Assess student's academic and attendance records.
- Assess need for homebound and/or hospital instruction.
- Assess need for modified physical education program.
- Assess fluid requirements and restroom privileges.
- Assess needs for health assessment, medication, and management of symptoms in th school setting, including off-campus school activities.
- Assess need for an IEP.
- Determine need for modifications in the school environment.
- Determine need for Emergency Care Plan (ECP).

Nursing Diagnoses (N.D.)

N.D. 1 (Risk for) altered tissue profusion—renal, cerebral, cardiopulmonary, gastrointestinal, or peripheral vascular (NANDA 1.4.1.1)

N.D. 2 (Risk for) fluid volume deficit (NANDA 1.4.1.2.2.2)

N.D. 3 (Risk for) altered urinary elimination (NANDA 1.3.2)

N.D. 4 (Risk for) infection (NANDA 1.2.1.1)

N.D. 5 (Risk for) ineffective thermoregulation (NANDA 1.2.2.4)

N.D. 6 (Risk for) altered role performance (NANDA 3.2.1) (student) related to absence from school/class due to sickle cell disease symptoms

N.D. 7 (Risk for) altered comfort, pain (NANDA 9.1.1)

N.D. 8 (Risk for) knowledge deficit (NANDA 8.1.1) and self-care deficit related to cause, treatment, and diagnosis of sickle cell disease

N.D. 9 (Risk for) altered growth and development (NANDA 6.6)

N.D. 10 (Risk for) altered health maintenance (NANDA 6.4.2)

N.D. 11 (Risk for) activity intolerance (NANDA. 6.1.1.3)

N.D. 12 (Risk for) altered thought processes (NANDA 8.3) related to pain management and risk of cerebral vascular accidents

N.D. 13 (Risk for) impaired skin integrity (NANDA 1.6.2.1.2.2) related to peripheral vascular complications

N.D. 14 (Risk for) injury (NANDA 1.6.1) if complications of stroke or seizures occur

N.D. 15 (Risk for) impaired mobility (NANDA 6.1.1.1) if complication of aseptic necrosis of joints occurs

N.D. 16 (Risk for) altered sensory perception (NANDA 7.2) related to increase risk of visual disturbances

N.D. 17 (Risk for) impaired gas exchange (NANDA 1.5.1) related to increased risk of pulmonary infections and pulmonary emboli

N.D. 18 (Risk for) noncompliance (NANDA 5.2.1.1) with health maintenance activities related to:
- knowledge deficit
- perceived ineffectiveness of interventions
- denial of need for interventions
- poor self-care skills
- difficult access to care
- poor decision-making and/or problem-solving skills

Goals

- Attain and maintain adequate hydration. (N.D. 1-3, 7, 11, 13, 16, 18)
- Prevent / decrease the number of painful sickle cell events. (N.D. 1-7, 18)
- Attain and maintain current immunizations as recommended for student with sickle cell disease. (N.D. 1, 4, 6, 10, 17, 18)
- Increase age-appropriate knowledge of diagnosis, symptoms, prescribed interventions, and medication. (N.D. 8, 18)
- Increase self-care skills. (N.D. 10, 18)
- Improve decision-making/problem-solving skills. (N.D. 8, 10, 18)
- Demonstrate good school attendance pattern. (N.D. 6)
- Demonstrate good class attendance and participation. (N.D. 6)
- Develop and implement an action plan for each potential complication of sickle cell disease, including an emergency care plan for life-threatening symptoms. (N.D. 1-7, 10-17)
- Participate in regular school/class activities, including physical education, with modifications made as necessary. (N.D. 1- 3, 5-7, 11, 12 14-16, 18)
- Demonstrate compliance with sickle cell health management program. (N.D. 8, 18)

Interventions

Develop an individualized sickle cell action plan. (N.D. 1-5,7,11,12,15-17)
- include student, parent/guardian, teacher, and healthcare providers in the development process.
- coordinate with and incorporate the sickle cell home management plan with parent/guardian and healthcare providers.

- list and describe management measures to follow for each type of potential sickle cell-related problem.
- include considerations for field trips and other extracurricular school activities.
- establish guidelines for seeking assistance, include what to do with early warning signs, if medications or interventions have been used within the last hour, if symptoms subside and reappear, when to notify parent/guardian and/or healthcare provider, include telephone numbers.
- establish criteria for handling medical emergencies related to sickle cell disease.
- modify plan as needed.

Obtain medical orders for medications and/or interventions needed at school, including modifications needed in the school program. Work with parent/guardian and healthcare provider. (N.D. 1-7, 11-17)
- for preventive management of sickle cell
- for management of sickle cell events
- anticipate needs for homebound and/or hospital instruction

Keep accurate records of sickle cell events. (N.D. 1-7,11-17)
- time of onset of symptoms
- time symptoms were reported to teacher, health office, or other school personnel and who reported the information
- describe presenting symptoms—pain and location, not feeling well, difficulty breathing, change in behavior or level of consciousness
- action taken—temperature, fluids, medication, rest, relaxation techniques, notification of parent and/or healthcare provider, emergency response
- effectiveness of intervention used
- name of person notified of the event, time of notification, who made the contact and what was the response or further instructions

In-service teachers and other appropriate school personnel. (N.D. 1-7, 11-17)
- what is sickle cell disease
- what increases risk of problems with sickle cell disease
- what are the preventive measures needed at school
- note importance of acknowledging and recognizing early warning symptoms
- what to do in the event of symptoms
- describe importance of prompt management
- detail problems related to pain management

Work with physical education teachers to modify physical education requirements as indicated. (N.D. 1-7, 11-17)
- consider contract with older children to self-limit activities only when needed

Assist parents/guardians, teachers, and healthcare providers in understanding the need for student to participate in regular classroom activities. (N.D. 1-7, 11-17)
- consider classroom and restroom privilege modifications that may be needed
- consider modifications to promote self-care and maintain self-esteem

Encourage and assist parents/guardians to talk with the student's teachers about the child and his/her sickle cell disease. (N.D. 1-7, 11-17)
- what previous problems the child has experienced
- what preventive measures are used at home

- what treatment/interventions the child requires
- how to handle symptoms that occur at school
- any modifications in the classroom/school/field trips the child may require (seat near door to facilitate needed restroom facilities, access to sports bottle for fluid requirements during day, avoidance of extreme temperatures, ability to self-limit physical activities as needed)
- discuss criteria for when child will not be able to attend school and how teacher(s) will be notified
- need for assignments if child is absent, possible need for intermittent homebound or hospital-based instruction

Assist the student to administer prescribed medications and/or interventions appropriate for his/her knowledge and skills according to school district policy and legal mandates. (N.D. 1-5, 7, 8, 11-18)
- fluids and restroom facilities will be easily accessible
- medications will be easily accessible and administered according to prescribed orders and school district policy and procedures (controlled substances will be handled according to legal mandates as well)
- physical activities will be self-limited according to symptoms
- these activities will be done with the least amount of disruption to promote optimum participation in the school program
- these activities will be monitored and/or supervised by the school nurse

Discuss with the student: (N.D. 1-5, 7, 8, 11-18)
- importance of participating in class activities and physical education as much as possible
- responsibilities for fluid intake and appropriate use of restroom privileges
- symptoms that he/she should report to appropriate adult for further   evaluation/intervention
- responsibilities of notifying appropriate adult(s) when symptoms first appear
- what to do if a sickle cell event begins

Provide health education opportunities for individual or group instruction related to: (N.D. 1-18)
- what is sickle cell disease
- how is sickle cell transmitted
- what are signs and symptoms of sickle cell disease
- what can be done to reduce the risk of some of these problems
- what to do when symptoms occur
- relaxation and guided imagery techniques for mild pain management
- what may be needed to handle moderate and severe pain
- psychosocial issues related to pain management
- options for recreational activities/travel
- growth and development issues
- counseling on career choices
- how to get help, if needed

Assist the student to identify motivators and barriers to self-care. (N.D. 8-10, 18)

Assist the student to select motivators and implement them to promote self-care. (N.D. 8, 18)

Remove as many barriers to self-care as possible. (N.D. 8, 18)

Assist the student to develop self-care skills. (N.D. 8, 18)
- discuss fluid requirements
- discuss responsibility with restroom privileges
- discuss hygiene including rest and nutrition
- discuss activity levels and physical education participation
- discuss pain management including self-rating pain scale, relaxation techniques, nonsteroidal pain relievers, and controlled substances
- discuss adolescent changes when age appropriate
- discuss factors to consider in decision-making process
- monitor self-care skills, encourage appropriate actions, reinforce areas needing improvement

Assist the student to develop appropriate decision-making skills. (N.D. 8, 18)

Assist the student to participate in his/her sickle cell management measures. (N.D. 8, 18)
- allow the student to have control over designated areas

Discuss with the student: (N.D. 8, 18)
- the need to take medications as prescribed (on time, at designated intervals, proper dose, method and documentation)
- the need to implement interventions as recommended to decrease risk factors for potential problems
- the importance of his/her participation in the management of medications and interventions
- benefits of compliance
- consequences of noncompliance
- motivators and barriers to compliance

Assist the student to choose and implement motivators for compliance. (N.D. 18)Remove as many barriers to compliance as possible. (N.D. 18

Monitor student's compliance with medications and interventions as prescribed. (N.D. 18)

Monitor classroom and physical education activity tolerance. (N.D. 1, 7, 11, 12, 15)

Assist the teacher to adjust activity participation based on activity tolerance and current problems. (N.D. 6)

Monitor attendance patterns and reasons for absences. (N.D. 6)

Monitor need for and use of hospital or homebound services. (N.D. 6)

Monitor utilization of alternative instruction arrangements, if needed. (N.D. 6)

Monitor academic performance. (N.D. 6)
- refer for evaluation as appropriate
- participate in IEP development as indicated

Expected Student Outcomes

The student will:
- participate in regular classroom activities, with modifications made as necessary (hospital or homebound instruction when needed)
- participate in regular physical education activities, with modifications as needed

- define what sickle cell disease is (at a developmentally appropriate level)
- list his/her risk factors
- list his/her preventive measures
- list his/her warning signs of a sickle cell event
- maintain adequate hydration as defined in the prescribed health maintenance plan
- recognize his/her warning signs of a sickle cell event and stop activity
- describe what to do if this occurs
- inform his/her teacher (and/or other personnel) when he/she is having sickle cell symptoms
- initiate and perform his/her action plan (dependent on demonstrated knowledge, skill, school district policy and legal mandates)
- name the medications, fluid requirements and interventions he/she uses for management of his/her sickle cell disease
- explain why he/she needs each of the above medications, fluids, or interventions
- demonstrate use of self-rating pain scale
- demonstrate proper procedure for administering medication as prescribed according to school district policy and legal mandates (check label, dose, interval, time, documentation)
- demonstrate alternative pain management techniques (rest, relaxation, guided imagery)
- describe how he/she participates in his/her sickle cell disease management
- participate in his/her sickle cell disease management (dependent on demonstrated knowledge, skill, school district policy, and legal mandates)
- describe the benefits of each intervention
- describe the consequences of not using these interventions
- list motivators and barriers to compliance with prescribed medications and interventions
- demonstrate compliance with his/her sickle cell management plan (maintenance and emergency)
- demonstrate a good attendance pattern (number of days absent depends on severity of child's disease, would hope to have a decrease in number from preceding school year)
- have minimal disruptions in his/her educational program due to sickle cell disease

Table 1. SICKLE CELL CRISES ACTION PLAN

VASO-OCCLUSIVE EPISODE OR PAINFUL CRISIS
ALTERED PERIPHERAL/VASCULAR TISSUE PERFUSION

SYMPTOMS	PLAN OF ACTION

Pain in hands or feet: may have edema (younger children)	• Acetaminophen as prescribed for pain (no aspirin)
	• Encourage fluids; daily fluid requirements for weight are:
	  0-25 pounds = 1-1/2 to 1-3/4 quarts
	  26-50 pounds = 2 to 2-1/2 quarts
	  51-75 pounds = 2-1/4 to 3 quarts
	  76-100 pounds = 2-1/2 to 3-1/2 quarts

Bone pain in arms, legs, back or chest (older children)	

Abdominal pain	• Heating pad or warm compress may be used at site if helpful
	• Rest until medication takes effect
	• Acetaminophen with codeine if needed - a small amount may be kept on hand and used as prescribed
	• Use coping strategies for pain management
	  - divert attention from pain
	  - use calming self-statements
	  - reinterpret pain sensations (do not discount pain)
	• Return to class if pain is controlled
	• Notify parents of episode, treatment, and results

FEVER AND/OR INFECTION
POTENTIAL FOR INFECTION

Fever over 101°F	• Notify parent to seek medical attention • Assist parent to access medical care if needed

PULMONARY MANIFESTATIONS/ACUTE CHEST SYNDROME
ALTERED CARDIOPULMONARY TISSUE PERFUSION

Cough, pain in chest, fever, bone pain, hypoxia	• Notify parent to seek medical care • Anticipate child being absent approximately 2 weeks; arrange for schoolwork appropriately • Expect 1 week of limited activity when child returns to school; make necessary arrangements for schedule or activity modifications

INABILITY TO CONCENTRATE URINE
ALTERED URINARY ELIMINATION

Urinary frequency, enuresis	• Adequate fluid intake is essential; refer to daily requirements provided above • Access to restroom as needed • Communication among teacher, nurse, parent and child may be necessary to avoid abuse of these privileges

STROKE
ALTERED CEREBRAL TISSUE PERFUSION

Loses balance, falls more than usual, weakness in a limb or limbs on one side, altered gait, c/o headache, visual disturbances, change in behavior, unexplained change in academic performance, first seizure	• Contact parent to seek medical evaluation • In the event of neurological or physical impairment, provide appropriate individualized school services as needed

APLASTIC EPISODE, SEVERE ANEMIA
ALTERED PERIPHERAL TISSUE PERFUSION

Pallor (nail beds, conjunctiva), lethargy (often accompanies viral illness)	• Notify parent to seek medical evaluation

SPLENIC SEQUESTRATION
ALTERED CARDIOVASCULAR TISSUE PERFUSION

Pallor, weakness, lethargy; swollen, painful abdomen; perspiration May go into shock and die	• MEDICAL EMERGENCY. Activate EMS plan for this child

Reprinted, with permission from Holman.[7] For educational materials that may be used in the school setting, contact your local Sickle Cell Disease Association or: National Association for Sickle Cell Disease, 3345 Wilshire Boulevard, Suite 1106, Los Angeles, CA 90010-1880, (800) 421-8453.

Table 2. SUMMARY OF PRIMARY CARE NEEDS FOR THE CHILD WITH SICKLE CELL DISEASE

Growth and development

These children tend to weigh less and be shorter than their peers; weight is affected more than height, and males are affected more than females.

Puberty is delayed for both sexes.

Developmental impairment varies.

Immunizations

Routine standard immunizations are recommended.

Haemophilus influenzae type b vaccine is given at 2, 4, and 6 months; immunogenic response is not reliable.

Pneumococcal vaccine is given at 24 months, with boosters given every 3 to 5 years thereafter.

Hepatitis vaccine is strongly recommended.

Influenza vaccine given annually is strongly recommended.

Screening

Vision

Routine screening is recommended until 10 years of age, then an annual retinal examination is recommended to rule out sickle retinopathy.

Hearing

Yearly audiologic examination is recommended.

Dental

Routine screening is recommended.

Blood pressure

Blood pressure should be measured every 6 months after 2 years of age.

Hematocrit

Hematocrit is deferred because of condition specific screening.

Urinalysis

Urinalysis is deferred because of condition specific screening.

Tuberculosis

Routine screening is recommended.

Condition-specific screening

Hematologic screening

A CBC with differential, reticulocyte count, and RBC smear should be checked every 6 months.

Renal function screening

The BUN and creatinine levels should be checked and a urinalysis done on a yearly basis.

Lead poisoning

Lead screening using the EP level is unreliable; the serum lead level must be determined.

Scoliosis

Screening should be extended to the late teens because of delayed puberty.

Cardiac function

Both ECG and ECHO should be used every 1 to 2 years after age 5.

Liver function

Serum liver function tests should be done yearly, The gallbladder should be assessed using ultrasound every 2 years after age 10.

Drug interactions

Antihistamines and barbiturates may potentiate narcotics.

Diuretics and bronchodilators, which may have diuretics effects, may cause dehydration and sickling.

Differential diagnosis

Fever

Age 5 years or less

TEMPERATURE LESS THAN 38.5°C

Outpatient management may be considered if the source of the fever can be identified, appropriate antibiotics are given, and follow-up is ensured.

TEMPERATURE MORE THAN 38.5°C

The child should be admitted to the hospital for fever work-up, parenteral antibiotics, and observation.

Age 5 years or more

The child's condition, compliance with therapy, and ability to obtain follow-up determine whether or not he or she should receive inpatient or outpatient care.

Table 2. SUMMARY OF PRIMARY CARE NEEDS
FOR THE CHILD WITH SICKLE CELL DISEASE — cont'd

Acute gastroenteritis

Significant dehydration may occur quickly and lead to acidosis and sickling. If oral intake is inadequate, IV hydration is needed.

Abdominal pain

Abdominal pain crisis may be differentiated from surgical problems by evaluating fever, hematologic changes, peristalsis, and response to symptomatic, supportive therapy.

Anemia

Hemoglobin and hematocrit levels significantly lower than baseline levels may reflect aplastic crisis, hyperhemolytic crisis, or splenic sequestration. Splenic sequestration may be life threatening.

Respiratory distress

It is important to evaluate the patient for acute chest syndrome, which may be fulminant and require exchange transfusion.

Neurologic changes

Neurologic changes may indicate stroke. Rapid, through evaluation is critical. Exchange transfusion should be performed as quickly as possible if stroke occurs.

Developmental issues

Safety

Ingestion of narcotics could lead to respiratory depression.

Alcohol may dehydrate and potentiate narcotics.

Narcotics may impair driving or safe use of machinery.

Recreational activities that involve prolonged exposure to cold, prolonged exertion, or exposure to high altitudes should be avoided. Ice should not be used to treat injuries.

A medical alert bracelet may be helpful.

Diet

Diet should be well balanced with a generous amount of fluid; fluid intake should be increased during illness. Supplemental folate requirements may be met with folate tablets, 1 mg daily. Children who are receiving chronic transfusions should limit their oral intake of vitamin C-rich foods to limit iron overload.

Child care

The care giver needs to be mindful of fluid requirements and the importance of maintaining normal body temperature and must be able to administer medicines.

Discipline

Expectations should be consistent, fair, and similar to those of peers and siblings.

Toileting

Enuresis is frequently a long-term issue because of a large volume of dilute urine.

Nocturia may persist.

Sleep patterns

Routine care is recommended.

School issues

The child may have frequent, unpredictable absences. While at school, the child needs access to fluids and liberal bathroom privileges. He or she may participate in mainstream physical education.

Sexuality

Puberty may be delayed. Men may have fertility problems. Women usually have normal fertility but have some special contraceptive concerns.

Special family concerns

Because sickle cell disease is genetically transmitted, there is a need for genetic counseling, as well as support for feelings of guilt and responsibility.

Reprinted, with permission, from Jackson and Vessey. [5]

CASE STUDY

James Arnold is a 9-year-old black male with sickle cell disease. His date of birth is 9/5/89, height 57 inches, weight 48 pounds (both are slightly below the fifth percentile for age), blood pressure is 106/66 mmHg, which is within normal limits for age. Immunizations are up to date, including hepatitis B series, MMR booster, and pneumococcal booster. His primary care provider is Dr. Sam Jones and his pediatric hematologist is Dr. Tom White. Mother talks with Nancy Brown, the nurse practitioner at Dr. White's office (Sickle Cell Center) if she has questions or if problems arise during office hours.

Mrs. Arnold states that James has never been hospitalized for sickle cell events. He was treated in the emergency department for diarrhea and vomiting last year. He had several ear infections as a preschool child but they resolved with antibiotic therapy. He is no longer on prophylactic antibiotics unless he goes to the dentist. He eats a well-balanced diet with the rest of the family (parents and two older brothers). He is not on folate or other medications at this time.

His fluid requirements are approximately 3 1/2 quarts a day. He prefers cranberry juice, orange sports drink, and water. He has marked containers in the refrigerator at home, and he is responsible for his fluid intake through the day (summertime). He tries not to drink anything after 6 PM so he will not have problems with nocturnal enuresis. He likes to feel "in control" of this since he "wants to be like his older brothers and take care of himself."

The only symptoms he has experienced so far are painful events (vaso-occlusive episodes) in his arms and legs. Several episodes were precipitated by hot weather, poor fluid intake, and increased outdoor activity (playing basketball with his older brothers). His pain management plan includes: resting, taking three acetaminophen chewable tablets, and increasing fluid intake. He had to use Tylenol #2 with codeine on one occasion last summer.

James has not missed many days of school. He is doing well with his studies. He has never had an IHP before. He enjoys his friends and joined the Cub Scouts at church last year. His maternal grandparents live nearby and help with after-school activities since both parents work outside the home. They try to treat him like all the other grandchildren and don't make a fuss over his health condition.

Individualized Healthcare Plan*
Sickle Cell Disease

Assessment Data	Nursing Diagnosis	Goals	Nursing Interventions	Expected Outcomes
ND1 Mother reports history of sickle cell events, usually occurring in summer or extremely hot weather with increased activity.	Risk for alternation in tissue perfussion related to sickle cell disease resulting in need to decrease participation in activities to prevent or manage a sickle cell event (NANDA 1.4.1.1 and 1.4.1.2.2.2)	Prevent/ decrease sickle cell events. Maintain adequate hydration.	Obtain medical orders for interventions needed at school including modifications needed in his school program. Develop a sickle cell action plan to manage events that occur at school. Keep accurate records of sickle cell events. In-service teachers and other identified school personnel regarding sickle cell disease and what to do if a sickle cell event occurs. Collaborate with the physical education teachers to modify physical education requirements, as indicated. Assist parents, teachers and healthcare providers in understanding the need for James to participate in regular classroom activities.	James will attend school unless symptoms are present that indicate he should not attend (according to criteria established by physician, parents, and school.) Teacher/ other school personnel will initiate action plan if an episode occurs at school. James will participate in regular physical education activities, with modifications made as needed. James will have minimal disruptions in his educational program due to his health condition.

Interventions	Outcomes
Encourage and assist parents to talk with James about his sickle cell disease.	James will participate in regular classroom activities, with modifications made as needed.
Discuss with James: his responsibilities for fluid intake and use of the restroom; importance of participating in classroom and physical education activities; symptoms he should report to teachers, the school nurse or other school personnel if they occur; responsibility for notifying appropriate adult when symptoms first appear; what he should do when a sickle cell event begins.	James will participate in homebound or hospital-based instruction, if needed. James will drink 8 oz of fluids per hour while at school. James will recognize his warning signs for a sickle cell event, stop activity, and notify his teacher of they occur.
Provide health education opportunities for James— individual and group. Monitor classroom and physical education activity tolerance.	James will initiate sickle cell action plan if an episode occurs at school. James participates in sickle cell education opportunities.

Individualized Healthcare Plan*
Sickle Cell Disease (continued)

Assessment Data	Nursing Diagnosis	Goals	Nursing Interventions	Expected Outcomes
ND7 History of painful sickle cell events in arms and legs.	Risk for alteration in comfort/ pain, related to vaso-occlusive events associated with sickle cell disease (NANDA 9.1.1)	Improve and maintain good pain management during occurrences of sickle cell events at school.	Monitor classroom and physical education activity tolerance. Assist teachers in modifying activities based on tolerance. Obtain medical orders for medication to manage pain associated with sickle cell events. Discuss with James: signs and symptoms of sickle cell disease; what to do if the symptoms occur; relaxation and guided imagery techniques for mild pain management; medications that may be needed for moderate to severe pain management; responsibility for notifying an appropriate adult when symptoms first occur.	James will participate in regular classroom activities, with modifications made as needed. Medication is available in the Health Office for use during sickle cell episodes. James recognizes the signs and symptoms of sickle cell disease. James tells his teacher, of the school nurse if signs and symptoms occur at school. James identifies two methods to decrease pain/ discomfort during a sickle cell event. James utilized methods of decreasing pain/ discomfort during a sickle cell event.

				Assist James to practice guided imagery techniques in school to use for management of mild pain during sickle cell events.	James demonstrates the use of guided imagery to manage mild pain.
				Assist parents to provide medication for management of pain during school hours. Medication is stored and administered according to school policy and procedures.	James demonstrates proper administration of medication to manage moderate to severe pain.
				All doses of medication given are properly documented.	

EMERGENCY CARE PLAN

Date: 9/5/98

Student: James Arnold

Date of birth: 9/7/89   **Teacher:** Mrs. Mary Smith

Parents/Guardians: Paul and Mary Arnold   **Home telephone:** (123) 444-7896
Mother's work number: (123) 444-3434
Father's work number: (123) 454-7036

Primary Care Provider: Dr. Sam Jones   **Telephone number:** (123) 454-9988
Address: 342 General Street, Suite E, Timbuktu, MI 36937

Specialist: Dr. Tom White (ped. hematology) **Telephone number:** (123) 454-3421
          Contact: Nancy Brown, CRNP
Address: 342 General Street, Suite H, Timbuktu, MI 36937

Medical Diagnosis: Sickle Cell Disease

Symptom	Action
Pain in arms or legs (mild to moderate)	1. Stop activity—rest, James will rate pain with attached self-rating pain scale. (Document pain, time of onset, initial)
	2. Give fluids (juice, soft drink, or bouillon recommended). Maintenance for James is 8 oz per hour-catch up, if indicated (Document amount taken per 15 minutes, initial)
	3. Give 3 acetaminophen chewable tablets (80 mg/tab). They are labeled in locked medicine cabinet. (Document according to medication administration policy for school district, include effectiveness.)
	4. Use coping strategies for pain management -divert attention—quiet activity, reading, coloring, deep breathing
	5. Reevaluate pain at 30 minutes and 1 hour. James will rate pain with attached self-rating pain scale. (Document responses, initial)
	6. Return to class if pain controlled. (Document time, initial)
	7. If pain not improved after one hour, administer Tylenol #2 with codeine elixir (1 tsp=5 ml). Labeled medication is in locked medication cabinet. (Document according to medication administration policy for school district, include effec tiveness, initial)

Symptom	**Action**
	8. Notify parent of event, treatment, and outcome. Note: Parents will arrange for James to be picked up if Tylenol #2 was needed. Advise teacher of early dismissal. She will bring any homework assignments to him in the health room. (Document time and persons notified, initial) 9. Repeat steps 4 and 5 if Tylenol #2 with codeine was administered.
Fever over 101 degrees F	1. Notify parent to seek medical attention. (Document fever, time, who was notified, initial) 2. Give fluids (juice, soft drink, or bouillon recommended). Maintenance for James is 8 oz per hour-catch up, if indicated. (Document amount taken per 15 minutes, initial) 3. Keep in health room until parent picks up. 4. Notify teacher. 5. Assist parent access healthcare if needed.
Vomiting and/or diarrhea dehydration	1. Contact parent immediately since can occur rapidly in children with sickle cell thus precipitating a painful event.(Document time of onset, frequency, time parent notified, who was contacted, initial)

* These are the most likely symptoms you might see with James at this time. Attached is a summary of other problems that could arise due to his sickle cell disease. Please refer to this since some symptoms may be life threatening and require emergency measures.

Signature: Parents/Guardians_____
            School Nurse _____
            Teachers _____
            Principal _____

cc: Parents/Guardians, Primary care provider,
     Specialist, Health Room, Teachers, Principal   Other _____

Letter to Schools about Physical Education

Date: _____

Re: Patient's name   _____

       Medical record number   _____

       Date of birth   _____

To Whom It May Concern:

_____is currently under my care for sickle cell disease.

Please allow him/her to participate in the regular physical education program. It will be necessary for him/her to self-limit participation at times due to the effects of sickle cell disease. When this becomes necessary, please allow for alternate activities to promote participation.

Dehydration, extreme temperatures and heavy exercise may precipitate a sickle cell event. An individualized healthcare plan is on file in the school for this child, which should be helpful to you.

Please contact me if you have further questions or concerns regarding this student.

Sincerely,

_____

Phone number_____

REFERENCES

1. Sickle Cell Disease Guideline Panel. *Sickle Cell Disease: Screening, Diagnosis, Management, and Counseling in Newborns and Infants.* Rockville, Md: Agency for Health Care Policy and Research, US Dept of Health and Human Services, 1993:1-10, 37-46. US Public Health Service publication 93-0562. Clinic Practice Guideline no. 6.
2. National Heart, Lung and Blood Institute. *Management and Therapy of Sickle Cell Disease.* 3rd ed. Bethesda, Md: National Institutes of Health, 1995:3-11, 21-22, 26-42, 66, 77-88, 95-97. NIH publication 95-2117.
3. National Heart, Lung and Blood Institute, National Institutes of Health. *New treatment prevents strokes in children with sickle cell anemia.* Available at: www.pslgroup.com Accessed 1/26/99.
4. Ballas SK. Sickle cell disease. In: Rakel E, ed. *Conn's current therapy 1995.* Philadelphia, Pa: WB Saunders Company, 1995:318-327.
5. Jackson PL, Vessey JA. *Primary Care of a Child with a Chronic Condition.* St Louis, Mo: Mosby Year Book, 1992:485-513.
6. Sperhoff L, Darney P. *Clinical Guide for Contraception.* 2nd ed. Baltimore, Md: Wilkins and Williams, 1996:92, 177, 303.
7. Holman C. *Management of the Child with Sickle Cell Disease within the School Setting. J School Nurs.* 1997;13(5):29-34.

BIBLIOGRAPHY

Doenges ME, Jeffries MF, Moorhouse MF. *Nursing Care Plans: Nursing Diagnoses in Planning Patient Care.* Philadelphia, Pa: F A Davis, 1984:362-368.

Fithian JH. *Sickle Cell Disease: Handbook for the School Nurse.* Philadelphia, Pa: Comprehensive Sickle Cell Center, The Children's Hospital of Philadelphia, 1993.

Hacker N, Moore JG. *Essentials of Obstetrics and Gynecology.* 2nd ed. Philadelphia, Pa. WB Saunders Company, 1992:212-213.

North American Nursing Diagnosis Association. *NANDA Nursing Diagnoses: Definitions & Classification 1999-2000.* Philadelphia, Pa: North American Nursing Diagnosis Assn, 1999. (NANDA, 1211 Locust Street, Philadelphia, PA 19107. 800-647-9002; fax 215-545-8107; e-mail: NANDA@nursecominc.com)

Sickle Cell Pamphlets for Parents:

Lessing S, Vichinsky E, eds. *A Parent's Handbook for Sickle Cell Disease. Part I: Birth to Six Years of Age.* Oakland, Calif: Children's Hospital, Oakland Sickle Cell Center, State of California, Department of Health Services, Genetic Disease Branch, Rev 1991. (Oakland Sickle Cell Center, 747-52nd Street, Oakland, CA 94609. 510-428-3372)

Earles A, Lessing S, Vichinsky E, eds. *A Parent's Handbook for Sickle Cell Disease. Part II: Six to Eighteen Yeas of Age.* Children's Hospital, Oakland Sickle Cell Center, State of California, Department of Health Services, Genetic Disease Branch, Rev 1994. (Oakland Sickle Cell Center, 747-52nd Street, Oakland, CA 94609. 510-428-3372)

30 | IHP: Skin Disorders

Sue Boos

INTRODUCTION

The skin is the largest organ of the body and is the primary protective barrier to the outside environment.[1] Its main purpose is protecting of inner layers of the body from infectious organisms and from injury caused by temperature extremes and chemical burns, from mechanical damage causing scrapes, bruises, or cuts, and from perforations by foreign objects. Other purposes include sealing the body from outside chemicals and sealing the inner environment of the body from excessive fluid and electrolyte loss. The vascularity of the skin allows it to be the main temperature regulator of the body, as well as an organ of expression, as seen from blushing due to embarrassment or sweating due to fear. Also, the skin is a sensory organ where the perceptions of temperature, texture, and pain are felt. On different parts of the body, the skin differs in texture and color, with each variation being an adaptation to its particular location. Some areas, such as the bottom of the feet and the palms of the hands are thicker and tougher, whereas delicate areas, such as around the eyes, are thinner and therefore more fragile and pliable.

Pathophysiology

Skin structures include the outer layer, the epidermis, which itself is composed of

five layers. Skin cells are continually produced from its lowest level and progressively migrate to the surface where they thicken, eventually die, and are constantly sloughed off to be replaced by new cells approximately every 28 days.[1] The tough epidermis is nourished by blood vessels within the next lower level of skin, the dermis, which is the thickest skin layer. This layer is more firm than the epidermis and gives skin its flexibility. It has an elaborate network of blood vessels and nerves within its connective tissue mass. Below the dermis is the thick, subcutaneous fat tissue layer, which is the cushion for major vessels, nerves, and lymphatics. This is the layer that gives contour to the body and protects and insulates against cold and absorbs trauma.[1] Hair follicles, as well as sweat and sebaceous glands, originate within this layer.

Different structures, such as sweat glands and hair follicles are more concentrated in certain parts of the body and are very sparse in others. The concentration of various skin structures in different locations is often the determining factor regarding the type of skin disorder found on various parts of the body.[2]

Skin lesions have various causes. They may be the result of 1) trauma from injury, infectious organisms, temperature extremes, or toxic chemicals; 2) an allergic reaction due to an insect bite or from contact with an individual allergen or irritant; 3) a hereditary condition; or 4) a systemic disease with a skin manifestation.[2] Distinctive reactions may differ from child to child and from age to age with a specific child.

More than half of all dermatologic disorders constitute a variety of dermatitis.[2] Common and acute reactions cause erythema with or without vesicles, edema, and inflammation. The location and type of reaction are often distinctive to the particular disorder. Without subsequent infection from itching and scratching, they are often easily treated and the skin recovers with no lasting marks.[2] This may not be true of chronic conditions.

Wounds are the disruption of the integrity of the skin. They are classified as 1) partial-thickness, meaning that the epidermis and some portions of the dermis are compromised; 2) full-thickness, which is more serious, meaning that damage extends through the epidermis, the entire dermis, and into the subcutaneous tissue; and 3) complex, those which extend into muscle or bone.[2] Acute wounds are those that will heal uneventfully in an expected manner and time frame barring infection or other complications. Chronic wounds are those that fail to heal as anticipated due to other complications. Children with mobility problems, paralysis, or paresthesia are prone to skin breakdown when pressure from braces or wheelchairs presses on soft skin over bony protuberances.

Many factors influence the healing of wounds of all kinds. Good, overall health and the quality of nutrition, with sufficient protcin, calorics, and vitamin C, in particular, are necessary for the healing of serious assaults to the skin. An adequate intake of water and other fluids is needed to maintain skin hydration.[3] Certain

chemicals commonly used as antiseptics, such as hydrogen peroxide and povidone-iodine solutions, have been found to have only minimal disinfectant properties and may be damaging to healthy cells, and may possibly be absorbed through the skin.[2]

Because of the very large and visible nature of skin disorders, they can be a source of great emotional discomfort, as well as painfully and physically distressing. Other children may reject a child who "looks funny or strange" or fear that they may "catch" the disorder regardless of its cause. For acute, short-lived and, usually, easily treated conditions, this does not present a long-term problem. But for children who suffer from chronic or severely disfiguring conditions, the psychological effects may be more devastating than the physical.

Management

Treatment for skin disorders may be topical or systemic. Bland ointments are used topically to avoid further irritation and reduce absorption through broken or inflamed skin lesions. To reduce stimuli causing itching in many disorders, avoid hot or cold applications. Instead, tepid or cool applications of soaks or lotions soothe the skin surface and protect from external stimuli. The anti-inflammatory effects of glucocorticoids are used to ease minor allergic skin reactions. These topical over-the-counter ointments are often used incorrectly by families for all skin manifestations. Other topical treatments include antibiotics for localized and minor infections and antifungals for localized fungal infections.

Systemic treatment, usually corticosteroids and antibiotics, is often used as an adjunct to topical treatment for skin disorders.[2] To avoid excessive absorption, topical treatments are used cautiously for skin lesions of a serious nature and/or long-term nature or for those covering a large amount of body surface.[1]

If the offending causative factor is thought to be allergic in nature, it must be eliminated from the child's environment. Many common household remedies can further irritate dermatitis and must be identified and eliminated. If the skin disorder is chronic, nursing care must be sensitive to the ongoing regularity of treatment and the psychosocial disturbances caused by visible flare-ups.

Commonly used dressings serve many functions, including 1) protection from infection and further injury; 2) compression to stop bleeding and reduce swelling; 3) maintenance of a moist, healing environment; 4) reduction of pain; 5) absorption of drainage; and 6) application of medication.[2] Not only does the traditional sterile gauze pad used on an open wound offer little protection from infection, it also may cause further damage by allowing a wound to become dry and crusted, or by sticking to the wound itself, disrupting healing when the dressing is removed.

In the school setting, nursing management is directed toward preventing further damage, preventing infection or other complications, and providing pain relief and protection during healing.

INDIVIDUALIZED HEALTHCARE PLAN

Assessment

History

For wounds:
- How did the injury happen?
- How long ago did it occur?
- What has been done for it to this point?
- Has there been any medical or home management of the wound?
- Have similar skin problems occurred previously?
- Are other injuries associated with the wound?
- If serious, can the parent, caregivers, teacher, playground supervisor, or others, shed light on how the wound occurred?

For other skin manifestations:
- When was it first noticed?
- Has it spread since then?
- Has the appearance changed since it was first noticed?
- Does its appearance change from day to day or during the day?
- What were you doing when you first noticed it? Where were you?
- Did it start while you were taking any medication or over-the-counter drug?
- Had you eaten anything different from your usual diet shortly before it started?
- How does it feel? Does it: hurt? itch? burn? sting?
- Has it awakened you or kept you awake at night?
- Are you taking any medications, either prescribed or over-the-counter?
- Currently, are you putting anything on it? If yes, is it getting better or worse?
- Have you or anyone in your family or among your friends had a similar skin manifestation (sore, rash, lesions, etc.) recently? In the past?
- Have you ever had anything like this before? If so, when?
- Was a healthcare provider seen? If so, what was diagnosed?

- What was done for it then? How effective was the treatment? What side effects were noticed?
- Does anything at home or school make the skin disorder better or worse?
- What other symptoms are present?

Current Status and Management

- Describe the lesion(s) by color, size, shape, texture, exudate, odor, location, amount, and distribution pattern on the body. Are there any apparent "bite" or sting marks? Are all the lesions similar or different?
- Palpate the area gently to determine if the lesion(s) is painful, swollen, tender, weepy, warm, crusty, or otherwise different from adjacent skin. To the examiner, does the affected skin feel different from normal skin? If so, describe.
- Observe the behavior of the child for scratching, splinting, covering, or otherwise protecting the area. Is the child crying, irritable, distracted, and so on?
- Observe, question, and assess for other symptoms, such as fever, headache, malaise, sore throat, stiffness, joint pain, etc.
- Wounds are further assessed for depth of the injury into lower tissue levels, cleanliness and/or signs of infection, and any evidence of healing.[2]
- Observe for any skin indications of physical or sexual abuse, such as bruises in several stages of healing, patterns of marks, cuts, or bruises, frequent health room visits, designation as an "accident-prone student," etc.

Self-care

- What is the student's, parents'/guardians' knowledge level and insight into the cause, treatment, and prevention of the skin condition? Have specific triggers been noticed previously?
- Is there a previous history of skin problems for this student or other family members?
- What is the student's and/or parents'/guardians' ability to carry out a treatment regimen? What self-care skills are present?
- How motivated are the student and parents to follow through with what may be a long and frustrating clinical course of treatment?
- What has been the level of previous compliance with a healthcare regimen?
- Who in the family, in addition to the student, has been involved in the development and implementation of the treatment?
- What are the student's and family's barriers to self-care? Are there financial, housing, or privacy barriers that would make continuous treatment difficult at home or school?

Psychosocial Status

For chronic or seriously disfiguring skin disorders:
- What is the age and developmental level of the student?
- What is the developmental level of the family?
- What is the student's perception of his/ her skin disorder?
- What is the student's perception of what his/her friends and classmates think and feel about the skin condition?
- What is the psychosocial comfort level of the student with his/her peers? (Has there been a change in social relationships? Does the teacher describe the student as with-

drawn? Does the student avoid social relationships? Does the student try to hide the affected skin with cosmetics or by keeping the face or area covered with clothing or long hair?)

- What are the student's classroom, physical education class, cafeteria, and playground social behaviors? (Does the student try to avoid physical education participation or showers? Is the child a loner on the playground or in the lunchroom? Is the student a target of taunts by other students because of the skin condition?)
- What social support network/s has the student developed at school or in the community? Are support groups available?

Academic Issues

- Attendance patterns, specifically in relation to skin disorder breakouts
- Participation in physical education and extracurricular activities
- Need for special education (P.L. 94-142) or Sec. 504 accommodations (Federal Rehabilitation Act of 1973)
- Teacher's perception and knowledge of the student's abilities in relation to performance in school and classroom adjustment

Nursing Diagnoses (N.D.)

N.D. 1 Impaired skin integrity (NANDA 1.6.2.1.2.1) related to:
- environmental agents
  chemicals
  unclean water
- mechanical trauma
  repeated friction over skin surface (such as from braces or wheelchairs)
  scratching or picking at affected skin
- compromised immunologic factors
  other systemic chronic illness or disease
  recent viral illness
- infective agents
  childhood communicable disease (such as chickenpox, fifths disease, strep infection, etc.)
- allergens
  known food allergen for this student (such as peanuts, chocolate, milk, strawberries, etc.)
  known or suspected seasonal allergies (such as grass, molds, pollens, etc.)
  other symptoms thought to be allergic in nature (such as a runny nose, husky voice, scratchy throat, and/or hearing difficulties)
- inherited traits
  family history of allergies (to food, pets, dust mites, pollens, molds, etc.)
  family history of severe acne (at and during puberty)

N.D. 2 Risk for infection (NANDA 1.2.1.1) related to:
- presence of bacterial, viral, or fungal infective agents within school population (such as chickenpox, strep infection, plantar warts, athlete's foot, ringworm, etc.)
- pruritus (itching) and scratching

- inadequate hand washing and general hygiene
- ineffective or inadequate treatment plan
- noncompliance with treatment plan
- improper care of medications (such as not washing hands before opening ointments or salves, leaving medication containers open after use, etc.)

N.D. 3 Pain (NANDA 9.1.1) related to:
- skin lesions
- pruritus/itching
- underlying disease process
- secondary infection
- noncompliance with treatment plan

N.D. 4 Risk for body image disturbance (NANDA 7.1.1) related to:
- inaccurate perception of appearance
- avoidance of peer relationships (due to fear of reaction of others/peers and personal feelings about appearance)
- unpredictable nature of chronic skin outbreaks
- scarring from repeated lesions

N.D. 5 Risk for knowledge deficit (NANDA 8.1.1) related to:
- lack of knowledge of current management plans and information about healing
- continuous nature of treatment for chronic skin conditions
- importance of hand washing and general hygiene
- relationship of nutrition to healing
- ways to avoid or reduce contact with allergens
- pain reduction techniques (both pharmacologic and nonpharmacologic)1.

N.D. 6 Risk for ineffective management of therapeutic or medical management regimen, individuals (NANDA 5.2.1) related to:
- knowledge deficit
- improper use of medications
- perceived ineffectiveness of medication
- chronic nature of some skin disorders leading to necessity of long-term adherence to treatment plan
- complexity and regularity of treatments
- inability of student and/or family to demonstrate proper care skills and behavior
- noncompliance with management/ therapeutic/ medical plan
- perceived financial or transportation barriers

Student Goals

- Attain and maintain (normal) skin appearance and integrity. (N. D. 1)
- Demonstrate compliance with treatment plan. (N. D. 6)
- Demonstrate treatment self-care skills, including proper hand washing, glove use, and proper technique with medications and treatments. (N. D. 2, 3, 5, 6)
- Demonstrate proper disposal of medications/ointments/soaks, gloves, and any applicators and/or dressings. (N. D. 2, 5, 6)
- Identify and describe signs and symptoms of secondary skin infection, such as redness, increased temperature (systemically or at site of lesion), oozing, increased size or distribution of lesions, etc. (N. D. 2)

- Demonstrate knowledge and avoidance of known allergens. (N. D. 5, 6)
- Practice good nutrition choices. (N. D. 5, 6)
- Maintain an improved self-image. (N. D. 4)
- Maintain good school attendance.
- Participate, fully, in age-appropriate activities, including physical education. (N. D. 4)
- Maintain academic achievement. (N. D. 4)
- Resume and/or maintain active social participation with peers in school, extracurricular, community (church, groups, clubs, etc.) and home/ neighborhood activities during free time. (N. D. 4)
- Increase in ability to manage itching, soreness, and/or pain. (N. D. 3)

Nursing Interventions

Teacher/School Interventions:

Develop an IHP (N. D. 1-6)
- Include student, parents/guardians, teachers, and healthcare provider
- Coordinate IHP with student, family, and healthcare providers for coordinated home and school management
- Determine if known allergens or triggers are present at school
- Determine time and place for daily treatments needed at school
- Identify a place to keep medications and treatment supplies secure and clean
- Identify place and proper method of disposal for used gloves, treatment and/or dressing supplies
- Modify plan as needed

Keep accurate treatment records. (N. D. 1-6)
- Changes in skin appearance
- Treatments and medications, time, dose, route of administration
- History of effective and ineffective medications and treatments
- Supplies used and/or needed
- Psychosocial adjustment of student
- Pain management techniques

Provide in-services for teachers and other school personnel working with the student. (N. D. 1, 2, 4, 5, 6)
- General skin disorder information and skin disorder information specific to student
- Medication and treatments necessary on a daily basis
- Signs and symptoms of a secondary skin infection
- Importance of regular and continuing treatment, including medications and treatments that must be administered during the school day (allowing for input from teachers on how to avoid an impact on learning or social relationships for the time missed from the classroom and peer contact)
- Allergic components (if pertinent), including known triggers for this student.
- If food allergies are suspected or identified, ensure that classroom teacher and lunchroom personnel are notified.
- Detail importance of avoidance of known triggers
- Importance of good hand washing and good hygiene in general
- Importance of well-balanced nutrition to enhance healing. If severe acne is the diagnosis, stress that food is rarely implicated as a cause.

Observe and monitor medication and treatment administration. Teach and reinforce proper technique when needed. (N. D. 2, 5, 6)
- Periodically inspect affected skin.
- Have student practice and demonstrate proper technique.
- Discuss treatments, including proper storage, use, and disposal of medications and treatment supplies. Observe periodically.
- Modify treatment plan as needed.

Student/Family Interventions:

Refer for medical evaluation, diagnosis, and treatment. (N. D. 1, 2, 3)
- Assist parent and student to access health care.
- Assist parent to access skin specialist (dermatologist).
- Encourage periodic follow-up with healthcare provider.
- Assist family to decrease barriers (financial, transportation) to continued healthcare.

Obtain medication and treatment orders from student's healthcare provider and parental authorization. (N. D. 1, 2, 6)
- Administer medications and treatments in accordance with prescribed orders.
- Encourage positive skin care procedures and general hygiene measures to promote skin healing.
- Encourage compliance with prescribed treatments.
- Teach developmentally appropriate self-care with treatments, medications, and supplies.
- Assist student to prevent secondary infection.
- Obtain accurate information of known allergens.
- Assist student to maintain proper technique with treatments and medication.

Develop health education plan for student and family to encourage compliance with proper and continuing treatment at home and at school. (N. D. 1-6)
- Develop plan to increase student's and family's level of knowledge on causes of skin disorder and treatments needed.
- Assess student's knowledge about medications.
- Stress importance of and encourage regular school attendance and participation.
- Stress importance of social relationships and support.
- Stress importance of regular peer interaction.
- Monitor classroom performance and academic achievement. Refer as needed.

Assist student to properly treat skin condition at school and at home. (N. D. 2, 4, 5, 6)
- Assess level of skill with supplies and medications.
- Teach, encourage, and periodically monitor and reinforce proper hand-washing technique.
- Stress importance of keeping hands away from affected skin.
- Keep healthy skin which is near affected skin dry and clean to prevent its breakdown from moisture.
- Teach and periodically reinforce proper glove technique.
- Reinforce safe disposal of all dressings and supplies used, including gloves, to prevent possible spread of germs and infection to self or others.
- Insure privacy for treatments, with secure storage of medications.

- Determine how to decrease disruption of the regular school day as much as possible.

Discuss with student/family and periodically reinforce (N. D. 1, 2, 5, 6), as needed:
- Importance of regular school attendance.
- Regular and normal peer interactions and relationships.
- Full participation in school day activities, including physical education.
- Understanding the need to avoid known allergens.
- Importance of proper nutrition and diet to enhance and promote healing.
- Importance of adequate intake of water to enhance hydration.
- Modification of treatment plan, in collaboration with healthcare provider, student, family, and teachers.

Assist student/family to identify barriers to continued treatment. (N. D. 5, 6)
- Assist with removing barriers

Assist student to identify motivators to continued self-care. (N. D. 4, 6)
- Implement motivators

Discuss and periodically reinforce with student. (N. D. 1-6)
- Understanding of causes of disorder
- Knowledge of and responsibilities for self-care
- Identification of known allergens and ways to avoid or reduce contact with irritants
- Self-care skill level, acknowledging good care
- Knowledge and recognition of signs and symptoms of infection
- Importance of adherence to regular treatment protocols (when, where, how, proper medications and disposal of used supplies)
- Consequences of noncompliance
- Motivators and barriers to compliance
- Importance of participation in normal school and peer activities
- Perceptions of self-image

Assist student to participate in management of skin disorder treatment plan, as appropriate. (N. D. 4, 5, 6)
- Allow student input into daily schedule (dependent upon age, developmental level, and knowledge of and skill level for treatments).
- Increase student independence in medication and treatment administration, as appropriate.
- Monitor student, family, teacher perceptions of student's self-care ability and responsibility level to adhere to treatment protocol.
- Implement non-drug or medication pain reduction techniques (such as using lukewarm rather than hot water, loose clothing made from natural fibers [avoidance of wool], and washing irritants from skin quickly with cool water).
- Modify plan accordingly.

Assist student to recognize and verbalize positive social and peer interactions. (N. D. 4)
- Encourage increased participation in extracurricular activities.
- Recognize student achievement in classroom and social activities.

Promote confidence through emphasis on past successful coping. (N. D. 4)
- Identify and encourage use of past successful coping skills.
- Identify and eliminate unsuccessful coping skills.
- Assist student to learn and utilize coping strategies that are more successful.

Encourage persistence with treatments through frequent and regular interactions with the student and family. (N. D. 6)

Expected Student Outcomes

The student will:
- accurately describe steps in wound healing. (N.D. 5)
- correctly identify known allergens. (N.D. 5)
- independently avoid allergic irritants. (N.D 1 and 5)
- describe the signs and symptoms of infection. (N.D. 1, 2)
- verbalize absence, reduction, or control of pain or itching, and exhibit no evidence of discomfort or continued scratching. (N.D. 3)
- maintain regular school attendance. (N.D. 4)
- participate in age-appropriate activities with peers and family. (N.D. 4)
- verbalize and manifest positive self-image by active participation in management of, and compliance with, treatment modalities. (N.D. 4, 5)
- consistently demonstrate proper self-care, hand washing and glove technique. (N.D. 2, 5, 6)
- demonstrate good hygiene practices. (N.D. 2, 5, 6)
- make wise food choices to enhance healing. (N.D. 1, 2, 5, 6)
- continue treatment and medical care as needed. (N.D. 1, 5, 6)

The affected skin will:
- show signs of healing, lessening of allergic reaction, or maintenance of control of chronic or inherited condition. (N.D. 1, 2)
- show no signs of impaired skin integrity or evidence of secondary infection. (N.D. 1, 2)

CASE STUDY

Josh is a rough-and-tumble 11-year-old boy with a history of asthma and chronic atopic dermatitis (eczema) seen on the flexor surfaces of elbows and knees and on the backs of both hands. His type of manifestation and body distribution is the most common for his age. He lives in the sunny western part of the United States where the weather is frequently windy and dry with long hot summers. The dermatitis is exacerbated from mid spring to late fall when the boys and girls play soccer and football, with the attendant number of scrapes and cuts which occur from falls on the turf and rolling along the ground. Because of his age, careful hand washing usually is minimal, so secondary infection from scratching with dirty fingernails is common.

More than half of children with atopic dermatitis have a family disposition toward allergic conditions, including asthma. The skin of affected children usually has a strong inflammatory response to allergens or other irritants causing swelling and erythema that aggravate pruritus. Due to excessive scratching from intense itching, skin infections often accompany atopic dermatitis.

The typical appearance of the child is one of a tired and cranky child with dry and itchy skin that shows a pattern of exacerbation and healing. When infected, the skin may be oozing or crusted. A diagnosis is made by a positive family history, the type and body distribution of the lesions, intense itching and scratching, and the elimination of scabies as a cause. The goals of treatment are control of the itching, hydration, prevention or control of secondary infection, and avoidance of allergens or irritants.

Individualized Healthcare Plan*
Skin Disorder

Assessment Data	Nursing Diagnosis	Goals	Nursing Interventions	Expected Outcomes
ND1 J. has chronic, but periodic itchy weepy skin sores on his elbows and hands related to seasonal allergies.	Impaired skin integrity related to: a) Allergies and inherited traits; b) Sensitive and easily irritated skin; c) Frequent trauma to the skin related to rambunctious nature of J. (NANDA 1.6.2.1.2.1)	J. will learn age- and developmentally appropriate self-care. J. will appropriately avoid know allergic triggers. J. will drink water regularly to enhance hydration. J. will learn ways to avoid injuries on the playground.	Refer for complete medical work-up, if information is not current and available. Secure physician orders and parent authorization for medication and treatment. Determine known allergens.	Normal skin appearance and integrity will be seen. J's self-care will prevent further skin irritation. Playground injuries and other cuts and scrapes will decrease.
Family history of allergic symptoms and conditions.			Develop a plan of care for J. and coordinate efforts at home and school to promote healing. Keep accurate records of skin appearance and treatments, including effective and ineffective. Carry out prescribed treatments at school.	Avoidance of know allergic triggers and skin irritants will be routine for J.
J's skin is dry and easily becomes itchy, red, and weepy in response to many irritants, environmental contacts, and some food allergies and during seasonal allergies.			Periodically inspect all affected skin and chart appearance. Encourage compliance with continued treatment.	

J. is a very active boy who frequently has cuts and scrapes on his skin.			Provide in-service for school personnel with information specific to J. such as allergic triggers, food that must be avoided, importance of nutrition, enough water, clean hands, proper storage of medications, and importance of regular and extended treatment.	Skin will show no evidence of secondary infection. Good hygiene and proper hand washing are routine. J. will recognize and treat quickly and properly any secondary infection.
ND2 J. has frequent secondary infection from playing soccer and football during times of skin breakout. J.'s hands and fingernails don't appear clean. His hand washing skills are poor. J. frequently scratches his skin until it is open and bleeding.	Rick for infection related to: a) Itching and scratching, causing open sores that are easily contaminated with germs; b) Inadequate hygiene and hand washing; c) Non-use of gloves for treatment; d) Improper care and disposal of medication and treatment supplies; e) Frequent skin trauma due to J's rambunctious nature. (NANDA 1.2.1.1)	J. will learn signs and symptoms of skin infection. J. will learn and practice good hygiene in general, with hand washing being a high priority. J. will stop scratching behaviors to relieve itching.	Teach signs and symptoms of infection. Teach and encourage good hygiene, hand washing, and use of gloves for treatments. Teach and encourage proper storage, use, and disposal of treatment supplies.	

Individualized Healthcare Plan*
Skin Disorder (continued)

Assessment Data	Nursing Diagnosis	Goals	Nursing Interventions	Expected Outcomes
Medication tubes and bottles are left open and not kept n clean containers. J. doesn't understand that scratching with dirty fingernails will lead to secondary infection. J. doesn't know how to properly take care of and dispose of medications and treatment supplies, to minimize risk of secondary infection.		J. will practice age- and developmentally appropriate self-care to prevent infection. J. will keep medications and supplies clean and in closed containers.	Teach age- and developmentally appropriate treatment self-care. Explore behavior modification plan to acknowledge and reward NOT scratching.	Intact skin will show no evidence of scratching. Without prompting, proper use, storage and disposal of medication and supplies will be routine.
ND3 J. says skin is itchy and sore.	Pain related to: a) Weepy and itchy skin sores; b) Underlying disease process; c) Secondary infection; d) Incomplete treatment. (NANDA 9.1.1)	J. will comply with treatments. J. will stop scratching. J's itching will be relieved. J. will avoid allergies and irritants.	Teach nonpharmacologic techniques to avoid irritating skin. Teach age- and developmentally appropriate pain management techniques. Administer medication and treatment as prescribed. Encourage continued self-care to promote healing and lessen itchy lesions.	No more, or relieved itching and/or soreness. No evidence of secondary infection. J. will practice several non-pharmacologic pain reduction techniques, if needed.

ND4 J. expresses embarrassment over skin appearance. J. is aggressive due to anger and rejects his friends when skin disorder is present. J's school attendance is poor when disorder is apparent. J. avoids his friends and social activities.	Risk for body image disturbance related to: a) Inaccurate perception of appearance; b) Inaccurate perception of friends' thinking and feeling about J; c) Avoiding social activities; d) Poor school attendance. (NANDA 7.1.1)	Maintain a high self image. J. will attend school regularly and participate fully in class activities. Maintain normal peer relationships. Maintain normal social relationships.	Provide privacy and increasing independence with self-care. Allow age- and developmentally appropriate control over scheduling of treatments. Regularly monitor psycosocial adjustment, participation in and behavior during classroom activities. Regularly monitor academic performance. Encourage and promote positive coping skills.	J. freely verbalizes feelings and concerns appropriately. J. has regular school attendance and participates fully in activities.

Individualized Healthcare Plan*
Skin Disorder (continued)

Assessment Data	Nursing Diagnosis	Goals	Nursing Interventions	Expected Outcomes
ND5 J. doesn't understand why treatment must be continued for long periods. J. doesn't practice good food choices. J. forgets to wash his hands.	Risk for knowledge deficit related to: a) Underlying disease process; b) Chronic nature of treatment; c) Relationship of good nutrition, adequate hydration, and hygiene to healing; d) Identification and avoidance of allergens; e) Nonpharmacologic pain reduction (NANDA 8.1.1)	J. will demonstrate proper treatment self-care skills. J. will practice good hygiene and proper hand washing and gloving technique. J will demonstrate proper disposal of used supplies.	Develop educational plan for J. by first assessing knowledge level and deficits. Teach signs and symptoms of infection, disease process, technique for treatment and disposal of supplies.	Independently follows treatment regimen. Effective treatment management. Good hygiene and clean hands are the norm.
J. forgets to use gloves, and when he does, he forgets to dispose of them properly. J's skin is dry and scaly looking, with poor turgor.		J. will identify and avoid known allergens. J. will drink enough water and fluids for adequate hydration.	Teach importance of hand washing and good hygiene, proper nutrition, adequate hydration, and recognition and avoidance of allergens. Periodically monitor treatment technique and supply and medication usage and storage.	Proper food choices and adequate hydration are the usual behavior.

ND6 Because of periodic, but chronic nature of skin condition, treatment isn't continuos and frequently not followed until symptoms are resolved. J. doesn't understand that treatment may be complex and long-term. J. gets tired of constant treatment regimens. J. doesn't use good treatment technique and doesn't properly dispose of supplies.	Risk for ineffective management of therapeutic regimen related to: a) Chronic nature of allergic skin disorders; b) Improper use, storage and disposal of medication and supplies; c) Complexity, regularity, and continuity of treatment protocols; d) Poor self-care skills; e) Noncompliance. (NANDA 5.2.1)	J. will explain his skin condition and demonstrate understanding of complex and long-term nature of treatment. J. will demonstrate compliance with regimen. J. will demonstrate proper treatment technique and disposal of gloves and supplies.	Secure privacy for self-care treatments. Aid student to recognize barriers to continued treatment protocols. Aid recognition of and implement identified motivates to long-term treatment. Allow student input into daily schedule as much as possible. Give increasing independence in treatment regime as compliance increases. Encourage persistence with continued and frustrating self treatment	Compliance and age-appropriate management of medical regimen will be routine. J. will avoid allergic triggers and know allergens. J. independently uses proper self-care skills regularly.

REFERENCES

1. Betz CL, Hunsberger M, Wright S. *Family-Centered Nursing Care of Children.* 2nd ed. Philadelphia, Pa: WB Saunders Company, 1994:1623-1632, 1648-1660.
2. Wong D, DL, Hockenbery-Eaton M, Wilson D, Winkelstein ML, Ahmann E, Divito-Thomas PA, eds. *Whaley and Wong's Nursing Care of Infants and Children.* 6th ed. St. Louis, Mo: Mosby, 1999:820-838, 1338.
3. Bowden VR, Dickey SB, Greenberg CS. *Children and Their Families: The Continuum of Care.* Philadelphia, Pa: WB Saunders Company, 1998:1686-1712, 1724-1728.
4. Carpenito LJ. *Nursing Diagnosis: Application to Nursing Practice.* 7th ed. Philadelphia, Pa: JB Lippincott, 1997.

BIBLIOGRAPHY

Bryant R, Doughty D. *Acute and Chronic Wounds: Nursing Management* 2nd ed. St. Louis, Mo: Mosby, 1998.

Chauvin VG. Common skin rashes in children and adolescents. *School Nurse* 1989;5(1):23-38.

Forsdyke H, Watts J. Skin care in atopic eczema. *Prof Nurse* 1994;10(1):36-38, 40.

Garvin G. Wound healing in pediatrics. *Nurs Clin North Am.* 1990;25(1):181-192.

Hanifin JM. Atopic dermatitis in infants and children. *Pediatr Clin North Am* 1991;38(4):763-787.

Hunt TK. Basic principles of wound healing. *J Trauma.* 1990;30(12, suppl):S122-S128.

Hurwitz S. *Clinical Pediatric Dermatology: A Textbook of Skin Disorders of Childhood and Adolescence* 2nd ed. Philadelphia, Pa: WB Saunders Company, 1993.

Krasner D. The twelve commandments of wound care. *Nursing 92.* 1992;12:34-41.

North American Nursing Diagnosis Association. *NANDA Nursing Diagnoses: Definitions & Classification 1999-2000.* Philadelphia, Pa: North American Nursing Diagnosis Assn, 1999. (NANDA, 1211 Locust Street, Philadelphia, PA 19107. 800-647-9002; fax 215-545-8107; e-mail: NANDA@nursecominc.com)

O'Brien J. Common skin problems of infancy, childhood, and adolescence. *Primary Care.* 1995;22(1):99-115.

Romeo SP. Atopic dermatitis: the itch that rashes. *Pediatr Nurs.* 1995;22(2):157-163.

Rothe MJ, Grant-Kels JM. Atopic dermatitis. In: Arndt KA, Wintroub BU, Robinson JK,

LeBoit PE, eds. *Primary Care Dermatology.* Philadelphia, Pa: WB Saunders Company, 1997:48-51.

Singleton JK. Pediatric dermatoses: three common skin disruptions in infancy. *Nurs Pract.* 1997;22(6):32-50.

Spowart K. Childhood skin disorders. *Pediatr Nurs.* 1996;8(7):29-35.

Whaley LF, Wong DL. *Essentials of Pediatric Nursing.* 5th ed. St. Louis, Mo: Mosby, 1997.

Wysocki A. Skin structure. In: Bryant R, ed. *Acute and Chronic Wounds: Nursing Management.* St. Louis, Mo: Mosby, 1992.

31 | IHP: Spinal Cord Injury

Cynthia K. Silkworth

INTRODUCTION

Spinal cord injuries are not common in children. The occurrence in children, from birth to 15 years, is only 4.4% of all spinal cord injuries.[1] The majority of spinal cord injuries, about 80%, occur in young men, between the ages of 16 and 25.[2]

Causes of spinal cord injury vary with age. Birth injuries can produce traumatic cord damage, usually related to traction of the head and shoulders and hyperextension of the neck.[3,4] Motor vehicle accidents (including automobile-bicycle accidents and all-terrain vehicle accidents) are the leading cause of spinal cord injury in children and adolescents. Other known causes of spinal cord injuries in children and adolescents include falls from heights and horseback riding; recreational activities, such as diving accidents; and sports activities, such as gymnastics and downhill skiing.[4,5] Spinal cord injuries may also be caused by acts of violence, such as gunshot wounds.[1,5] Diseases, such as polio and spina bifida, and tumors may also cause spinal cord injury.

Pathophysiology

The spinal cord transmits motor and sensory signals between the brain and the body. An injury to the spinal cord affects the sending and receiving of signals across the site of the injury and results in a loss of motor and sensory function below the site. Depending on the level of the injury, a person who sustains a spinal cord injury may also experience impairments in regulating respiration, temperature, and blood pressure and bowel, bladder, and sexual function. Unless a head injury was also sustained, a person with a spinal cord injury will not have intellectual or cognitive impairment as a result of the injury.[4,6,7]

Spinal cord injuries can occur at any level on the spinal column or at multiple levels. They are described by the highest point of normal functioning of the cord in relation to the vertebra. For example: an injury at the level of the fifth cervical vertebra is described as a C5 injury.

Characteristics of spinal cord injury[5,6] depend on three factors:

1) **Level of the spinal cord at which the injury occured**—in general, the higher the level of injury, the greater the paralysis and loss of sensation.

2) **Damage to the cord**—whether or not the lesion cuts across the entire cord. Complete lesions usually lead to complete loss of functional motor movement and sensation below the level of injury. Incomplete lesions result in varying degrees of motor and sensory loss.

3) **Cause of the injury**—direct or indirect trauma, hyperextension, hyperflexion, or compression of the spinal cord.

Definitions associated with spinal cord injury[4,6]

Paralysis: loss of function, voluntary movement, and sensation

Paraplegia: paralysis of the lower portion of the body, involving both legs, due to injury to the spinal cord at thoracic vertebra 1 (T1) or below, common sites of injury are at thoracic vertebra 12 (T12) and lumbar vertebra 1 (L1)

Quadriplegia: paralysis, involving both upper and lower extremities with loss of bladder, bowel, and sexual function

Tetraplegia: high—injury to the spinal cord at cervical vertebrae 1-4 (C1-C4), with paralysis from the neck down. low—injury to the spinal cord at cervical vertebrae 5 and 6 (C5-C6), with paralysis from the shoulders down

Hemiplegia: paralysis on one side of the body

Flaccid paralysis: paralysis with low muscle tone

Spastic paralysis: paralysis with involuntary contraction of muscles associated with loss of muscle tone

Autonomic Dysreflexia

In autonomic dysreflexia, a stimulus, either internal or external, causes a generalized spread of sympathetic and parasympathetic activity in a person with a T-7 or higher spinal cord injury that leads to increased blood pressure. The body is unable to recognize or take the necessary action to decrease the stimulus and blood pressure because of the spinal cord injury. **Autonomic dysreflexia is a medical emergency that requires immediate intervention.**

Stimuli that may cause an episode of dysreflexia include:
- distended or spastic bladder
- bladder infection
- distended bowel or impaction
- pressure areas on skin, irritating clothing, skin temperature changes

Symptoms include:
- sweating (above the site of the spinal cord injury)
- sudden, periodic high blood pressure
- pounding headache
- tachycardia or bradycardia (abnormally fast or slow heartbeat)
- flushing of the face and/or red splotches on skin (above the site of the spinal cord injury)
- pallor (below the site of the spinal cord injury)

Management of an episode requires reducing or removing the stimulus, such as slow drainage of the bladder, loosening tight or constricting clothing, shifting position to relieve pressure area, and removal of stool or impaction.[4,8]

Management

A complex team of people, including the child or adolescent and the family, needs to work collaboratively to identity the child's or adolescent's needs and to plan and implement realistic interventions. Other members of the team include: physicians (primary and specialists), rehabilitation nurse, physical therapist, occupational therapist, respiratory therapist, dietitian, recreational therapist, social worker, psychologist, and vocational counselor.

Management measures[4] include:
- Respiratory care—maintenance of good airway and ventilation, child with a high level injury, C1-C4, will require ventilatory assistance, most often a tracheostomy and ventilator; other care may include positioning for optimal chest expansion, chest physiotherapy,

Functional Ability Associated with Spinal Cord Injury

Highest Intact Cord Level	Functional Ability
C1-3 Muscle innervation: head and neck muscles	No voluntary control below chin Respiratory paralysis, ventilator dependent May cause bradycardia or tachycardia Requires electric wheelchair
C4 Muscle innervation: intact sterno-cleidomastoid, trapezius, upper cervical paraspinous muscles	No voluntary function in upper extremities, trunk, or lower extremities All neck movements Respirator dependent Requires electric wheelchair
C5 Muscle innervation: partial deltoid, biceps, major muscles of rotator cuffs at shoulders, diaphragm	Abduction, flexion, and extension of arms, shoulder and bicep control Flexion and extension of forearms, no control at hand or wrist Unable to roll over or attain sitting position Abdominal respiration Poor respiratory reserve Requires electric wheelchair
C6 Muscle innervation: pectoralis major, serratus anterior, latissimus dorsi muscles, complete deltoid and brachioradialis muscles, partial triceps muscle	Significant increase in function over C5 level Adduction and medial rotation of arm Wrist extension, but no hand function Good elbow flexion Able to assist in dressing and transfers May be independent in wheelchair
C7 Muscle innervation: triceps and finger flexor muscles, shoulder depressor muscles	With elbow stabilized in extension, and intact shoulder depressor muscles, able to lift body weight Grasp and release still weak, low dexterity with hand and fingers Can roll over, sit up and eat independently Requires some assistance with transfers and lower extremity dressing
T1 Muscle innervation: hand intrinsic muscles	Full use of upper extremities, including hand muscles
T2-8 Muscle innervation: full innervation of upper extremity muscles, upper back and chest muscles	Poor trunk control May have difficulty in lifting sufficiently to put on lower extremity clothing May be braced for standing
T9-T12 Muscle innervation: full abdominal and lower back muscles	Good trunk control, good sitting balance Good respiratory reserve Ambulatory with bilateral long leg braces and four-point or swing-through crutches
L1-L5 Muscle innervation: leg muscles, partial gluteus muscles	Floppy ankles, ambulates well with short leg braces with or without a cane May be lumbar lordosis

Adapted from Wong DL, Hockenbery-Eaton M, Wilson D, Winkelstein ML, Ahmann E, Divito-Thomas PA, eds,[4] and National Spinal Cord Injury Association.[6]

breathing exercises
- Temperature regulation—maintenance of normal body temperature by use of clothing and environmental measures added or removed, depending on body temperature, and monitoring for fever and signs of infection
- Skin care—maintenance of clean and dry skin and monitoring for signs of pressure areas
- Autonomic dysreflexia—prevention of episodes and quick assessment and intervention to remove the causes and resolve the episodes
- Remobilization—use of wheelchair, walker or crutches, braces, orthoses

- Maintenance of bladder dynamics— prevention of overextension of the bladder and urinary retention; control of urinary tract infections
- Bowel training—control of defecation until in an appropriate, usually planned, time and place
- Physical rehabilitation—preparation of the child and family to resume and maintain life at home, in school, and in the community
- Psychosocial rehabilitation—expression of feelings; alteration of concepts about self and social roles; development of a realistic definition of interdependent living and vocational rehabilitation

INDIVIDUALIZED HEALTHCARE PLAN

Assessment

History

- Development and health prior to the spinal cord injury
- When the spinal cord injury occurred
- Age of the student when the injury occurred
- How the injury occurred
- Level of the spinal cord injury
- Initial care after the injury
- Rehabilitation program
- Complications or infections related to the spinal cold injury
- Prognosis
- Most recent reevaluation

Current Status and Management

- Level of function—motor and sensory
- Mobility—wheelchair use, orthoses, braces
- Respiratory care—need for ventilatory assistance, tracheostomy care, chest physiotherapy or breathing exercises, cough reflex and strength
- Autonomic dysreflexia—prevention, common causes, interventions used
- Skin care—skin breakdown prevention measures, monitoring of pressure areas
- Bladder elimination—pattern, during school hours, monitoring for urinary tract infections
- Bowel program—pattern, needs during school hours
- Temperature regulation—environmental needs
- Medications—at home, during school hours

- Nutrition—meal pattern, snacks, assistance needed with eating
- Growth—height and weight
- Daily activity schedule—energy use, need for rest
- Current therapy—physical, occupational, recreational, speech

Self-care

- Knowledge about current health status, abilities, and disabilities
- Student's perception of his/her abilities and disabilities and health status
- Parent's perception of student's abilities and disabilities and health status
- Student's decision-making skills
- Student's ability to participate in self-care activities—activities of daily living
- Participation in activities of daily living—at home, in school
- Independent skills—physical, psychosocial, cognitive
- Motivation to participate in self-care
- Barriers to participating in self-care

Psychosocial Status

- Student's contact and interaction with family, peers, and adults
- Student's locus of control
- Involvement with support persons, groups, and services
- Participation in family, peer, school, and community activities

Academic Issues

- Past and current academic achievement
- Schools the student has attended—including hospital-based and homebound educational programs
- Special educational services—past services, current needs
- School and classroom modifications needed - facilities; equipment—including computer utilization; transportation; assistance with locker, jacket, books, lunch, and getting between classes; management aide assistance in the classroom; schedule; assistance from peers; access to media center books and resource materials
- Specialized healthcare procedures required during the school day
- Emergency evacuation from the building

Nursing Diagnoses (N.D.)

N.D. 1 Impaired physical mobility (NANDA 6.1.1.1) related to paraplegia, quadriplegia.

N.D. 2 Risk for disuse syndrome (NANDA 1.6.1.5) related to spinal cord injury / neuromuscular impairment / paralysis.

N.D. 3 High risk for injury (NANDA 1.6.1) related to:
- paralysis / immobility
- sensory deficit (tactile)

N.D. 4 High risk for impaired skin integrity (NANDA 1.6.2.1.2.2) related to immobility.

N.D. 5   Ineffective breathing pattern (NANDA 1.5.1.3) related to paralysis/ immobility

N.D. 6   Inability to sustain spontaneous ventilation (NANDA 1.5.1.3.1) related to spinal cord injury / paralysis.

N.D. 7   High risk for dysreflexia (NANDA 1.2.3.1) related to autonomic nerve dysfunction.

N.D. 8   Ineffective thermoregulation (NANDA 1.2.2.4) related to autonomic nerve dysfunction.

N.D. 9   Alteration in urinary elimination pattern (NANDA1.3.2) related to neuromuscular impairment.

N.D. 10   Bowel incontinence (NANDA 1.3.1.3) related to lack of voluntary sphincter control due to neuromuscular impairment.

N.D. 11   Constipation (NANDA 1.3.1.1) related to neuromuscular impairment.

N.D. 12   Self-care deficit (NANDA 6.5.1,2,3 or 4) in feeding, bathing / hygiene, dressing/grooming, toileting, related to physical disability.

N.D. 13   High risk for disturbance in body image (NANDA 7.1.1) related to perception of physical disability.

N.D. 14   High risk for powerlessness (NANDA 7.3.2) related to:
  • physical impairment
  • dependence on others for activities of daily living at home and school

Goals

Be independent with mobility in the school setting. (N.D. 1,2)

Increase independence with mobility in the school setting. (N.D. 1,2,13)

Develop and implement an Emergency Evacuation Plan (EEP). (N.D. 1,2)

Prevent physical injuries. (N.D. 3)

Utilize prevention methods to prevent skin breakdown and pressure areas. (N.D. 4)

Prevent respiratory infections. (N.D. 5,6)

Maintain open airway, effective breathing pattern, and air exchange. (N.D. 5,6)

Develop Emergency Care Plan (ECP) for management of a dysreflexia episode at school. (N.D. 7)

Manage episodes of dysreflexia effectively. (N.D. 7)

Maintain optimal body temperature. (N.D. 8)

Dress appropriately for body temperature and environmental conditions. (N.D. 8)

Prevent bladder distention and incontinence during the school day. (N.D. 9)

Prevent urinary tract infections. (N.D. 9)

Maintain adequate dietary and fluid intake. (N.D. 9,10,11)

Prevent bowel incontinence during the school day. (N.D. 9)

Participate verbally and physically in: feeding, dressing, toileting, and bathing activities. (N.D. 12)

Increase self-care skills (specify what skills). (N.D. 12)

Maintain optimal hygiene with assistance. (N.D. 12,13)

Utilize healthy adaptation and coping skills. (N.D. 13)

Describe abilities, disabilities, and appearance realistically. (N.D. 13)

Make decisions regarding health management, assistive care, school, and peer activities. (N.D. 12,14)

Communicate effectively with parent(s) and teachers. (N.D. 14)

Identify and demonstrate responsibility and control of identified factors in his/her life (N.D. 14)

Nursing Interventions

Orient student to the school building, make note of rooms or areas that are inaccessible, such as the media center, band room, auditorium, etc., and modifications that need to be made to make them accessible. (N.D. 1,2)

With the student, check the time it takes to get from class to class, class to lunch, and last class to bus home, and make modification in release times if needed. (N.D. 1,2)

With the student, check all classrooms to make sure there are desks or tables that will accommodate the student's needs, such as the wheelchair being able to fit under the desks or tables. (N.D. 1,2)

Educate teachers and management assistants on assistive measures that will be needed in the classroom, such as accessing books and materials that are needed, assistance with writing for assignments and tests, assistance with completing special assignments or experiments, etc., based on student need and preference. (N.D. 1,2)

Develop an EEP that clearly indicates how the student will be evacuated from the building in case of an emergency situation. All persons who will be involved with the student during the school day, as well as the student, should be involved in developing and practicing the plan. (N.D. 1,2)

Assist the student to maintain proper body postioning in his/her wheelchair. (N.D. 1, 2, 3 and 4)

Discuss with the student: factors that increase risk of injury. (N.D. 3)

Instruct student to use safety equipment, properly, at all times, such as having the wheelchair belt securely fastened. Monitor use. (N.D. 3)

Utilize correct techniques for moving, transferring, and transporting the student. (N.D. 3)

Handle extremities carefully when turning and positioning. (N.D. 3)

Monitor for signs of contracture deformity. Inform parents if signs are noticed. (N.D. 3)

Monitor environment for possible contact with environmental hazards, such as chemicals, heat / cold, slippery floor or sidewalk surfaces, etc. Utilize measures to prevent exposure. (N.D. 3).

Discuss with student: (N.D. 4)
- what skin breakdowns are
- ways to prevent skin breakdown and pressure areas, such as shifting weight at least once every class period
- signs and symptoms of skin breakdown
- what to do if signs and symptoms are present

Assist student to notify parent(s) if signs or symptoms of a skin breakdown or pressure area occur. (N.D. 4)

Assist the student to keep skin and clothing clean and dry. (N.D. 4)

Inspect skin for signs and symptoms of skin breakdown, especially when putting on or removing braces or orthotic devices, doing catheterization procedures, when cleaning anal area after a bowel movement, or changing the student's clothing. (N.D. 4)

Inform teachers and others working with the student of tactile deficit and need to protect skin from pressure and harmful environments, such as chemicals, hot and cold. (N.D. 4)

Discuss with student: (N.D. 5)
- how regular breathing exercises can assist in maintaining good respiratory function
- signs and symptoms of a respiratory infection
- ways to minimize risk of contracting a respiratory infection
- what to do if signs and symptoms are present

Encourage the student and family to consult their healthcare provider about yearly influenza immunization. (N.D. 5,6)

Assist the student to demonstrate and utilize effective coughing. Utilize quadcough technique as needed. (N.D. 5)

Provide tracheostomy care as prescribed and as needed. (N.D. 6)

Maintain an adequate supply of tracheostomy care equipment and supplies. (N.D. 6)

If the student is ventilator dependent, develop knowledge and understanding of the function of the particular ventilator the student is on and what to do if a malfunction occurs. A manual ventilation bag must always be immediately available. (N.D. 6)

If the student has a diaphragmatic pacemaker, develop a knowledge and understanding of the function of the pacemaker and what to do if the pacemaker malfunctions. An extra supply of batteries for the student's pacemaker and a manual ventilation bag must always be available. (N.D. 6)

Develop an ECP to manage occurrences of ventilator or diaphragmatic pacemaker malfunction. (N.D. 6)

Develop an ECP to manage dysreflexia episodes at school with the student, parent(s), and healthcare provider. (N.D. 7)

Follow ECP if an episode occurs. (N.D. 7)

Provide inservices to the student's teachers and other staff who work with him/her regarding dysreflexia and what to do if an episode occurs. Include a copy of the ECP. (N.D. 7)

Discuss with the student: (N.D. 7)
- what causes dysreflexia episodes
- signs and symptoms of a dysreflexia episode, and how he/she feels when an episode occurs
- what to do if an episode occurs at school, during after-school activities, and on field trips

Encourage the student to dress appropriately for the weather and school environment. (N.D. 8)

If the student is exposed to significant temperature changes during the school day, assist the student to adjust clothing accordingly. Provide extra coverage with blankets if appropriate. (N.D. 8)

Encourage the student to maintain good hydration. (N.D. 8)

If the student has an indwelling catheter, assist the student to drain the bag at a mutually agreed upon time during the school day. (Note: color, amount and clarity of urine, patency of catheter.) (N.D. 9)

If the student requires sterile catheterization, provide a private area for the procedure to be done. Arrange for an adequate supply of equipment to be kept at school. (Note: color, amount and clarity of urine.) (N.D. 9)

If the student is able to self-catheterize, provide a private bathroom that is handicap accessible and easily accessible for the student. Provide a place for the student to store catheters and other supplies. (N.D. 9)

Inform the student's teachers of the student's need for catheterization and, if needed, extra time out of class for the procedure to be done. (N.D. 9)

Assist student to have and store extra clothing and supplies in school in case urinary incontinence / bowel incontinence occurs. (N.D. 9,10)

Provide a private space/bathroom for the student to use for cleaning and clothing change, if urinary incontinence or a bowel movement occurs at school. (N.D. 9,10)

Monitor for signs and symptoms of a urinary tract infection. (N.D. 9)

Discuss with the student: (N.D. 9)
- signs and symptoms of a urinary tract infection
- what to do if the signs and symptoms occur

Assist the student to notify his/her parent(s) if any signs or symptoms of a urinary tract infection occur. (N.D. 9)

Discuss the current bowel elimination program with the student and parent(s). (N.D. 10,11)

Discuss with student and parent(s): what to do if a bowel movement occurs at school. (N.D. 10)

Promote participation in feeding, hygiene, toileting, and dressing activities. (N.D. 11,14)

With the student and parents, determine areas for potential increase in participation in self-care activities. (N.D. 12,14)

Provide opportunities for the student to increase his/her self-care skills, such as choosing which clothes to wear, getting his/her own drink of water, opening his/her own locker after it has been unlocked by a peer or adult, etc.

(N.D. 12,14)

During care activities, provide choices and request preferences from the student. (N.D. 12,14)

Encourage the student to express how he/she feels and thinks or views him/herself, and to ask questions at home and school. (N.D. 13)

Clarify any misconceptions the student has about him/herself and his/her care and education. (N.D. 13)

Assist the student to ask for and accept assistance from others when it is appropriate. (N.D. 12,14)

Encourage good hygiene, grooming, and dress. (N.D. 12,13)

Encourage involvement with peers in school and community activities. (N.D. 13)

If the student's perception of body image is strongly distorted or negative, discuss it with the student's parents and refer them to their healthcare provider or community mental health resources for further assessment.

(N.D. 13)

Assist the student to maintain good communication with his/her parents and teachers. (N.D. 13,14)

Provide the student with opportunities to make decisions regarding health management, assistive care, and school and peer activities. (N.D. 14)

Respect and follow ithe student's decision if you have given him/her options. (N.D. 14)

Provide opportunities for the student to take on responsibility and control of identified factors in his/her life, such as relaying information to teachers or parents, getting homework done and turned in on time, getting missed assignments if he/she is absent, and being in class on time. (N.D. 14)

Emphasize the student's strengths and abilitities. (N.D. 12,13,14)

Expected Student Outcomes

The student will:
- demonstrate independent mobility in the school setting. (N.D. 1,2)
- demonstrate increase in independent mobility in the school setting. (N.D. 1,2)
- utilize adaptive devices to increase mobility in the school setting. (N.D. 1,2)
- help develop and implement an EEP, date: _____. (N.D. 1,2)
- maintain proper body positioning in wheelchair. (N.D. 3, 4)
- identify factors that increase the risk of injury. (N.D. 3)
- utilize saftey measures to prevent injury (specific measure). (N.D. 3)
- identify causes of skin breakdown and pressure areas. (N.D. 4)
- identify prevention methods that can be used to prevent skin breakdown. (N.D. 4)
- describe how regular breathing exercises can assist in maintaining good respiratory function. (N.D. 5)
- demonstrate proper technique and utilization of breathing exercizes. (N.D. 5)
- demonstrate effective coughing. (N.D. 5)
- maintain an open airway and effective breathing pattern and air exchange. (N.D. 5,6)
- help develop ECP for occurrence of ventilator or diaphragmatic pacemaker malfunction, date: _____. (N.D. 6)
- Emergency Care Plan (ECP) is developed and implemented for occurrence of a dysreflexia episode, date: _____. (N.D. 7)
- describe what causes dysreflexia episodes. (N.D. 7)
- identify symptoms of a dysreflexia episode. (N.D. 7)
- describe what to do if a dysreflexia episode occurs. (N.D. 7)
- demonstrate effective management of dysreflexia episodes. (N.D. 7)
- dress appropriately for the weather and school environment. (N.D. 8)

Self-catheterize every 4 to 6 hours. (N.D. 9)

See that catheterization is done every 4 to 6 hours. (N.D. 9)

Experience no urinary incontinence during the school day. (N.D. 9)

Identify the signs and symptoms of a urinary tract infection. (N.D. 9)

Describe what to do if signs and symptoms of a urinary tract infection occur. (N.D. 9)

Accurately report signs and symptoms of a urinary tract infection to his/her parent(s). (N.D. 9)

Maintain good dietary and fluid intake, as observed by parent(s) and reported by student. (N.D. 9,10,11)

Follow bowel elimination program, as reported by student and parent(s). (N.D. 10,11)

Experience no bowel incontinence during the school day. (N.D. 10)

Participate in feeding, hygiene, toileting, and dressing activities. (N.D. 12,14)

Make choices and request preferences with caregivers, as observed by school personnel and parent(s). (N.D. 12,14)

Demonstrate increase in self-care skill(s) (specify skill). (N.D. 12)

Demonstrate good hygiene and appearance in school, with assistance as requested or needed. (N.D. 12,13)

Describe, realistically, his/her abilities, disabilities, and appearance, as observed by: school staff, peers, parent(s). (N.D. 13)

Ask for and accept assistance, when needed. (N.D. 12, 13,14)

Participate in one activity with peers in school, in the community (specify number and organization). (N.D. 13)

Make decisions regarding school and peer activities in school, as observed by teachers and other school staff. (N.D. 14)

Demonstrate good communication with parent(s), as reported by student and parent(s). (N.D. 14)

Demonstrate good communication with teachers, as reported by student and teachers. (N.D. 14)

Identify factors in his/her life over which he/she has control. (N.D. 14)

Demonstrate responsibility for _____ (identify the factor). (N.D. 14)

CASE STUDY

Karen is an 11-year-old girl who will begin at Central Middle School this fall. Karen is a bright, articulate sixth grader who has quadriplegia caused by a birth injury. She uses an electric wheelchair for mobility. She has recurrent urinary infections and bronchial stenosis, which places her at higher risk for respiratory infections. Karen also has severe osteoporosis, especially in her legs and hips due to quadriplegia and no weight-bearing activities.

Karen will be placed on a mainstream sixth grade team. Other than assistance with setting up the materials she needs for her classes and adapted physical education, Karen does not require any direct academic assistance. She will need assistance getting her lunch and opening her milk carton and with her coat and locker at the beginning and end of the day.

Karen and her parents came to visit the school yesterday. In meeting with them, several health-related issues and concerns were discussed:

1. Karen will need to be catheterized after lunch every day. The parents want the school nurse to use sterile technique and they will provide all the supplies that are needed in school. Because she has a history of recurrent urinary tract infections, her parents would like the school nurse to report any signs of an infection to them as soon as possible so appropriate antibiotic therapy can be initiated.

2. Because Karen has quadriplegia, she has a potential for developing autonomic dysreflexia (sudden increase in blood pressure). It is a medical emergency and requires immediate action.

3. Central Middle School is a multifloor building. Karen will use the elevator to get between floors of the building as needed. However, if she is on the second floor and there needs to be an emergency evacuation of the building, she will not be able to use the elevator. Plans for safe and expedient evacuation from the building are a big concern to both Karen and her parents.

4. Due to her severe osteoporosis, Karen should remain in her wheelchair throughout the school day, except for during catheterization and as needed to evacuate the building. When she is rolled to remove her thoracic lumbar sacral orthosis (TLSO) for catheterization, she needs to be logrolled to prevent twisting of joints that may lead to fractures. She must also remain properly positioned in her wheelchair.

5. Due to her bronchial stenosis, Karen's respiratory status can change quickly if she has a respiratory infection. Karen will receive an influenza vaccine again this year; however, her parents would like to be notified if there are numerous cases at school or if school personnel notice Karen coughing or having other respiratory symptoms.

Individualized Healthcare Plan*
Spinal Cord

Assessment Data	Nursing Diagnosis	Goals	Nursing Interventions	Expected Outcomes
ND7 C7 quadriplegia related to birth injury dysreflexia episodes—usually caused by bladder distention and need for bowel movement.	High risk for dysreflexia episode, related to autonomic nerve dysfunction (NANDA 1.2.3.1)	Develop an Emergency Care Plan (ECP).	Develop an ECP with Karen and her parents. Meet to discuss the ECP with Karen's teachers.	ECP is developed, date: (see attached ECP).
		Karen describes what causes her episodes and what the signs and symptoms are.	Discuss with Karen: potential for and actual causes of dysreflexia episodes for her, the signs and symptoms of a dysreflexia episode.	Karen identifies three causes of dysreflexia episodes, including her two most common reasons. Karen describes how she feels (the signs and symptoms) when a dysreflexia episode occurs.
		Karen describes and demonstrates what to do if a dysreflexia episode occurs.	Discuss with Karen what to do if an episode occurs during school, during an after-school activity, and on a field trip.	Karen describes and demonstrates what to do when a dysreflexia episode occurs at school, during after-school activities, and on field trips. Karen follows the ECP when an episode occurs.

ND3 Severe osteoporosis, especially in hips and legs related to quadriplegia and no weight bearing on legs. Twisting of joints may lead to fractures.	High risk for injury, especially in lower extremities, related to severe osteoporosis (NANDA 1.6.1)	Develop Emergency Evacuation Plan (EEP). Karen is able to evacuate the building quickly and safely. Karen will have no fractures of her lower extremities. Karen will maintain proper positioning in her wheelchair. Karen describes how she needs to be transferred and log rolled to prevent lower extremity fractures.	Develop EEP with Karen, her parents, and school staff. Hold trial evacuation and make changes as needed. Staff are in-serviced on what to do if an emergency evacuation is needed. Karen wears her TLSO brace every day at school to provide proper trunk support. Parents will position Karen properly in her wheelchair before she leaves for school. Karen will remain in her wheelchair during the school day, except when she is catheterized. Karen's wheelchair belt will remain securely fastened at all times. Karen is transferred from her wheelchair to the cot maintaining proper alignment. Karen is log rolled, when she is lying down, maintaining proper alignment.	EEP is developed, date: (see attached EEP). In an EEP trial, Karen successfully evacuates the school building in a safe and timely manner. Karen has no fractures of her extremities during the school year. Karen maintains proper positioning in her wheelchair. Karen wears her wheelchair belt securely fastened at all times. Karen accurately describes how she needs to be log rolled and transferred.

Individualized Healthcare Plan*
Spinal Cord (continued)

Assessment Data	Nursing Diagnosis	Goals	Nursing Interventions	Expected Outcomes
			nform Karen's teachers of her increased risk for fractures, interventions being used to minimize the risk of fractures, and what to do if Karen does not have proper positioning or falls out of her chair.	
ND4 Stays in wheelchair throughout the day except during catheterization. Wears orthoses on trunk and lower legs, ankles and feet to maintain proper alignment.	High risk for alteration in skin integrity related to tactile deficit due to quadriplegia and need to wear orthoses (NANDA 1.6.2.1.2.2)	Karen will prevent pressure areas by shifting her weight at least once per class period.	Discuss with Karen the importance of shifting her weight to prevent pressure areas from forming. This should be done once per class period. Have Karen demonstrate how to shift her weight to prevent or remove weight in a particular area.	Karen shifts her weight at least once per class period, as reported by Karen and observed by her teachers.
		Karen describes what causes skin breakdown and what to do if she or someone notices it is occurring.	Discuss with Karen: what skin breakdowns are, what the signs and symptoms are, and what to do if it occurs.	Karen describes what skin breakdowns are pressure areas are, the signs and symptoms of skin breakdowns, and what to do if they occur.

Nursing Diagnosis	Goal	Intervention	Expected Outcome
		Check skin under TLSO every day when it is removed for catheterization. Smooth clothes under TLSO prior to putting it back on. Assist Karen to notify her parents of changes in her skin condition. Inform teachers of Karen's tactile deficit and the need to protect her skin form pressure and harmful environments (e.g. hot and cold).	Karen demonstrates what to do if she or others notice skin breakdown or pressure areas. Parents are notified by Karen when any skin breakdowns or pressure areas occur.
ND8 Doesn't always wear appropriate clothing for outside weather conditions, especially in the winter. Ineffective thermoregulation related to autonomic nerve dysfunction. (NANDA 1.2.2.4)	Karen wears appropriate clothing to maintain her body temperature and for environmental conditions.	Before Karen leaves school each day, check to determine if she is dressed appropriately for outside weather.	Karen wears appropriate clothing for outside weather conditions.
ND9 C7 quadriplegia recurrent urinary tract infections (UTI). Sterile urinary catheterization after lunch, at school, every day. Alteration in urinary elimination pattern related to quadriplegia requiring the need for urinary catheterization and resulting in frequent UTIs. (NANDA 1.3.2)	Karen will have sterile urinary catheterization done at school, every day, after lunch.	Sterile urinary catheterization procedure done at school, by the school nurse, every day, after lunch. Parents will provide all sterile catheterization and diapering supplies.	Karen will independently come to the health office, every day, after lunch.

Individualized Healthcare Plan*
Spinal Cord (continued)

Assessment Data	Nursing Diagnosis	Goals	Nursing Interventions	Expected Outcomes
		Karen will not experience a UTI due to incomplete emptying of the bladder, distention or introduction of pathogenic organisms.	Discuss with Karen: signs and symptoms of a UTI and what to do if they occur. Daily observation by the school nurse for signs and symptoms of a UTI. Assist Karen to notify her parents if signs and symptoms of a UTI occur. Inform Karen's teachers of her need to be catheterized during the school day, which will cause her to miss the first ten minutes of her sixth mod class.	Karen lists the signs and symptoms of a UTI. Karen describes what to do if the symptoms occur. Karen does not develop a UTI. Karen notifies her parents if she has any signs or symptoms of a UTI.
ND5 Decreased pulmonary function due to bronchial stenosis and C7 quadriplegia.	High risk for respiratory infections related to decreased pulmonary function due to bronchial stenosis and quadriplegia. (NANDA 1.2.1.1 and 1.5.1.3)	Karen will have fewer than two upper respiratory infections which lead to complications, such as pneumonia, this school year.	Daily observations for signs and symptoms of a respiratory infection. Encourage Karen to cough, with quad-cough technique, when she does have a respiratory infection.	Karen has fewer than two respiratory infections which lead to complications this schools year.

Karen will increase her knowledge about and recognition of the signs and symptoms of respiratory infections.	Discuss with Karen: signs and symptoms of a respiratory infection, ways to minimize the risk of contracting a respiratory infection at school and at home.	Karen lists the signs and symptoms of a respiratory infection. Karen states three ways to prevent/minimize contracting a respiratory infection.
Karen will report signs and symptoms of respiratory infection to her parents or the school nurse when she notices them.	Assist Karen to notify her parents if signs or symptoms of a respiratory infection occur.	Karen reports signs and symptoms of a respiratory infection to her parents of school nurse when they occur.

*See Appendix for student profile information to include on an IHP form.

EMERGENCY EVACUATION FOR STUDENTS WHO ARE HANDICAPPED

1. Please circulate to concerned personnel and return to case manager.
2. Case manager to attach form to student's I.E.P.
3. Give parents a copy.
4. Any suggested changes should be discussed with the Child Study Team and Principal, if necessary

---

STUDENT'S NAME: Karen Larson   DISABILITY AREA: PI

SCHOOL BLDG.: Central Middle School   GRADE: 6

CONCERNED PERSONNEL: Teachers   Administrators   Student
                                    Counselor   Parents   Social Worker
                                    Management Assistant

CONCERN: Karen is physically impaired (quadriplegia) and may have difficulty
          evacuating the building in an emergency situation. She uses an electric
          wheelchair for mobility around school and uses the elevator to get between
          first and second floor. (The elevator cannot be used in an emergency
          evacuation.)

PLAN: For emergency evacuation from first floor (mods 2-10):
              Karen, accompanied by school nurse (or designated person), will
              exit the building by her wheelchair, out the front door or annex door.
          For emergency evacuation from second floor (mod1):
              Karen will go to the main stairway at the north end of the building.
              The School Nurse and a teacher will carefully remove Karen from her
              wheelchair and place her in the carrying sling, transport her down the
              stairs and out the door. (The wheelchair will be left in the building.)
          On cool days, a space blanket will be placed over Karen for warmth.
              The psychologist will cover for the school nurse when she is out of
              the building.

CASE MANAGER_____School Nurse

cc: Case Manager, Parents(s), Management Assistant, Health Services,
    Classroom Teacher, Principal

REFERENCES

1. National Spinal Cord Injury Statistical Center (NSCISC). *Spinal Cord Injury: Facts and Figures at a Glance.* Birmingham, Ala: University of Alabama, Spinal Cord Injury Care System, 1997.
2. National Spinal Cord Injury Association (NSCIA). *Factsheet #2: Spinal Cord Injury Statistical Information.* Cambridge, Mass: NSCIA, 1995.
3. Behrman RE, Kliegman RM. *Nelson Essentials of Pediatrics* 2nd ed. Philadelphia, Pa: WB Saunders Company, 1994.
4. The child with neuromuscular or muscular dysfunction. In: Wong DL, Hockenbery-Eaton M, Wilson D, Winkelstein ML, Ahmann E, Divito-Thomas PA, eds. *Whaley and Wong's Nursing Care of Infants and Children* 6th ed. St. Louis, Mo: Mosby, 1999:chap 40.
5. Bigge JL. *Teaching Individuals with Physical and Multiple Disabilities.* New York, NY: Macmillan Publishing Company, 1991.
6. National Spinal Cord Injury Association (NSCIA). *Factsheet #1: What Is Spinal Cord Injury.* Cambridge, Mass: NSCIA, 1995.
7. *Understanding spinal cord injury, advanced.* [online] Available at: http://www.spinalcord.uab.edu/docs/05.htm. Accessed March 1996.
8. Autonomic hyperreflexia. In: Larson G, ed. *Managing the School Age Child with a Chronic Health Condition.* Wazata, Minn: DCI Publishing, 1988:chap 33. (Available from Sunrise River Press, 11605 Kost Dam Road, North Branch, MN 55056, 800-895-4585; fax 651-583-2023.)

BIBLIOGRAPHY

Autonomic hyperreflexia. Larson G, ed. *Managing the School Age Child with a Chronic Health Condition.* Wazata, Minn: DCI Publishing, 1988:chap 33. (Available from Sunrise River Press, 11605 Kost Dam Road, North Branch, MN 55056, 800-895-4585; fax 651-583-2023.)

Behrman RE, Kliegman RM. *Nelson Essentials of Pediatrics*, 2nd ed. Philadelphia, Pa: WB Saunders Company, 1994.

Bigge JL. *Teaching Individuals with Physical and Multiple Disabilities.* New York, NY: Macmillan Publishing Company, 1991.

Carpenito LJ. *Handbook of Nursing Diagnosis*, 7th ed. Philadelphia, Pa: JB Lippincott Company, 1997.

Graham P. School reintegration: a rehabilitation goal for spinal cord injured adolescents. *Rehab Nurs.* 1991;16(3):122-128.

National Spinal Cord Injury Association (NSCIA). *Factsheet #1: What Is Spinal Cord Injury.* Cambridge, Ma: NSCIA, 1995.

National Spinal Cord Injury Association (NSCIA). *Factsheet #2: Spinal Cord Injury Statistical Information.* Cambridge, Ma: NSCIA, 1995.

North American Nursing Diagnosis Association. *NANDA Nursing Diagnoses: Definitions & Classification 1999-2000.* Philadelphia, Pa: North American Nursing Diagnosis Assn, 1999. (NANDA, 1211 Locust Street, Philadelphia, PA 19107. 800-647-9002; fax 215-545-8107; e-mail: NANDA@nursecominc.com)

Panzarino C, Lash M. *Rebecca Finds a New Way.* Woburn, Mass: National Spinal Cord Injury Association, 1994.

Stover SA, Whiteneck GG, DeLisa JA. *Spinal Cord Injury: Clinical Outcome from the Model Systems.* Gaithersburg, Md: Aspen Publications, 1995.

Wong DL, Hockenberry-Eaton M, Wilson D, Winkelstein ML, Ahmann E and Divito-Thomas PA, eds. *Whaley and Wong's Nursing Care of Infants and Children.* 6th ed. St. Louis, Mo: Mosby, 1999.

Wong DL. *Clinical Manual of Pediatric Nursing.* 4th ed. St. Louis, Mo: Mosby – Year Book, 1996.

ORGANIZATIONS

National Information Center for Children
and Youth with Disabilities
P.O. Box 1492
Washington, DC 20013
Phone: (800) 695-0285
E-mail: nichcy@aed.org

National Parent Network on Disabilities
1130 17th Street, NW, Suite 400
Washington, DC 20036
Phone: (202) 463-2299
E-mail: NPND@cs.net

National Rehabilitation Information
Center
8455 Colesville Road, Suite 935
Silver Spring, MD 20910-3319
Phone: (800) 227-0216

National Spinal Cord Injury Association
8300 Colesville Road, Suite 551
Silver Spring, MD 20910
Phone: (301) 588-6959
E-Mail: nscia3@aol.com

National Spinal Cord Injury Statistical
Center (NSCISC)
1717 6th Avenue South, Room 544
Birmingham, AL 35233-7330
Phone: (205) 934-3320
E-mail: NSCISC@sun.rehabm.uab.edu

32 | IHP: Traumatic Brain Injury

Judy F. Harrigan

INTRODUCTION

The 1992 *Federal Register* defines traumatic brain injury (TBI) as an acquired injury to the brain caused by an external physical force, resulting in total or partial functional disability or psychosocial impairment, or both, that adversely affects a child's educational performance. The term applies to open or closed head injuries resulting in impairments in one or more areas, such as cognition; language; memory; attention; reasoning; abstract thinking; judgement; problem solving; sensory, perceptual, or motor abilities; psychosocial behavior; physical functions; information processing; and speech. Generally, classification of the severity of head injuries is based on the duration of unconsciousness, the period of time of posttraumatic amnesia, and the amount of documented neurologic damage. However, even injuries that do not lead to unconsciousness can have significant cognitive and behavioral consequences. [1]

The federal definition of traumatic brain injury includes only those children who have an injury to the brain caused by external physical force (open/closed head injury or near drowning). However, a number of internal acquired brain injuries can occur in children. While internal brain injuries are not covered by the federal definition of TBI, it is important to mention these because children who have acquired brain injuries caused by internal occurrences often present with many of the same characteristics as those children who have TBI caused by external forces. Furthermore, these children require the same specialized planning as those students who have TBI caused by external forces. [2]

1. **Internal Occurrences**—Internal occurrences causing brain injuries include cerebral vascular accidents (i.e., vascular occlusions, hemorrhages, aneurysms), ingestion of toxic substances (i.e., inhalation of organic solvents or ingestion of heavy metals such as lead), brain tumors, hypoxia, or infections of the brain (i.e., abscesses, meningitis, encephalitis). Treatment of tumors and cancer with chemotherapy and/or radiation may also affect the long-term replication of brain cells and cause diffuse brain damage. [2]

2. **External Physical Force**—Two major types of external injuries to the brain can occur. An open head injury occurs as a result of an object penetrating the skull (i.e. bullet, missile-like object). A closed head injury occurs when the head is struck by a moving object or the moving head encounters a stationary barrier (as in a car accident). In addition, a skull fracture can occur as a complication of a

closed head injury. The most frequent type of head injury among children is a closed head injury.[2]

Annually, one to two million children and adolescents receive head injuries. 200,000 of these injuries (1 out of 500 school-aged children) are severe enough to require hospitalization. The incidence of TBI is greater than the rate for spinal cord injury, multiple sclerosis, cerebral palsy, and muscular dystrophy combined. It should also be noted that the incidence of TBI is approximately twice as high for boys as compared to girls. With improvements in medical technology, the number of children who survive TBI and return to school is increasing.[3]

Effects of Traumatic Brain Injury

The effects of TBI are many and diverse. Each child has a unique pattern, rate, and degree of symptomatology and recovery. Final consequences of the brain injury may not be apparent for years. While initial physical effects of the injury often resolve quickly, long-term cognitive, behavioral, and sensorimotor difficulties are often present and result in significant and complicating effects on a child's school and social successes.[2]

Physical effects that may persist as the child is ready to return to school include reduced stamina, fatigue, seizures, headaches, hearing and vision losses, tactile deficits and occasionally, difficulty maintaining a consistent body temperature. Since these physical effects are addressed in healthcare plans elsewhere in this book or in Volume I, they will not be considered in detail in this section. The focus in this chapter will be on cognitive and social deficits that may result from traumatic brain injury.

Long-term cognitive effects are typically experienced by children with TBI and can affect memory, intellectual functioning, attention, academic functioning,

and psychosocial adjustment.

• **Memory**—Memory deficits are among the most common and long-lasting effects of TBI and are a serious consequence because memory problems affect educational progress. Material the child learned before the injury may be lost and learning new material may be difficult, especially when new material is presented quickly or in great amounts or in great detail. Memory problems may affect adjustment to noninstructional aspects of the child's life. For example, a student may not remember the day's schedule, classroom locations, class routines, organizational skills, or routine activities of daily living.

• **Intellectual Functioning**—Children with TBI usually suffer a decline of intellectual functioning. There may be progressive improvement in IQ for up to five years after the injury with some children able to return to preinjury level and others experiencing only partial recovery. Despite recovery of IQ scores, children may continue to experience difficulties with skills not measured by these tests, such as problem solving, reasoning, organizational skills, and capacity for new learning.

• **Attention and Concentration**—A student who has suffered TBI is likely to experience problems focusing and sustaining attention for long periods of time. They may be unable to filter out distractions and selectively attend to important stimuli. This can result in "overload," agitation, confusion, and inability to shift smoothly from one topic or activity to another.

• **Academic Functioning**—A student may experience difficulties in specific academic subjects such as math and reading for a variety of reasons:
  - inability to establish realistic goals
  - planning and organizational difficulties
  - difficulty in focusing and sustaining attention

- computational deficiencies
- reading comprehension deficits
- difficulty initiating new tasks

• **Psychosocial Adjustment**—Psychosocial problems are complex and are often more debilitating than other problems. Some behavior problems stem from the injury itself and some behavior problems represent a reaction to the new disabilities. Students may exhibit affective problems (i.e., depression, social withdrawal, lowered self-esteem, helplessness, guilt) or personality disturbances (i.e., anger, impulsivity, lack of motivation, irritability, inappropriate social behavior).

Students may be unable to predict the outcome of behaviors and understand the effect of a behavior on another person. They often have difficulty in perceiving the nature of problems and considering various solutions or transferring new skills to alternate settings. This wide range of behaviors contributes to the multitude of difficulties that students who have suffered brain injury experience as they try to reintegrate into their preinjury activities.[2]

The interrelatedness of cognitive, social/behavioral, and motor difficulties has a significant and complicating effect on a student's success in school. An understanding and appreciation of the effects of and relationships between various sequelae are fundamental to the assessment, planning and program implementation for children with TBI.

Management

Management of the needs of the child with traumatic brain injury must be symptomatic depending on the body systems involved and the severity of symptoms. An interdisciplinary team approach will usually be essential with representatives from the school, the healthcare community, and the family included in planning sessions. Members of the team may include teachers, parents, student, school nurse, other healthcare personnel, school counselor, psychologist, speech and language therapist, physical and occupational therapists, vocational counselor, and educational specialists. It is essential to identify a case manager to coordinate services. Depending on the child's symptoms, the school nurse or any other member of the team may assume this role.

Planning for management of the child's reintegration into school should begin as soon as possible after the brain injury occurs. Assessment, tutoring, and communication with school staff and peers can begin while the child is in the hospital and continue during the rehabilitation phase and during the reintegration into school. These ongoing connections are helpful to the psychosocial health of the child and can be comforting and supportive to family members.

INDIVIDUALIZED HEALTHCARE PLAN

Assessment

History

- Date of the incident
- History of loss of consciousness; duration of loss of consciousness
- Duration of posttraumatic amnesia
- History of surgical procedures
- Length of hospitalization in acute and rehabilitative phases
- Previous level of cognitive function or requirements for special education services

Current Status and Management

- Physical effects including:
  weakness or paralysis
  vision loss in all or part of a visual field
  double vision
  decrease in hearing acuity
  headaches
  fatigue/ need for rest
  seizures
  hydrocephalus, including presence of shunt
- Ability to provide self-care in activities of daily living and management of medications and treatments
- Level of compliance with treatment regimes
- Recommendations for physical, occupational, or speech therapy
- Need for adaptive equipment such as wheelchair, braces, etc.
- Activity restrictions
- Medications

Psychosocial Status

- Student's understanding/acceptance of disability, treatments, etc.
- Family's understanding/acceptance of the child's disabilities, prognosis, and needs
- Family's ability to provide care and support
- Behavioral issues
- Problems with social adjustment and self-esteem

Academic Issues

- Current level of cognitive function
- Memory problems
- Need for adaptations/modifications such as note takers, computers, extended time for test taking to optimize academic performance
- Need for classroom and school building modifications
- Need for special education services (OT, PT, speech, program aide, health services)
- Safety issues related to orientation (ability to get from class to class, bussing issues)
- Prevention of trauma to head (especially physical education class, activity restrictions)

Nursing Diagnoses (N.D.)

N.D. 1 Impaired thought processes (NANDA 8.3) related to:
- Acquired learning problems
- Deficit in short-term memory
- Difficulty concentrating
- Shortened attention span

N.D. 2 Risk for alteration in student role (NANDA 3.2.1) related to:
- Prolonged absence from school during rehabilitation phase
- Cognitive/memory deficits resulting in disorganization, poor retention of information and instructions

- Risk for school failure resulting from cognitive/memory deficits
- Problems with fine motor coordination resulting in slowness/illegibility in writing, inability to take notes
- Speech impairment

N.D. 3 Self-esteem alteration (NANDA 7.1.2) related to:
- Changes in physical/mental abilities
- Lifestyle changes related to brain injury
- Grieving over loss of physical and/or psychosocial well-being
- Feelings of powerlessness
- Loss of school time
- Inability to interact at previous level with peers

N.D. 4 Alteration in activities of daily living (NANDA 6.1.1.2) related to:
- Acquired physical disabilities
- Cognitive/memory deficits

N.D. 5 Sensory perceptual alteration (NANDA 7.2) related to:
- Hearing deficit
- Vision deficit
- Tactile deficit

N.D. 6 Risk for injury (NANDA 1.6.1) related to:
- Seizures
- Mobility impairment and/or decreased coordination

N.D. 7 Risk for alteration in family process (NANDA 3.2.2) related to:
- Perceived loss of "previously perfect child"
- Family inability to cope with changes resulting from brain injury
- Financial stresses
- Inability of family to allow/process/express emotions

N.D. 8 Risk for social isolation (NANDA 3.1.2) related to:
- Lengthy hospitalization
- Inability to participate in activities at same level as prior to brain injury because of:
  mobility impairment
  cognitive/memory problems
  socially unacceptable behaviors
  speech impairment
- Discomfort of peers to relate to student because of changes in abilities

Goals

Student will achieve academic success appropriate to chronological age and cognitive abilities. (N.D. 1, 2)

Student will maintain good school attendance pattern. (N.D. 1, 2)

School activities will be based on student's level of tolerance and ability. (N.D. 1, 2)

A broad-based system of social, emotional, and health-related support will be available to the student and family. (N.D. 2, 7, 8)

Student will participate in appropriate social activities/relationships, with modifications as necessary. (N.D. 2, 3, 8)

Student will develop a realistic self-image and demonstrate adaptation to and comfort with changes related to brain injury. (N.D. 3)

Student will be successful in activities that foster self-esteem. (N.D. 3)

Student will be encouraged to express feelings to others. (N.D. 3)

Student will use positive, effective coping measures to decrease stress and anxiety. (N.D. 3, 8)

Student will acquire adaptations necessary to achieve mobility and success in school. (N.D. 3, 4)

Student will achieve maximum independence in school and classroom and activities of daily living. (N.D. 1, 3)

Student will make appropriate decisions on when to accept assistance from others. (N.D. 4)

Adaptive devices to improve/remedy visual and auditory deficits will be in place. (N.D. 5)

Student will be safe in the school environment and remain free from physical injury. (N.D. 6)

Family integrity and support will be maintained. (N.D. 7)

Family will be able to communicate openly and effectively. (N.D. 7)

Family will encourage and allow student to maintain independence and make decisions. (N.D. 7)

Student will develop and maintain meaningful social relationships with similar age peers. (N.D. 8)

Barriers to social contact with peers will be minimized and peers will be comfortable interacting with and helping student. (N.D. 8)

School staff and peers will help student to develop positive social relationships and increase self-esteem. (N.D. 3, 8)

Interventions

Refer to Committee on Special Education (CSE) or 504 Committee for evaluation of academic program needs. (N.D. 1, 2)

Develop IHP that addresses student's physical and academic needs. (N.D. 1, 2)

Arrange for assistance/modifications as necessary for daily school activities, i.e. note-taker, computer, extended time for test taking, etc. (N.D. 1, 2)

Participate as a member of the interdisciplinary team, which will develop an individualized education program (IEP). (N.D. 1, 2)

Monitor student's ability to perform self-management skills and collaborate with OT/PT staff to instruct him/her in methods to improve ability and maximize potential. (N.D. 1, 2)

Assist family and school staff to identify barriers and implement modifications in academic program, home and school environment, and scheduling. (N.D. 1, 2, 4)

Encourage student to ask questions and share feelings about his or her condition, its management requirements, limits, the stigma it imposes, and the prognosis with family members, school staff, peers, and healthcare providers. (N.D. 3, 8)

Encourage student to identify his or her strengths and weaknesses and signs that he/she is coping effectively/ineffectively. (N.D. 3, 8)

Reinforce student's positive abilities, interactions, etc. (N.D. 3, 8)

Refer student and family to support groups, counseling, family therapy, and/or clergy as indicated. (N.D. 3, 7, 8)

Collaborate with OT/PT staff for use of appropriate assistive devices to increase independence in self-care and classroom activities and monitor use in the classroom. (N.D. 4)

Identify and remove as many barriers to self-care as possible. (N.D. 4)

Assist in making arrangements for appropriate transportation to and from school if needed. (N.D. 4)

Monitor student's ability to perform self-management skills and instruct him or her in methods to improve skills and maximize potential. (N.D. 4)

Refer to and/or collaborate with vision specialist, audiologist, and/or speech pathologist due to need for and appropriate use of assistive devices and techniques to improve vision, auditory, and speech deficits. (N.D. 5)

If a tactile deficit is present, monitor school environment for possible sources of injury, especially for extreme hot or cold, i.e., science lab equipment, cooking class stoves, heaters, etc. (N.D. 5)

Monitor student's orientation and memory skills, especially in regard to safety within the school building, i.e., ability to follow schedule, get from class to class, assistance needed from staff to assure success. (N.D. 6)

Assess school environment for accessibility and facilitate the installation of equipment such as ramps, railings, etc. to allow safe access. (N.D. 6)

Maintain regular communication with student and family about healthcare plan. (N.D. 7, 8)

Listen to student and family and encourage expressions of concern, grief, fear, and anxiety. (N.D. 7, 8)

Identify family's developmental stage. (N.D. 7)

Promote wellness for student and family with teaching and support. (N.D. 7, 8)

Encourage continued and age-appropriate peer relationships. (N.D.8)

In collaboration with others, assist the student to develop appropriate social skills. (N.D. 8)

Provide educational opportunities for the student and peers to increase knowledge about traumatic brain injury and its prevention. (N.D. 8)

Expected Student Outcomes

- Student will be referred to and assessed by CSE or 504 Committee and an IEP will be developed to address academic program needs. (N.D. 1, 2)
- An IHP will be in place that addresses physical and health-related academic needs. (N.D. 1, 2)
- Appropriate adaptations/modifications will be in place to assure optimal success in academic program. (N.D. 1, 2)
- Student will utilize assistive devices at school and home to achieve an optimal level of independence. (N.D. 1, 2, 4)
- Student and family will participate in problem solving and decision making in relation to student's care, academic program, and physical needs. (N.D. 1, 2, 4)
- Student will verbalize feelings about his/her concerns, grief, anger, anxiety, fears and limitations, and others' reactions to his/her disability to appropriate adults. (N.D. 3, 8)
- Student will verbalize positive feelings about him/herself and identify individual strengths. (N.D. 3, 8)
- Student will develop answers and will use them to explain to others about his/her disability and limitations. (N.D. 3, 8)

- Student and family will participate in counseling/support group as appropriate to increase understanding and acceptance of the student's disability and to assist the student to develop and maintain appropriate social skills. (N.D. 3, 7, 8)
- OT/PT schedule will not interfere with classroom schedule. (N.D. 4)
- School and home environments will be assessed for barriers to self-care and adaptations/ modifications will be introduced as appropriate. (N.D. 4, 6)
- Appropriate referrals will be made and interventions introduced to correct/improve vision, hearing, or speech deficits. (N.D. 5)
- A routine of regular communication between school personnel and family will be established. (N.D. 7, 8)
- Family members will be encouraged to play a supportive role in assisting/managing student's care and academic needs. (N.D. 7)
- Student will describe his/her roles and responsibilities in the family and the roles and responsibilities of other family members. (N.D. 7)
- School staff will collaborate with student and family to develop a program that will enable the student to achieve academic and social success. (N.D. 7, 8)
- Student will participate with peers in activities and functions that he/she enjoys and that give him/her positive feelings and enhanced self-esteem. (N.D. 8)
- Program of head injury prevention and bicycle safety will be implemented in the school. (N.D. 8)

CASE STUDY

John is an 11-year-old boy who was injured in a fall from his bicycle 4 months ago. He suffered a closed head injury when the unbuckled bicycle helmet he was wearing flew off. He slowly regained consciousness after 3 days in a coma. He was hospitalized for 3 weeks in an acute-care hospital, then transferred to a rehabilitation center 90 miles from his home. Because of the distance from home, job responsibilities, and financial stresses, his family has been able to visit him only on weekends. John will be discharged from the rehab center in about 2 weeks. Prior to the accident, John was a healthy, popular and active sixth grader who was academically successful and participated on several youth sports teams. He had many friends and was out going and cooperative.

A number of physical and mental deficits are currently present. He has a right-sided hemiparesis that has necessitated his wearing a below-the-knee brace on his right leg and using a cane when ambulating. This hemiparesis interferes with the strength and coordination in his right hand. Psychological testing reveals that his IQ is about 10 points lower than prior to the accident and his speech is halting and slow. Memory of the accident and for recent events is poor. He has had frequent outbursts of tears and anger while in the rehab center. He has participated in individual counseling, family counseling, and a support group with other children for the last 8 weeks of his stay at the center. He has expressed frustration and anger at the unfairness of his situation.

Staff at the rehab center have been meeting regularly with school personnel to plan for his reintegration into school and to develop an IEP and an IHP. This team includes John's mother, his teacher, the school principal, the school nurse, members of the occupational, physical, and speech therapy departments, an educational specialist, the nurse practitioner from John's primary care practice, and the counselor who will counsel John and his family. The group has been facilitated by the social worker who is currently providing counseling at the rehab center. It has been determined that, upon John's return to school, the educational specialist, in collaboration with John's mother, will become the case manager. Each member of the team has had a part in planning for John's reentry and will be responsible for specific aspects of follow-up during the upcoming months. The team has decided to continue meeting weekly during the first few weeks after John returns to school.

Plans have been made to provide an aide to assist John in moving around the school building and in reintegrating back into school. He is returning to a self-contained regular education classroom, but will need assistance getting from the bus to the class and to special classes such as art, and music and to the lunchroom. A transportation aide has been assigned to ride his bus and to assist as needed for the first several weeks. John will participate in physical education with his peers and a decision will be made prior to each unit about the need for modifications. John's teacher will work with the classroom aide to see that he has notes and assignments for all subjects. There has been discussion about the need for a full-time note-taker once he moves into the junior high school. He will be provided a computer to use at school and training in keyboarding skills. His family has a computer at home. Speech, physical, and occupational therapy will be provided during the school day.

John's peers have been communicating with him by way of e-mail, videos, and tape recordings. Some have accompanied his family on their weekend visits. A schoolwide assembly has been held to discuss bicycle safety and included a videotaped message from John stressing the importance of properly wearing a helmet. A local Kiwanis Club has offered to provide free bicycle helmets to children who cannot afford them.

Individualized Healthcare Plan*
Traumatic Brain Injury

Assessment Data	Nursing Diagnosis	Goals	Nursing Interventions	Expected Outcomes
ND1 and ND8 Previous cognitive function. Current cognitive function. Ability to participate in activities as prior to TBI.	Self-esteem alteration related to changes in physical/mental abilities, grieving over loss of physical and/or psychosocial well-being, and feelings of powerlessness (NANDA 7.1.2)	Student will participate in social activities with modifications as necessary. Student will develop and maintain meaningful social relationships with similar age peers.	Encourage student to ask questions & share feelings about his condition, its management requirements, limitations, the stigma it imposes and the prognosis with family, school staff, peers & healthcare providers.	Student will verbalize feelings about his concerns, grief, anger, anxiety, fears and limitations and others' reactions to his disability to appropriate adults.
Understanding/ acceptance of disability, limitations, etc.	Risk for social isolation related to inability to participate in activities at same level as prior to TBI, and discomfort of peers in relating to student because of changes in abilities (NANDA 3.1.2)	Student will develop a realistic self-image and demonstrate adaptation to and comfort with changes related to TBI.	Encourage student to identify his strengths and weaknesses and signs that he is coping effectively/ ineffectively.	Student will verbalize positive feelings about himself and identify individual strengths. Student will develop answers about his disability and will use them to explain to others about his disability and limitations.
Available support systems within family, school, and community		Student will be successful in activities that foster self-esteem. Student will be encouraged to express feelings to others.	Reinforce student's positive abilities, interactions, etc. Refer student and family to support groups, counseling, family therapy, and/or clergy as indicated.	Student and family will participate in counseling to increase understanding and acceptance of the disability and to assist student to develop and maintain appropriate social skills.

| Behavioral issues | Student will use positive, effective coping measures to decrease stress and anxiety.

Student and family will communicate feelings to one another. Barriers to social contact with peers will be minimized.

Peers will be comfortable interacting with and helping student | Identify student's developmental stage and assure that expectations are real for that stage. In collaboration with others, encourage student to develop appropriate social skills.

Encourage continued and age-appropriate peer relationships and activities. Provide educational opportunities for student and his peers to increase knowledge about TBI, its prevention, and implications. | Student will participate with peers in activities that he enjoys and that give him positive feelings and enhanced self-esteem.

Student will demonstrate improved social skills with peers. Student will demonstrate increase in appropriate behavior in the school/ classroom setting.

Student will identify activities in which he is not able to participate as well as prior to the TBI. Student will identify activities in which he can fully participate.

Student will interact positively and successfully in classroom, small groups, lunchroom, hallways, etc.

Student will demonstrate positive coping strategies to decrease stress and anxiety. |

Individualized Healthcare Plan*
Traumatic Brain Injury (continued)

Assessment Data	Nursing Diagnosis	Goals	Nursing Interventions	Expected Outcomes
ND2 History of loss of consciousness. Duration of post traumatic amnesia.	Risk for alteration in student role related to cognitive and or memory deficits resulting in disorganization, poor retention of information and instructions.	Student will achieve academic success appropriate to chronological age and cognitive abilities.	Refer to CSE or 504 Committee for evaluation of academic needs. Participate as member of interdisciplinary team to develop IEP.	IEP will be developed to address academic program needs.
Previous level of cognitive function or requirements for special education services.	Risk for school failure. Problems with fine motor coordination (NANDA 3.2.1)	School activities will be based on student's level of tolerance and ability.	Develop IHP that addresses physical and academic needs. Assist family and school staff to identify barriers and implement modifications in academic program, home and school environment, and scheduling.	IHP that addresses physical and health-related academic needs will be in place.
Results of psychological testing. Current level of cognitive functioning		A system of social and emotional support will be available to the student.	Arrange for assistance/modification for daily activities: full-time aide; computer; extended time for test taking; note-taker; someone to carry materials when moving within building or to school bus.	Student will actively and successfully participate in his academic program.

Documented memory problems. Identified need for adaptations or modifications to optimize academic performance	Collaborate with OT/PT to monitor self-care, improve ability, and maximize potential and independence.	Student will increase academic achievement, with modification in curriculum, assignments, and grading as needed.
Behavioral issues	Instruct and encourage school staff to optimize independence in self-care, academics, and decision making.	Student will utilize assistive devices at home and school to achieve optimal success.

*See Appendix for student profile information to include on an IHP form.

REFERENCES

1. *Traumatic Brain Injury.* 57 *Federal Register* 44802 (1992).
2. DeLorenzo JP, Geary PJ. *Traumatic Brain Injury: A Guidebook for Educators.* Albany, NY: The University of the State of New York, State Education Department, 1995.
3. Blosser JL, DePompei R. *Pediatric Traumatic Brain Injury: Proactive Intervention.* San Diego, Calif: Singular Publishing Group, 1994.

BIBLIOGRAPHY

Blosser JL, DePompei R. *Pediatric Traumatic Brain Injury: Proactive Intervention.* San Diego, Calif: Singular Publishing Group, 1994.

DeLorenzo JP, Geary PJ. *Traumatic Brain Injury: A Guidebook for Educators.* Albany, NY: The University of the State of New York, State Education Department, 1995.

Haas MB. *The School Nurse's Source Book of Individualized Healthcare Plans* Vol I. North Branch, Minn: Sunrise River Press, 1993. (Available from Sunrise River Press, 11605 Kost Dam Road, North Branch, MN 55056. 800-895-4585; fax 651-583-2023)

North American Nursing Diagnosis Association. *NANDA Nursing Diagnoses: Definitions & Classification 1999-2000.* Philadelphia, Pa: North American Nursing Diagnosis Assn, 1999. (NANDA, 1211 Locust Street, Philadelphia, PA 19107. 800-647-9002; fax 215-545-8107; e-mail: NANDA@nursecominc.com)

Traumatic Brain Injury. 57 *Federal Register* 44802 (1992).

33 | IHP: Tuberculosis

Margarita Fernan Granthom

INTRODUCTION

In a child with a healthy immune system, primary tuberculosis usually does not progress immediately to disease. Children with tuberculosis infection or disease can attend school and daycare if they are receiving chemotherapy, clinical symptoms have disappeared, and an acceptable plan for completing the course of chemotherapy has been developed and begun.

Most children recover from the primary infection. Screening high-risk populations for tuberculosis and treating those with infection has been shown to be a cost-beneficial component of a comprehensive tuberculosis elimination strategy.[1] Routine source case investigations for young children with tuberculosis disease are an effective way of identifying individuals with active tuberculosis and others requiring treatment. [2]

Pathophysiology

Tuberculosis (TB) is an airborne communicable disease caused by *Mycobacterium tuberculosis*, or the *tubercle bacillus.* A primary infection usually goes unnoticed clinically, but sensitivity to tuberculin protein (skin tests) usually appears within three to six weeks following primary infection. Infection begins with the multiplication of *tubercle bacilli* in alveolar macrophages, some of which spread through the bloodstream; however, the immune system response usually prevents the development of disease. Persons who are infected, but who do not have TB disease, are asymptomatic and not infectious; such persons usually have a positive reaction to the tuberculin skin test. Most infected people have a positive reaction to the tuberculin test within two to ten weeks after infection.

Symptoms of pulmonary tuberculosis include:	Systemic symptoms consistent with tuberculosis include:
cough chest pain hemoptysis	fever chills night sweats easy fatigability loss of appetite weight loss

The specific symptoms of extrapulmonary TB depend on the site of the disease. Tuberculosis of the spine may cause pain in the back; TB of the kidney may cause blood in the urine. Tuberculosis infection usually begins in the lungs (the most common site for TB disease) and spreads to the hilar lymph nodes, then to the bloodstream. Approximately 85% of TB cases are pulmonary; extrapulmonary TB is rarely contagious.[3]

Common sites of TB disease include:
- lungs (85 % of all cases)
- pleura
- central nervous system
- lymphatic system
- genitourinary system
- bones and joints
- disseminated (miliary TB)

Infection can progress to disease very quickly or many years after infection. In the United States, in approximately 5% of persons who have been recently infected with *M tuberculosis*, TB disease will develop in the first year or two after infection. In another 5%, disease will develop later in their lives. The remaining 90% will stay infected but free of disease for the rest of their lives.[3] Infection with human immunodeficiency virus (HIV) is the most important risk factor for TB infection progressing to active disease.[4]

Children are susceptible to both the human (*M tuberculosis*) and the bovine (*M bovis*) organisms. In those locations where tuberculosis in cattle is not controlled or pasteurization of milk is not practiced, the bovine type is a common source of infection in children.

Other factors that influence development of tuberculosis include the following:
- heredity (resistance to the infection may be genetically transmitted)
- sex (higher in adolescent girls)
- age (lower resistance in infants; higher incidence during adolescence)
- stress (emotional or physical)
- nutritional state
- intercurrent infection (especially human immunodeficiency virus, measles, and pertussis)

The lung is the usual portal of entry in human beings; the organism enters less often by ingestion. In the lungs a proliferation of epithelial cells surround and encapsulate the multiplying bacilli in an attempt to wall off the invading organisms, thus forming the typical tubercle. After primary infection, lesions may become inactive or progress to active pulmonary tuberculosis. Extension of the primary lesion at the original site causes progressive tissue destruction as it spreads within the lung, discharges material from foci to other areas of the lungs, or produces pneumonia. Erosion of blood vessels by the primary lesion can cause widespread dissemination of the *tubercle bacillus* to near and distant sites.

Tuberulosis is spread person to person by airborne particles that contain *M tuberculosis*, called droplet nuclei. Droplet nuclei may be expelled when a person with infectious TB coughs and sneezes. Persons at the highest risk of becoming infected with *M tuberulosis* are close contacts, those persons who often spend time with someone who has infectious TB, such as family members, roommates, friends, coworkers, or others. The source of infection in children is, in most situations, an infected adult or a teenager, usually a member of the household.[5] The probability that TB will be transmitted depends on three factors:
- the infectiousness of the person with TB
- the environment in which exposure occurred
- the duration of exposure

The incubation period is four to twelve weeks, at which time the primary lesion appears. Communicability persists as long as living tubercle bacilli are being discharged, usually by coughing. Appropriate chemotherapy can reduce communicability within several weeks.

Diagnostic Evaluation

All screening activities should be accompanied by a plan for follow-up care for persons with infection or diseases and should always be carried out in consultation with the health department. False-

Classification System for Tuberculosis [3]

Class	Type	Description
0	No TB exposure Not infected	No history of exposure Negative reaction to tuberculin skin test
1	TB exposure No evidence of infection	History of exposure Negative reaction to tuberculin skin test
2	TB infection No disease	Positive reaction to tuberculin skin test Negative bacteriologic studies (if done) No clinical or radiographic evidence of TB
3	Current TB disease	*M tuberculosis* cultured (if done) or Positive reaction to tuberculin skin test and Clinical or radiographic evidence of current disease History of episode(s) of TB or Abnormal but stable radiographic findings Positive reaction to the tuberculin skin test
4	Previous TB disease	Negative bacteriologic studies (if done) and No clinical or radiographic evidence of current disease

positive reactions may be caused by factors where infection with mycobacteria other than *M tuberculosis* and vaccination with bacille Calmette-Guérin (BCG).

Limited immunity can be produced by administration of the only successful vaccine to date, BCG (bacille Calmette-Guérin). It contains the bovine bacilli with reduced virulence and is injected intradermally. The vaccine is not used extensively and distribution is controlled by local or state health departments. Anergy, a condition in which there is absence of a reaction to the tuberculin test may lead to false-negative reactions. [3]

Tuberculin skin test is the single most important test to determine whether a child has been infected with the *tubercle bacillus*. Two types used for skin tests: OT (old tuberculin) and PPD (purified protein derivative of tuberculin). The PPD is most widely used and standard dose is 5 TU in 0.1 ml solution, injected intracutaneously.

Techniques for injection are:
1. Mantoux tuberculin test (standard and preferred method)
   Intradermal injection of .01 ml of puri-

fied protein derivative (PPD) tuberculin containing 5 TU into either the volar or dorsal surface of the forearm. Injection should be made with a disposable tuberculin syringe, just beneath the surface of the skin, with the needle bevel facing upward. This should produce a discrete pale elevation of the skin (a wheal) 6 to 10 mm in diameter. Reaction should be read by a trained healthcare worker 48 to 72 hours after injection.

2. Multiple-puncture tests: tine, Heaf, SclavoTest, Sterneedle, or MonoVac. A positive reaction indicates that the individual has been infected and has developed sensitivity to the protein of the *tubercle bacillus* but it does not confirm the presence of the actual disease.

Manifestations of pulmonary tuberculosis in children are extremely variable and most children have no symptoms when first infected. A history of possible contact would be helpful and radiographic examinations. Diagnosis is confirmed by isolation of the tubercle bacilli by culture from sputum, gastric washings, and/or pleural fluid.

Diagnosis of active TB requires other procedures, such as a chest x-ray (abnormalities often occur in the apical and posterior segments of the upper lobe). or in the superior segments of the lower lobe. Lesions may appear anywhere in the lungs and may differ in size, shape, density, and cavitation. In some instances, other views or additional studies (e.g., computed tomographic scans) may be necessary.

Management

People in whom TB develops and who have been treated for at least two weeks with appropriate drugs are usually not infectious. [6]

In children, management consists of adequate nutrition, chemotherapy, general supportive measures, and avoidance of unnecessary exposure to other infections. The need for hospitalization varies, although it may serve as an excellent opportunity for family education regarding the importance of medication and follow-up care.

Chemotherapy is the most important therapeutic modality. The most commonly used combination of drugs include:
- INH (isoniazid) 10-15 mg/kg body weight in children, not to exceed 300 mg/dose
- rifampin: usual therapeutic dose should be given
- pyrazinamide: treatment regimen may be either six-month or nine-month.
- ethambutol (EMB) or streptomycin (SM)

Children should receive at least nine months of preventive therapy. New, short regimens of preventive therapy (e.g., rifampin and pyrazinamide for two months and rifampin alone for four months) are currently being evaluated. The initial regimen for treating TB disease should include four drugs and can be adjusted when results of drug susceptibility become available. The major determinant of the outcome of treatment is patient adherence to the drug regimen. The TB control program in the health department should assist in evaluating the patient for causes of nonadherence and should provide additional services to enable completion of recommended therapy. [3]

The American Academy of Pediatrics (1991) recommends annual tuberculin testing of high-risk children. For children from areas where there is low prevalence of the disease, testing is recommended at 12 to 15 months of age and before entry to school (4 to 6 years of age) and in adolescence (14 to 16 years of age). Children with risk factors, such as recent immigration, institutional residence, incarceration, or exposure to adults at high risk for TB, should be tested with greater frequency. [7]

In children and adolescents, a specific treatment and monitoring plan should be developed in collaboration with local health departments and should include a description of treatment regimen, methods of assessing and ensuring adherence, and methods of monitoring for adverse reactions.

If schools require screening for tuberculosis:

- the goals of any screening should be clearly defined and mechanisms must be in place to ensure that students receive any follow-up (e.g., chest radiographs, medical evaluation, preventive therapy) that is needed.
- widespread screening of the general student population should not be done.

Instead, students at high risk for infection, for example, international or foreign-born students from countries with high rates of tuberculosis, students working in healthcare settings, and immunocompromised students, should be targeted for screening.

- only the Mantoux method for skin testing should be used.
- students vaccinated with BCG should not be excluded from screening.
- results of screening (all skin test results and demographic, clinical, and follow-up information) must be collected and periodically analyzed to evaluate the usefulness of screening and ensure that the goals of screening are met.

The modification and/or continuation of any screening program should be based on these analyses. [8]

INDIVIDUALIZED HEALTHCARE PLAN

Assessment

History

- When was tuberculosis diagnosed
- Previous TB testing (including x-rays): dates and results
- Healthcare providers involvement in management of the student's TB
- Illness symptoms: fatigue/weakness, anorexia, weight loss, night sweats,
- Fever, hemoptysis, aching, tight chest
- Known exposure to TB lived in TB-endemic community /country
- Involvement of support persons/systems
- Experience with self-medication at home
- Tuberculosis management plan: medications, child and family education, counseling
- Compliance with medical management plan
- Previous medical treatment for TB, including prophylaxis
- History of immunocompromised status

Current Status and Management

- Knowledge about TB (student, parents/guardians, teachers)
- Current symptoms: cough, fever, thick/bloody sputum
- Current treatment plan, including medication and follow-up
- Student's health, school, family, and activities of daily living

Self-care

- Self-care skills
- Ability to self-administer medication
- Motivation for self-care, self-medication
- Barriers to self-care, self-medication
- Parent perception of student's ability for self-care

Psychosocial Status

- Student's perception of his/her health and TB
- Parent's perception of the student's health and TB
- Decision-making skills
- Impact to activities of daily living
- Impact of diagnosis/health status on: peer relationships
  ability to participate in activities with peers

Academic Issues

- Health needs at school — medications
- Individualized Education Program (IEP) is developed and implemented as appropriate
- Section 504 services and accommodations, as needed
- Activity tolerance in the school setting

Nursing Diagnoses (N.D.)

N.D. 1 Risk for infection (NANDA 1.2.1.1) related to:
- Exposure to infectious person
- Immunocompromised health status

N.D. 2 Knowledge deficit (NANDA 8.1.1) related to:
- Cultural beliefs
- Cognitive limitations
- Lack of interest/motivation in learning
- Lack of information

N.D. 3 Knowledge deficit (NANDA 8.1.1) concerning:
- Spread of this infectious disease
- Hand washing
- Prevention and treatment measures

N.D. 4 Altered health maintenance (NANDA 6.4.2) related to:
- Denial of chronic disease (infections)
- Lack of medical health assessment/ healthcare
- Noncompliance with medical treatment plan
- Cultural beliefs

N.D. 5 Risk for alteration in self-esteem (NANDA 7.1.2) related to:
- Chronic infectious disease

N.D. 6 Risk for noncompliance (NANDA 5.2.1.1) with prescribed medications related to:
- Knowledge deficit
- Denial of need for medications
- Inability to access medication

Goals

Increase knowledge about tuberculosis. (N.D. 2.3)

Comply with prescribed tuberculosis management plan. (N.D. 4.6)

Develop tuberculosis self-care skills. (N.D. 3, 4, 6)

Participate in school/class activities, including physical education class with modifications made as necessary. (N.D. 4, 5)

Demonstrate good school attendance pattern and classroom participation. (N.D. 2, 4, 5)

Interventions

Review assessments, observations, and recommendations with student and parent. (N.D. 4,7)

Exclude student suspected of having TB for medical assessment (N.D. 1-3) referral to:

- healthcare provider
- community resources

For student diagnosed with TB (N.D. 1-4, 7)

- advise school staff that student may return to school when the healthcare provider determines that the student is not contagious and is able to participate in school activities.
- reinforce healthy practices of covering nose and mouth when coughing or sneezing.
- assist staff to obtain answers to questions they have.

Medication administration in schools (N.D. 1-3)

- obtain medication orders and authorization for medications needed at school.
- ensure compliance with the drug regimen by instructing student/parents and staff regarding the importance of giving the medication as often and for as long as it is ordered.
- monitor student's medication compliance. (N.D.6)

Provide inservice for school staff, (N.D. 1-7) covering:

- signs and symptoms of TB
- infection vs disease
- causes
- preventive measures
- treatments
- preventive therapy
- demonstration of appropriate technique to prevent droplet spread
- hand washing—the most critical infection control practice

Assist physical education teachers to modify physical education requirement, if necessary. (N.D. 1-7)

In collaboration with local public health agency, assist in identification of possible contacts and notification of students/parents as recommended by health officer regarding possible exposure to tuberculosis and medical management as well as provision of TB screening and consultation with health department's TB control program. (N.D.1)

Expected Student Outcomes

The student will:

- participate in regular classroom activities, with modifications made when necessary (N.D. 1-7)

- define what tuberculosis is (N.D. 1-7)
- describe the benefits of taking medications as prescribed (N.D. 5,6)
- describe the consequences of not taking medications as prescribed (N.D.6)
- demonstrate a good school attendance pattern (N.D.7)
- demonstrate compliance with medication management plan (N.D.6)
- follow through, with family, on medical management of tuberculosis (N.D. 1-6)

CASE STUDY

You are a school nurse in a school district of 5,000 students. You are responsible for five school buildings—four elementary schools and a combination elementary/middle school. It is the first week of January and you get a call from the principal asking you to make a phone call to the parents of a ninth grader. The principal says that Cici, 15 years old, has been diagnosed with tuberculosis. The principal wants you to figure out what the school needs to do and expresses safety as well as health education concerns for other students and teachers in the school building.

Cici is a 15-year-old student at White Mountain Junior High. She has just been diagnosed with tuberculosis. She lives with her mother and father and is an only child. They had a relative visit their home who has had a history of tuberculosis. Cici's mother took her to the community health nursing office due to frequent coughing, night sweats, and fever with thick, bloody sputum. They do not have any medical insurance and her father had just gotten laid off from work. A local physician diagnosed her with tuberculosis and chemotherapy has been initiated and continued for over two weeks. Cici tells her school counselor that she is embarrassed to let her friends know she has been diagnosed with tuberculosis. She does not understand a lot of things about tuberculosis and would like to know more about it.

What can you do to help Cici and her family? Who else needs to be involved? What is your priority? What kinds of nursing care will Cici need for the rest of the school year? What additional data do you need? What outcomes do you want to achieve? What should Cici's IHP look like? How can the school nurse collaborate with the community health nurse?

It is important to develop the IHP with input from the parents and the student. For an older student, being a partner in the planning process and participating in her care is important for her self-esteem. The school nurse writes up a draft of the plan and gives Cici a copy to go over with her parents and physician. The school nurse will identify and assist in dealing with cultural and communication/language barriers. Signing the IHP may indicate their agreement and willingness to participate. The IHP will be shared with appropriate school staff as needed. Using the nursing process, confidentiality will be maintained in line with the standards of practice and school policies

Individualized Healthcare Plan*
Tuberculosis

Assessment Data	Nursing Diagnosis	Goals	Nursing Interventions	Expected Outcomes
ND1 Frequent coughing, night sweats, and fever with thick/bloody sputum. A relative visited their home and said he used to have tuberculosis.	Risk for infection (NANDA 1.2.1.1) related to exposure to infectious person	Increase knowledge about tuberculosis	Review assessments, observations, and recommendations with student. Exclude student, until referral to community resources or local healthcare provider is completed.	Student will define what tuberculosis is. Student is evaluated by physician to determine if infection has occurred.
ND2 States that her parents have no medical insurance and no financial resources to see a healthcare provider	Health maintenance altered (NANDA 5.6.4.2) related to lack of medical resources/access	Access healthcare community resources.	Assist parents to access financial resources for healthcare.	Student and family will follow through on medical management of tuberculosis.
ND3 States she is embarrassed to let her friends know her recent diagnosis	Potential for self-esteem disturbance (NANDA 7.1.2) related to having chronic infectious disease	Increase ability and comfort in talking with friends about her disease	Discuss concerns regarding others knowing she has TB. Give her the opportunity to discuss her feelings. Meet with nurse weekly.	She will feel comfortable asking questions regarding TB and sharing information with friends.
ND4 Has difficulty understanding why she has to cover her nose and mouth when coughing and sneezing	Knowledge deficit (NANDA 8.1.1) related to diagnosis	Develop self-care skills and demonstrate skill: covering nose and mouth when coughing, sneezing	Reinforce healthy practices. Explain to student: What tuberculosis is, its causes, preventive measures, preventive treatments, and practices	She will describe, understand, and demonstrate the appropriate technique to prevent droplet spread.

*See Appendix for student profile information to include on an IHP form.

REFERENCES

1. Mohle-Boetani JC Miller B Halpern M et al. School-based screening for tuberculous infection. *JAMA*, 1995;274:613-619.
2. Besser R, Pakiz B, Haverkamp J, Schulte J, Moser K, Onorato I, *Source Case Investigations of Children with Tuberculosis Disease in San Diego,* Department of Pediatrics, University of California, San Diego and San Diego County Department of Health Services, Atlanta, Ga: Centers for Disease Control, September 1998.
3. Centers for Disease Control. *Core Curriculum on Tuberculosis: What the Clinician Should Know.* 3rd ed. Atlanta, Ga: Centers for Disease Control, 1994: chap 2.
4. Huebner R, Villarino M, Snider D. Tuberculin skin testing and the HIV epidemic. *JAMA.* 1992;267:409-10.
5. Wong DL. *Whaley & Wong's Essentials of Pediatric Nursing.* 4th ed. St. Louis; Mo: CV Mosby, 1993; 729.
6. Huang M, Fighting tuberculosis. *JAMA,* 1998;280(19):1724.
7. Pong A, Anders B, Moser K, Starkey M, Gassmann A, Besser R. Tuberculosis screening at two San Diego high schools with high-risk populations. *Arch Pediatr Adolesc Med.*1998;152:646-650.
8. Hennessey K, Schulte J, Cook L, Collins M, Onorato I, Valway S. Tuberculin skin test screening practices among US colleges and universities.*JAMA.* 1998;280(23):2008-2012.

BIBLIOGRAPHY

American Academy of Pediatrics. School Health Policy and Practice. Evanston, Ill: American Academy of Pediatrics, 1993.

American Thoracic Society/CDC.Treatment of tuberculosis and tuberculosis infection in adults and children. *Am J Respir Crit Care Med.* 1994;149:1359-1374.

Behrman RE, Vaughan VC III. *Nelson Essentials of Pediatrics.* 2nd ed. Philadelphia; Pa: WB Saunders Company, 1994.

Benenson AS, ed. *Communicable Diseases in Man.* 15th ed. Washington, DC: American Public Health Association, 1990.

Boyles S, Primary school teacher in Amsterdam infects 19 students. *Infect Dis Weekly.* December 1995,17-19.

Brady M. Tuberculosis in children: primary care prevention and managment. *J Pediatr Health Care*, 1990;4.

Carpenito LJ. *Nursing Diagnosis: Application to Clinical Practice.* 5th ed. Philadelphia; Pa: JB Lippincott, 1993.

Centers for Disease Control. Essential components of a tuberculosis prevention and control program. *MMWR.*1995;44(11):1-34.

Centers for Disease Control. The role of BCG vaccine in the prevention and control of tuberculosis in the United States. *MMWR.*1996;45(4):921-925.

Centers for Disease Control. Tuberculosis and human immunodeficiency virus infections: recommendations of the Advisory Committee for the Elimination of Tuberculosis. *ACET). MMWR,* 1989;38: 236-8,240-250.

Committee on Infectious Disease. Update on tuberculosis skin testing of children. *Pediatrics.* 1996;97:282-284.

Hootman J. *Quality Nursing Interventions in the School Setting: Procedures, Models, and Guidelines.* National Association of School Nurses, III-TUB-1. 1996.

Kenyon T, Driver C, Schneider E, et al. Immigration and tuberculosis in young children, San Diego. In: *Abstracts of the 35th Interscience Conference on Antimicrobial Agents and Chemotherapy,* San Francisco: American Society for Microbiology,1995.

Marx E,Wooley S, Northrop D, eds. *Health is Academic: A Guide to Coordinated School Health Programs.* New York, NY: Teachers College Press. 1998;169-194.

North American Nursing Diagnosis Association. *NANDA Nursing Diagnoses: Definitions & Classification 1999-2000.* Philadelphia, Pa: North American Nursing Diagnosis Assn, 1999. (NANDA, 1211 Locust Street, Philadelphia, PA 19107. 800-647-9002; fax 215-545-8107; e-mail: NANDA@nursecominc.com)

Peter G, ed. 1997 *Redbook: Report of the Committee on Infectious Diseases.* 24th ed. Grove Village, Ill: American Academy of Pediatrics; 1997:541-562.

Whaley LF, Wong DL. *Nursing Care of Infants and Children.* St Louis, Mo: CV Mosby, 1999.

Wong DL, Whaley LF. *Clinical Manual of Pediatric Nursing.* St. Louis, Mo: CV Mosby, 1990.

INTERNET RESOURCES

http://www.state.hi.us/doh/aboutpress/p9_tb.htm

http://www2.northstar.k12.ak.us/schools/ndl/faculty/smith/chronic.html

http://www.uah.edu/pedinfo/index.html/SubSpec_Other2.html#School

http://indy.radiology.u10ua.edu/cgi_bin/bglimpse/39/var/web/vh

http://www.nationaltbcenter.edu

http://www.nationaltbcenter.edu/pediahtml

http://www.cpmc.columbia.edu/resources/tbcpp/

http://www.lungusa.org/diseases/pedtbfac.html

APPENDIX
Individualized Healthcare Plan

Name: Birthdate:

Address: School:
Home Phone: Teacher/Counselor:
Parent/Guardian: Grade:
Day/Work Phone: IHP Date:
Healthcare Provider: IEP Date:
Provider's Phone: Review Dates:
IHP Written By: ICD-9 Codes:

Assessment Data	Nursing Diagnosis	Goals	Nursing Interventions	Expected Outcomes

Index